Principles
and Methods
of Pharmacy
Management

Principles
and Methods
of Pharmacy
Management

Harry A. Smith, Ph.D.

Professor of Pharmacy Administration,
College of Pharmacy,
University of Kentucky,
Lexington, Kentucky

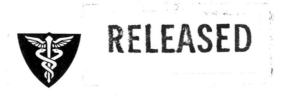
LEA & FEBIGER · 1975 · PHILADELPHIA

Library of Congress Cataloging in Publication Data

Smith, Harry A   1925–
  Principles and methods of pharmacy management.

  1. Pharmacy management.   I. Title.   [DNLM: 1. Pharmacy
administration.   QV704 S649p]
RS100.S57   1975   658′.91′6154   74-18448
ISBN 0-8121-0507-9

Published in Great Britain by Henry Kimpton Publishers, London
Printed in the United States of America

Preface

A textbook on Pharmacy Management must of necessity draw on many disciplines and apply many and varied concepts, principles, and methods to the practice of pharmacy. At the time this book was begun and until the final manuscript was completed, there was not a textbook on Pharmacy Management that met the needs of students and practitioners of pharmacy. These needs had been apparent for several years, since the one established textbook had not been revised since 1960.

This book is designed for teachers and undergraduate students of Pharmacy Management, and to serve those practitioners of pharmacy who wish to improve their managerial practices. The text is primarily a basic one, which will serve both students and practitioners who intend, or are at present, practicing in *any* practice environment. While some five or six chapters are designed to serve the needs of community or retail pharmacists more specifically, this is not a weakness, in my opinion, because over 80 percent of pharmacists practice in this type of environment.

While the text emphasizes basic concepts and principles that will be valid and applicable to the various types of practices for the present and the future, many techniques and methods have been incorporated to make the book a useful tool for the everyday management of a pharmacy.

It is recommended that students have an understanding of the basic principles of accounting and a working knowledge of its terminology—the language of business—as a prerequisite to the study of this text. In addition, it is highly desirable that students have a prior course in the social, behavioral, and economic aspects of health care in general, and specifically, the practice of pharmacy.

The author realized that where statistical information has been included, it is outdated even before it is published. This, of course, is unavoidable. New techniques and methodologies will be developed, and thus, this aspect of the text will become outmoded in time. Revisions are necessary and are anticipated.

As is true with any author, I owe a multitude of acknowledgements and thanks. First, gratitude is expressed to the many researchers and writers whose works have been acknowledged and cited as references. The author wishes to thank those people whose works have been used with their permission. To the many colleagues and students who have contributed to my fund of knowledge and have encouraged me, I am most appreciative.

A special thanks goes to the following: Dean Joseph V. Swintosky, who encouraged the use of regular working hours while writing the original draft of the manuscript; Mr. Robert L. Barnett, Jr., who assisted in the selection of relevant topics; Dr. D. C. Huffman, Jr., who provided some original material and helpful criticism; Mrs. Susan Janecek, who typed the original draft and provided valuable assistance; Mr. Kenneth Scrogham, who provided valuable editorial assistance and whose firm, Master Services, typed the final manuscript.

A very special thanks to my wife, Norma, and children, Elizabeth Ann and Harry (III), who have made my home life so easy and a blessing for many years and especially during the preparation of the manuscript; and to Mr. and Mrs. Alton McAnelly, whose encouragement and assistance made my professional career a possibility. Finally, a humble acknowledgement of the grace of God, who provided me with the talent and time to write this book.

I hope that those who use this book will gain a measure of the satisfaction and professional growth that I have gained while writing it.

Harry A. Smith

Lexington, Kentucky

Contents

3. ORGANIZATIONAL STRUCTURES

4. ALTERNATIVES IN THE PRACTICE OF PHARMACY

5. PLANNING FOR CAPITAL REQUIREMENTS

6. LOCATION ANALYSIS AND EVALUATION

7. PHARMACY LAYOUT DESIGN

8. PERSONNEL ADMINISTRATION

12. PHARMACY PATRONAGE

13. PROMOTION

1. *Historic Overview of Pharmacy*

The general purpose of this chapter is to provide the pharmacy student with a sociohistoric perspective of his profession, in order that he may better understand the diversities of practices and organizations and the conflicts of vested interests, as well as personal or internal conflicts, and thus be better prepared to make sound choices as he pursues his life's work. Sufficient reason for including this brief historic sketch of the pharmacy profession in a course in pharmacy management can be seen in the following quote from the preface of *Kremers and Urdang's History of Pharmacy.*[1]

> The history of pharmaceutical science and technology has the cumulative, progressive quality that characterizes the history of science at large; the history of the pharmaceutical profession shows the character of social history, with its unforeseen regressive turns of events, its conflicts of interests, and their resolution by trends and forces that would elude comprehension solely in terms of science, or conviction, or effort, circumscribed by a given time or group.

Origin of Pharmacy

Pharmacy, as well as other professions and sciences, had a common origin in primitive civilizations. The witch doctor possessed the only perceived source of help in solving all of the problems that beset mankind.

This concentration of power was the direct result of ignorance and superstition, which were prevalent among primitive people. As civilizations progressed, the various areas of authority and sources of help were divided among various "specialists." The priests were sought for religious matters; physicians were the source of healing; and wise men or judges were given political power and authority to dispense justice. In most societies, these three groups of authority and sources of ministration were combined into a single politico-religious system or order at the early stages of development. With the advancement of knowledge and specialization within the priesthood, these three major areas of human endeavor were separated and came to be known as the three learned professions.

Up to a point in time, pharmacy and medicine were not separate occupations. In fact, after the two professions became separated, the practice of medicine resembled the early practice of pharmacy more than it did the practice of medicine as we know it today. During the ninth to the thirteenth centuries, much of the Arabian contribution to medicine was more pharmaceutical than medical in its contents and techniques. However, it was not until the edict of Frederick II, the German Emperor, in 1240, that pharmacy was recognized officially as a profession separate from medicine.[1]

Separation of Pharmacy from Medicine

The edict of Frederick II contained three regulations that provided the legal basis for the separation of pharmacy as an independent branch of health services: (1) separation of the pharmaceutical profession from the medical profession; (2) official supervision of pharmaceutical practice; and (3) obligation by oath to prepare drugs reliably, according to skilled art, and in a uniform, suitable quality.

The first regulation is self-explanatory. The second provided the historic and legal basis for the control of the practice of pharmacy and the enactment of our various pharmacy laws. The third regulation provided the basis for official pharmacopeias.

Two other principles of the edict greatly affected the future practice of pharmacy in many European countries, but had negligible effect on the practice in Anglo-Saxon countries, especially the United States: (1) the limitation of the number of pharmacies within a designated geographic and political entity; and (2) the fixing of the prices of drugs by the government. Both principles have been adopted in several countries in which health care is under the control of government. The second principle, but not the first, is applied in England and, with the advent of third-party payment arrangements, is becoming fairly common in the United States.

English Conflicts and Organizations

A brief sketch of the history of English pharmacy has been included because American pharmacy was influenced more directly by English practices than by those of any other single country. The development of English pharmacy was different from that of European countries and, thus, the same is true of American pharmacy. The separation of pharmacy from medicine did not occur early or by direct edict or regulation. It evolved slowly through much conflict, negotiation, civil suits, and, finally, regulation and legislation. The delayed separation of the two professions paralleled the slow development of both professions. This slow development was the result of the various conquests of England, the slow amalgamation of the various peoples with different cultural backgrounds, the relatively small percentage of educated people, and, probably most importantly, the philosophy of *laissez faire.*

In the beginning no distinction was made between the physician, the apothecary, and the surgeon. Over the years a trade developed in spices, peppers, herbs, and other items of small weight but great value. Those dealing in these wares at the retail level were known as "spicers," and at the wholesale level as "peppers." Their stock in trade was called "spicery." Gradually the wholesalers developed a guild, known as the Grocers' Company, for their social and economic protection. Meanwhile, the spicers developed unique skills and knowledge in the preparation of their wares and became known distinctively as "apothecaries." The latter enjoyed the protective benefits of the Grocers' Company as a division of the guild, with official status, but not independence, granted by King James I in 1607. In 1617 they finally formed the separate Society of the Art and Mysteries of the Apothecaries. Meanwhile, the first regulation defining the functions of the physician and the apothecary was issued by Henry VIII in 1511. After the formation of the College of Physicians (later know as the Royal College of Physicians) in 1540, the apothecaries were placed under the more direct regulation of the College. This did not last long, and by 1543, an act was passed giving the right of "every person being the King's subject having knowledge and experience of the nature of herbs, roots and waters to use and minister, according to their cunning, experience, and knowledge."[1]

It was common practice for the apothecaries to practice as "minor physicians" and for the physicians not only to dispense medication, but to operate dispensaries. Under the authority of the 1543 Act, many people with less training practiced both medicine and pharmacy within certain limits. The major reason for this development was the small number of trained, certified physicians.

The feuds continued for centuries. By the eighteenth century, the dealers in herbs, spices, and medical remedies came to be known as "druggists" and "chemists," the chemists performing certain operations of a pharmaceutical nature. Ironically, the chemists took the place in the Grocers' Company formerly occupied by the apothecaries. As a result of the Great Plague (1665-66), during which most physicians died or fled London, the apothecaries gained official sanction to practice medicine when the House of Lords overruled a court decision in 1703. The fight did not end, but continued for many more years. Finally, apothecaries became the general practitioners of medicine and the chemists became the pharmacists. After many attempts, adequate laws were passed to regulate the practice of pharmacy and that of medicine. The Pharmaceutical Society of Great Britain became the official organization of pharmacists and ultimately became the licensing and regulating agency. Pharmacists were usually called chemists by the public. The pharmacies, or drugstores as we sometimes call them, were known as chemists' shops in England. The transformed apothecaries-physicians retained the Royal College of Physicians as their official organization and regulatory agency.[1]

Pharmacy in the Colonies

The brief historic sketch of pharmacy in England is similar to the development of pharmacy in the United States, with perhaps less direct legal confrontation among the various interests in the United States. The early settlers, and most immigrants, came to this country for political, economic, and religious freedom. They came from many different countries. As in the early history of Great Britain, there were (1) an amalgamation of people with varied cultural backgrounds, (2) a small percentage of educated people trained in the "arts and mysteries" of pharmacy or medicine, and (3) certainly people who subscribed to the philosophy of *laissez faire.* The primary consideration of the settlers was survival, which meant basically food, clothing, and shelter.

At the outset, the early settlers borrowed heavily from the Indians for remedies to treat the various and numerous illnesses. In fact, Indian drugs contributed nearly as much to European medicine as European medicine contributed to medicine in the New World. The settlers did bring with them some of their favorite recipes and materia medica (and seeds) to supplement the Indian remedies. This led to the fundamental principle of the "right to self-medicate." When people trained in the arts of physicks began to immigrate, it was much more practical to encourage those who were trained in both the arts of the apothecary and of the physician than to encourage those trained in only one art. Why pay the fare for two people when a single person would suffice?

During the first 200 years of colonization, medicine and pharmacy were practiced by housewives, barbers, governors, the clergy, and educators, in addition to trained apothecaries, surgeons, and physicians who were in the minority. As a result of this intrusion into the practice of pharmacy and medicine, when larger numbers of apothecaries and physicians later arrived in the New World many were forced to seek a livelihood in other occupations, such as teachers, ministers, or politicians.

The first apothecary to immigrate to North America was Louis Hebert, landing first in Nova Scotia in 1604 and later moving to Quebec in 1617.[1] He pursued husbandry in addition to providing his pharmaceutical skills and drugs to the members of the fur company. The first pharmacist in America was William Davice, who established a pharmacy in 1646.[1] One of the earliest American drugstores on record, actually a general store with a stock of drugs, was established in the colonies by a Dutch surgeon, Gysbert van Imbroch, in Kingston, New York, in 1663.[1]

There were letters sent to the Virginia Company with headquarters in London requesting "foure honest and learned Ministers, two Surgeons, two Druggists," indicating a need for educated people in the colonies. A later letter asked the Company to "send them some Phisitians and Apothecaries of which they stand much in need of."[1] A few, perhaps three, apothecaries came to the colonies during the seventeenth century. According to Blanton,[1] a medical historian, "there is no further record of apothecaries living in the colony in this century, the physician being for the most part his own apothecary." This represented the dominant factor influencing the development of pharmacy throughout the period of colonization.

There were at least four significant events during the eighteenth century that began to influence the development and practice of pharmacy in the United States. First, there was a great influx of English "patent medicines" into the colonies. These were widely advertised with greatly exaggerated claims, a practice that continued after the passage of the United States Patent Act and still exists under considerably more regulation today. These remedies provided an economical means to ameliorate diseases in view of the shortage of qualified physicians, and apothecaries, and nourished the practice of self-medication.

Second, the first hospital pharmacy was established in the Pennsylvania Hospital founded on the initiative of Benjamin Franklin. Jonathan Roberts, the pharmacy's first apothecary, was directed to compound medicines and make up prescriptions of physicians only, and this pharmacy was one of the early concrete examples of the separation of pharmacy and medicine in the colonies.

Third, Robert's successor, John Morgan, resigned after only one year to study medicine. After becoming a physician, Morgan was a strong advocate of the separation of the two professions and of restriction of the practice to those trained in the respective professions.

Fourth, an Act was passed in Virginia in 1736 to regulate and restrict the practice of medicine.

However, the progress toward the professionalization of pharmacy was slow, following the precedent set in England.

Early American Wars and Their Influence

Wars, by their requirement of greater productivity, stimulate a society to develop its resources, science, technology, and economic capabilities. Although the destructive effects of a war often outweigh the benefits, there are positive results.

THE REVOLUTIONARY WAR

The Revolutionary War caused pharmacy to be recognized officially as a separate and distinct profession when Andrew Craigie was appointed Apothecary-General. Much credit for this distinction of pharmacy goes to John Morgan, the Director General of the military hospitals and Chief Physician of the Army. Sonnedecker summarized the significance of the War:

> Eight years of successful pharmaceutical activity, separate from medicine but equally recognized and given the same official status; the first known American manufacture of pharmaceutical products on a large scale; the first practical attempt at a uniform and obligatory formulary as a basis for satisfactory and reliable pharmaceutical work (in this case, military pharmacy); and the meeting of American pharmacists with European colleagues who were more advanced professionally.[1]

With the end of the Revolutionary War, the colonists enjoyed a newly found freedom and an opportunity to develop a new society not tied to a monarchy or any oppressive political code or system. This climate was conducive to experimentation and rapid technologic and economic growth. It also deterred the enactment of laws that greatly restricted trade and the professions. However, one important law, the Patent Act, fostered the development of a flourishing trade in "patent medicines" or proprietary drugs independent of medicine. In addition, it provided the legal foundation for several medical practices such as the "Thomsonian," "Eclectic," and "Homeopathic" branches of medicine. Special remedies were developed and patented, based on the theories and practices of these various branches of medicine. The practical significance of the patent law was to promote a degree of monopoly for the various medical practices, including the dispensing of their special remedies. Also, the general public generally was ignorant of the nature of the various patented remedies and purchased these remedies wantonly in the hope of miraculous cure perpetrated by the vendors, physicians included.

Sonnedecker[1] named three classes of people involved in the drug field:

1. Persons who had served a more-or-less lengthy apprenticeship with a medical practitioner, and had learned to compound prescriptions; not infrequently, these people seem to have had a greater interest in their commercial talents and prospects than in their medical accomplishments.

2. Those who had trained as apothecaries, chemists, or druggists, and all who had pharmaceutical education, such as the apothecaries or Apotheker in their native countries. However, most of these people preferred medical practice combined with dispensing.

3. Storekeepers who specialized in drugs to some extent without having any special pharmaceutical training.

To this list should be added the dispensing physicians and physicians operating their own apothecary shops or dispensaries. And as the people migrated westward, the competition of the storekeepers was provided first by the proprietors of the trading posts and later the general stores. The competitive condition was enhanced by the itinerant peddlers and medicine shows selling their dubious remedies. Thus, not unlike their English counterparts, the trained American apothecaries or pharmacists faced vigorous competition from both ends of the professional-commercial continuum—the physicians at the professional end who had a distinctive monopolistic advantage, and the ordinary storekeepers and peddlers at the commercial end, who also had the advantage of being less scrupulous in making exaggerated claims for the drugs they sold. Both categories of competition far outnumbered the true apothecary shops until the latter part of the nineteenth century.

The legitimate pharmacists were forced to sell many lines of goods other than drugs to make a livelihood. Other commodities included spices, tobacco, pigments, paints, brushes, oils, glass, and various chemicals. Some, especially during the early years, became drug and spice importers and wholesalers providing raw materials to physicians, other apothecaries, and even general stores—especially those in the rural areas. Some of these pharmacists became manufacturers, for example Schieffelin, Wm. S. Merrell, and Smith Kline and French.

On the brighter side was the gradual development of professional pharmacy. Local associations were organized and many of them established colleges of pharmacy, the first being the Philadelphia College of Pharmacy in 1821. By 1860, six colleges were established and each organization later became an educational institution. In 1852 the American Pharmaceutical Association (APhA) was organized. It fostered the organization of state associations, which in turn, with the assistance of the APhA, enacted state pharmacy laws. The APhA adopted a code of ethics and sponsored a number of national pharmaceutical associations, including the National Association of Retail Druggists and the American Society of Hospital Pharmacists. Ironically, the latter group and the APhA disaffiliated by a series of individual actions in late 1972 and early 1973. The Pharmacopoeia of the United States was published in 1820 by "authority of the medical societies and colleges." Pharmacists were utilized in the first revision, and by 1860 pharmacists constituted one-half of the Revision Committee.

Meanwhile, several truly professional apothecary shops were established, principally in the large cities—New York, Philadelphia, Cincinnati, Louisville, St. Louis, and New Orleans. This development was fostered by the European trained physicians, both immigrants and United States citizens, who were trained to write prescriptions to be compounded by professional apothecaries. The greater number of pharmacies, however, were the traditional type, selling various non-drug commodities. Some drugstores were closer in character to general stores than they were to pharmacies, especially in the frontier towns.

THE CIVIL WAR

The Civil War had a dramatic effect on the political, social, and economic structure of our society and provided the impetus for the rapid industrialization of our country. This industrialization affected all trades and industries, including pharmacy, and had a direct effect on the American pharmacy.

First, the development of the textile industry reduced the demand for dye-stuffs in the drugstores since the production of clothing was shifted from the home, and drugstore purchases to the factory. Similarly, the paint, glass, and oil trade was shifted to the building trade industry. Retailers in paint, general building materials, and/or hardware absorbed much of this business, which had previously belonged to the general store or drugstore. The third direct effect on pharmacy was the gradual shifting of the compounding function from the drugstore to the emerging pharmaceutical industry. As Sonnedecker observed,[1] the shifting of the preparation of drugs to large manufacturers had a lesser effect in the United States than it did in Europe because most of the prescriptions were compounded by physicians or their apprentices. However, competition in the form of dispensing by physicians and physician ownership of pharmacies continued well into the twentieth century and still exists to a significant degree in many locales.

Deterrents to Professionalization

The question may be asked why pharmacy did not seize the opportunity to develop a strictly professional type of practice as the sale of several of the traditional lines of goods was transferred to other trades. The answer is manifold: The deterrents to professionalization of pharmacy include: (1) the demise of the general store, (2) competition of various types, (3) the introduction of the soda fountain, (4) inadequate regulations, (5) prohibition, and (6) Fair Trade laws.

DEMISE OF THE GENERAL STORE

As indicated earlier, the general stores and the drugstores were similar in the frontier towns; however, the typical pharmacy in the larger cities was quite different and was distinctly a different institution. It was not as highly specialized and professional as the German Apotheke, but was more specialized than the larger diversified general store, a true *American institution*. As the country became more settled and urbanized, the general stores gradually faded from the scene, although they still can be found in some rural areas today. Other lines of trades absorbed certain lines common to the general store, for example, clothing in the dry goods store and tools and nails in the hardware stores. Because of their accessibility and convenience—large numbers and long hours—the drugstores were the logical choice to carry many of the smaller items common to the general stores. These items collectively came to be referred to as "sundries." These include chemicals used as pesticides, veterinary drugs and implements, needles and thread, stationery and writing accessories, magazines and books, tobacco and accessories, toiletries, and confectioneries. It should be realized that the greatest motivation for stocking these sundry items was economic survival in the face of the competitive conditions facing pharmacy.

COMPETITION AND DIVERSIFICATION

Competition can assume several forms. Basically these are the number and types of business units or establishments vying for patronage with price and services. It should be obvious that the latter two forms derive from the first, the large numbers of establishments competing for the consumers' patronage and dollars.

Competition through diversification may be classified into two categories: within the drug trade and from outside the drug trade. This distinction is difficult to make today because of mergers. The supermarkets, variety chains, and other trades have entered the pharmaceutical business. Historically, competition has always come from both within and outside the traditional pharmaceutical businesses. During the early years, competition came from the general stores and physicians' apothecary shops, which have been discussed already. As the general stores faded from the scene, mail order houses, beginning with Montgomery and Ward in 1872, provided considerable competition, especially in the rural areas.

Meanwhile, drugstore chains were being established as indicated in Table 1-1.

According to the *Chain Store Age/Drug Executive Edition,*[2] chain stores in 1972 derived an average of 17.3 percent of their total revenue from prescriptions and 21.7 percent from proprietary drugs. The two departments combined occupied only 17.7 percent of the total space. In contrast, independent pharmacies derived an average of 44.5 percent of the revenue from prescriptions.[3] It has been estimated that the typical independent pharmacy realizes 67 percent of its total revenue from health-related activities.[4]

The department store, which is an organization of many single-line stores under one roof and management, naturally would sell many products in competition with the traditional drugstore. To provide a historic perspective, Macy's, one of the biggest and best-known department stores, was established in 1858.[5] However, recently Macy's has discontinued some of its pharmacy departments. Some department stores have professional pharmacies located within their establishments.

In the year 1859 the Great Atlantic and Pacific Tea Company (A&P) was founded. Later the Kroger Company was established in 1882. While these chain grocery companies provided little real competition in the beginning, after World War II, the health and beauty aid departments of the grocery stores began to compete significantly with the drugstores. These departments were stocked with limited lines and sizes with a high

Table 1-1. *Early Drugstore Chains*

Date Founded	Name	Location
1850	Schlegal Drug Stores	Davenport, Iowa
1852	Meyer Brothers Company	Fort Wayne, Indiana
1879	T. P. Taylor & Company	Louisville, Kentucky
1879	Jacobs Pharmacy Company	Atlanta, Georgia
1883	Read Drug & Chemical Co.	Baltimore, Maryland
1884	Marshall Drug Co.	Cleveland, Ohio
1885	Skillern's Drug Stores	Dallas, Texas
1889	Cunningham Drug Stores	Detroit, Michigan
1890	Bartell Drug Company	Seattle, Washington
1892	Owl Drug Company	San Francisco, Calif.
1898	Eckerd Drug Stores	Erie, Pa.
1899	Standard Drug Stores	Cleveland, Ohio
1901	Walgreen Drug Co.	Chicago, Illinois
1907	Louis K. Liggett Co.	New York City

Source: Lebhar, G. M.: *Chain Stores in America, 1859–1962,* 3rd ed. New York: Chain Store Publishing Corp., 1963, pp. 43–44.

turnover rate. The competition became more direct and vigorous when Kroger established its Super X Drug Corporation in 1961.[6] This period marked the vigorous expansion of price reduction and advertising of selected prescription drugs. This practice was not restricted to any one company, but it became prevalent among many drug chains and large discount stores with prescription departments.

The variety, or "Five and Dime," stores provided a degree of competition for the traditional drugstore from the inception of the variety stores. Woolworth, the first variety store chain, was established in 1879. Woolworth was followed by McCrory in 1881, Kress in 1896, and S. S. Kresge in 1899. The J. C. Penney Co., which was established in 1902, was somewhat unique in that it combined some of the features of both dry goods and variety stores, a sort of junior department store. Its real significance relative to drugstore competition is that the company has recently entered the pharmaceutical business with its Thrift Drugs, Treasury Drugs, and leased prescription and drug departments.

Some of the most persistent and effective competitors were the "pine-board drugstores." Their origin dates from the early part of this century.[7] They were characterized by: (1) location in low rent areas; (2) furnishings of inexpensive fixtures—usually pine boards nailed to the wall or placed on bricks which supported them; (3) stock limited to fast-selling products and popular sizes; and (4) sale prices of products at low gross margins. The "pine-board drugstore" flourished during the early part of the Great Depression and had its counterpart in the grocery trade.

It appears that the "pine-board drugstores" were the forerunners of the so-called "discount stores." The "pine-board drugstore" disappeared from the scene by the end of World War II. Although some form of discount merchandising had existed throughout history, the large, vigorously merchandised discount stores really began to develop and grow in the 1950s. The discount stores differed from the "pine-board stores" in the following aspects: (1) the discount stores were much larger and carried a greater variety of merchandise lines; (2) their fixturing was better and more attractive, but still not expensive; (3) they were located along a high traffic street or highway, but usually not in major shopping centers; and (4) they advertised vigorously and attempted to establish the one-stop-shop concept in the minds of the public—a "shopping center" under one roof. Of course, drugs and prescription departments were included and were used as "loss leaders" to promote greater traffic and sales volume.

Competition in pricing is as old as commerce itself, and it certainly is as old as pharmacy in this country. T. W. Dyatt is considered to have been the "father of price-cutting" in American pharmacy when he established a patent medicine warehouse in Philadelphia in 1806. The George A. Kelly Company, which later became Beckham and Kelly, was the forerunner of the chain drugstore concept in this country. The Company operated four drugstores in Pittsburgh around 1860, which used the sign "Cut-rate Drugstores."[1]

Price-cutting, a practice used by certain independents even more than the older chains, became prevalent in certain cities by the 1880s, and several steps were taken to combat this practice.

First, pharmacists began to manufacture, or have manufactured for them, exclusive private label drugs with controlled distribution and prices. Several of these co-ops were organized, but they gradually faded from the scene. Approximately six of these cooperative ventures existed over a period of fifty years. One such company, the United Drug Company, under the leadership of L. K. Liggett, became a permanent national organization. It began as a manufacturer of proprietary drugs and toiletries under the label of "Rexall" for franchised independent pharmacies, serving about 10,500 pharmacies by 1960. Meanwhile, the Company established a chain of drugstores reaching a total of 550 units, the largest drug chain in the United States in 1947.[1] This large diversified organization demonstrated that the economic interests of the chain drug industry and the independent pharmacists can merge. The Walgreen Drug Company represents a similar type of organization, which developed in the reverse order. The Company first organized a chain of drugstores and then established a large number of franchises among independent pharmacists to obtain a wider distribution of the Company's private label drugs and other products. Now, the Walgreen Drug Company is the largest drug chain organization.

Another attempt to combat price-cutting was the formation of mutual wholesale drug companies. Beginning as buying groups, some of these were initiated by pharmacists, while others were organized by regular wholesalers to establish a system of franchise dealers to promote and sell a controlled line of drugs and other products.

THE SODA FOUNTAIN AND PHARMACY

The soda fountain had a significant impact on the practice of pharmacy in the United States and became an integral part of the typical pharmacy in this country. "Soda water" was used as a medicinal preparation in the latter part of the eighteenth century. The first soda fountain probably was operated in Philadelphia around 1825. Soda fountains became common by 1860 to the extent that some were adorned with ornate fixtures. The soda fountain came into its own in the 1880s when the anti-whiskey movement resulted in the passage of local prohibition laws. This movement culminated in the Volstead Act in 1919 and the soda fountain reached its peak of popularity.

The impact of the soda fountain on pharmacy practice was dramatic and is hardly debatable, but the value to the professional practice of pharmacy *is* debatable. The extra income derived from fountains was significant and saved many proprietors from economic failure. It also revolutionized the nature of the drugstore, changing it from a sober professional-business institution to one that emanated a relaxed atmosphere where people gathered to "indulge" in a refreshing drink or repast, to share local news or gossip, or to consult with "Doc" privately about matters of a more serious nature. The latter purpose may not always have been health related. This feature, together with the diversified merchandising practice, has caused several writers to observe that "the American Drugstore is a unique social institution" peculiar only to the United States.

There were other concrete changes in the characteristics of the drugstore brought about by the complementary effects of the soda fountain and diversified merchandising.

1. The size of the drugstore increased to accommodate the increased merchandise and activities.

2. The business hours of the drugstore increased to take advantage of attracting patrons to the soda fountain in the evenings.

3. The location of the drugstore shifted from lower-rent sites to the high-rent, busy-corner locations, again to maximize traffic, sales, and profits.

4. All of the above changes increased investment and operating expenses, thereby increasing the risk of establishing a pharmacy practice.

5. Overall, the practice of pharmacy became more a commercial venture and less a professional venture. Of course, this was not always the case. One must keep in mind that the practice of pharmacy in the United States had been commercially oriented from the earliest years.

The positive financial results of the combined merchandising and soda fountain activities are shown in Table 1-2.

There was a sharp decline in the number of soda fountains during World War II. It has been reported that one out of every six stores closed their fountains during the war because of the shortage of personnel and materials, especially sugar and syrups.[8] In a survey of approximately 1700 pharmacies conducted by the National Association of Retail Druggists and *The Saturday Evening Post,* the percentage of pharmacies operating fountains showed a decrease from 81.5 percent to 74.8 percent.[9] Some of the fountain closings during the War may have been temporary, but a permanent trend of closing fountains coincided with the large-scale remodeling of pharmacies after World War II. Today, less than one-half of the pharmacies operate soda fountains.

INADEQUATE REGULATIONS

There was a definite parallel between the formation of state pharmaceutical associations and the passage of state pharmacy laws, with the

Table 1-2. *Relationship of Sales Volume to Presence of Soda Fountain*

Item	Pharmacies with fountain			Pharmacies without fountain			All pharmacies		
	1939	1935	1929	1939	1935	1929	1939	1935	1929
No. of pharmacies	39,452	38,431	34,844	18,451	17,966	23,414	57,903	56,697	58,258
Total sales millions of $	1,205	950	1,149	357	282	541	1,563	1,233	1,690
Avg. yearly sales in $	30,542	24,528	32,695	19,362	16,253	23,111	26,983	21,740	29,015
Avg. daily sales in $	84	67	89	53	44	63	74	60	80

Source: Publications of the Bureau of the Census.

laws usually following the associations by a few years. The major failing in the pharmacy acts and regulations was their trade or product orientation in contrast to a professional and personal orientation. Had more thought and effort been directed toward certifying highly competent pharmacists and less effort toward regulation of the drug trade, pharmacy would have benefited from self-regulation via an enforced code of practice.

Pharmacy was about three decades behind in the passage and amendment of the pharmacy acts. For example, if a college degree had been a requisite for licensure as a pharmacist by 1900, the flooding of the market with poorly trained graduates of the "cram schools" could have been avoided. This would have reduced the severe competition, elevated the practice of pharmacy to a higher plane, and caused physicians to accept pharmacists as co-equal colleagues in providing health services. Many of the conflicts within the ranks of pharmacy could have been avoided by a more enlightened body of practitioners. Comradeship would have largely replaced predatory competition. Given the nature of pharmacy even under nearly ideal conditions, wholesome competition probably would have existed.

PROHIBITION AND PHARMACY

The Volstead Act, previously alluded to in the context of its influence on an increase in fountain patronage, also had other effects on pharmacy. During the prohibition era, the pharmacy was the only legitimate source for alcoholic beverages. This, of course, provided yet another source of revenue for proprietors of drugstores. The incentive was such that some people were induced to establish pharmacies primarily for that purpose. Some, no doubt, were induced to study pharmacy in order to obtain a license to practice and dispense prescriptions, including those for whiskey. As a consequence, the number of pharmacies rose to an all-time high of 58,258 in 1929—before the stock market crash, the depression of the thirties, and the *repeal of prohibition.*

During the prohibition era, a pharmacy could be found at nearly every major intersection in the large cities. Many drugstores continued their liquor departments after prohibition. On balance, the so-called great American experiment (prohibition) did little, if anything, to further professional pharmacy; some pharmacists contend that it even exerted a negative effect.

"FAIR TRADE" LAWS

"Fair Trade" laws represented the greatest concerted effort to combat price-cutting. Earlier efforts to maintain prices had failed for various reasons. The Campion plan, a rebate for not undercutting the regular retail price, failed for a lack of an enforcement mechanism. The tripartite plan was a mutual agreement among the National Association of Retail Druggists (NARD), the National Wholesale Druggists Association (NWDA), and the Proprietary Association (PA). This plan, in essence, was to limit the distribution and sale of many of the nationally known products to those drugstores who maintained the suggested retail price. This plan was declared illegal under the Sherman Antitrust Law in a United States Circuit Court in Indiana in 1907.

It was not until the 1930s, when the Great Depression caused many business failures, that public sentiment turned in favor of laws and regulations to preserve American business, especially small businesses. The National Recovery Act (NRA), which was later declared unconstitutional, was a significant measure for this very purpose. Beginning with California in 1931, many states passed "fair trade" laws with the assistance of the NARD. By 1949, all of the states except Texas, Missouri, and Vermont had enacted fair trade laws. It should be noted that the old-line chain drugstores supported fair trade completely.

It would assist in the understanding of fair trade laws and some of the socioeconomic aspects of pharmacy if we briefly reviewed the social and legal bases for the fair trade laws. The social theory of fair trade supported the concept of pure or perfect competition. This is a classic economic theory that perfect competition can exist only when there are numerous small suppliers and buyers, and both have a complete knowledge of the market relative to price, quality, and other factors. The price is determined by the market through the interactions of the suppliers and purchasers. Fair trade laws helped to maintain a large number of small suppliers; there were numerous small buyers (consumers); and the price of a fair trade product became familiar to most purchasers even though it was fixed by the manufacturer and not by the market. The main purpose was the preservation of small businesses.

The legal basis for fair trade was quite different. It was based on the protection of property rights, the good will associated with trademarked or branded products. The product had to meet the following three criteria: (1) the product had to be in free and open competition with products of the same general class (use); (2) the product had to have a trademark or a trade name identifiable with the producer; and (3) the producer had the option of establishing the minimum resale price. It should be noted that price maintenance was legally binding vertically and not horizontally (among retailers) and enforceable only by the producer. Three conditions when the minimum resale price could be disregarded were: (1) if the product was damaged or deteriorated; (2) if the product was sold by order of a court; and (3) if the product was sold in a genuine closing-out sale.

The first fair trade laws did not contain the so-called "nonsigner" clause, which meant that each retailer had to sign a contract with each supplier and/or manufacturer. These early laws were amended, and the later laws incorporated the "nonsigner" clause, which caused the fair trade law to be binding on all retailers provided one retailer signed a fair trade contract in each state.

The fair trade laws were fortified by two legal developments at the federal level. The United States Supreme Court in 1936 upheld the constitutionality of the Illinois Fair Trade Act.[10] The Miller-Tydings Federal Enabling Act amended the Sherman Anti-trust Act, which enabled states to pass fair trade laws applicable to interstate commerce without being in violation of the Anti-trust Laws.

The fair trade laws received a severe setback in the famous Schwegman case.[11] The United States Supreme Court ruled the "nonsigner" clause unconstitutional for interstate commerce. This defect was quickly remedied with the passage of the McGuire Amendment to the Federal Trade Commission Act in 1952, and the "nonsigner" clause was reinstated for interstate commerce. From this point in time, fair trade laws lost ground rapidly, primarily through court decisions at the state level. It was mostly the "nonsigner" clause that was declared invalid; however, in some states the entire law was invalidated. Also, manufacturers became weary of enforcing the fair trade contracts. Today fair trade laws are of little or no effect except in the liquor and milk trades.

The fair trade laws had a favorable economic impact upon pharmacy by decreasing the number of business failures, and the laws, obviously, were construed favorably by a number of practitioners. However, the fair trade laws had a negative aspect from a strictly professional viewpoint. The net effect was a reduced sales volume per pharmacy for prescriptions and health-related products reflecting reduced revenues from professional activities. As late as 1939, Nolen reports that prescriptions accounted for only 13 percent of the total sales and 19.3 percent of the gross margin of sales.[12] Under these conditions, pharmacists were forced to offer a wider variety of products and services, and as a result pharmacy became more business-like than professional in character.

REFERENCES

1. Sonnedecker, G.: *Kremers and Urdang's History of Pharmacy.* 3rd ed. Philadelphia: J. B. Lippincott Co., 1963.
2. *Chain Store Age/Drug Executive Edition. 49*: 75-209, May, 1973.
3. *The Lilly Digest 1971,* Indianapolis: Eli Lilly & Co., 1971.
4. The estimate was derived from references 2, 3, and *Drug Topics, Chain Edition,* Sept. 25, 1972, pp. 21 and 22.
5. Lebhar, G. M.: *Chain Stores in America 1859-1950.* 1st ed. New York: Chain Store Publishing Corporation, 1952, p. 13.
6. Fletcher, F. M.: *Market Restraints in the Retail Drug Industry.* Philadelphia: University of Pennsylvania Press, 1967, p. 175.
7. Sonnedecker, *op. cit.,* p. 271.
8. *Drug Topics' Drug Trade Marketing Guide.* New York, 1961, p. 57.

9. *The Independent Druggist, Report #1.* NARD and Curtis Publishing Company, 1945, p. 64.
10. *Old Dearborn Co. v. Seagram Corp.* 299 U.S. 183, 1936.
11. *Schwegman Bros. v. Calvert Distillers.* 341 U.S. 384, 1951.
12. Nolen, H. C., and Maynard, H. H.: *Drug Store Management.* New York: McGraw-Hill Book Co., 1941, p. 7.

REVIEW

1. Explain why pharmacy and medicine did not begin as separate professions.

2. What were the regulations of the edict of Frederick II?

3. Identify the three socioeconomic factors that deterred the early development of pharmacy in both England and the United States.

4. What were the two pre-Revolutionary War factors and the one post-Revolutionary War factor that promoted the principle of self-medication in the United States?

5. Discuss the influence of the Revolutionary War on the development of pharmacy, and name the two important men involved.

6. Describe the three classes of drug vendors and their manner of competing for the drug business during the early history of this country.

7. Discuss the effects of the Civil War on the practice of Pharmacy.

8. Discuss the three major professional developments in pharmacy during the early part of the nineteenth century.

9. Discuss in detail how each of the following deterred the professionalization of pharmacy: demise of the general store; competition and diversification; the soda fountain; inadequate regulations; prohibition; and fair trade laws.

10. Discuss the positive effects, if any, of the six factors enumerated in Question 9.

11. Describe the economic impact of the early drugstore chains and the pineboard drugstores on pharmacy.

12. Contrast and explain the social and legal theories or bases of the fair trade laws.

2. Nature and Principles of Management

What Is Management?

The *classic definition of management* is the art and science of planning, organizing, directing, and controlling human effort and resources for the general good within the organizational framework and economic environment of the firm. The essence of management is *decision-making*. Its unique function is choosing between alternative means of moving toward an objective. The decision-making process involves the following: (1) identifying and defining the problem; (2) analyzing it; (3) developing alternate solutions; (4) deciding upon the best solution; and (5) converting the decision into effective action. In carrying out this mandate, the manager has to weigh the risks of every course of action against the expected gains. Then, having decided, he must clearly communicate the orders and provide the necessary leadership to get results. Many people shun this sort of responsibility. Only a few seek it, and they become leaders, knowing that there is a possibility that a decision may be wrong, but also knowing that this chance may be minimized if some basic rules and procedures are followed.

Management and administration are often considered synonymous by many employed in the field. However, with the changing characteristics of business—especially the changing economic environment, the vast size of many businesses, and the evolving bureaucracy in business—authorities now make a distinction between the two. The *administrator* is one who adapts to his environment in order to survive in it and obtain sustenance from it. The *manager* relates to his environment. He is more risk-oriented and relates directly to his resources in order to control, manipulate, and direct them for gain.[1]

Administration or management of a business is a network in which every decision is connected in some way with every other decision that has preceded it and will have a bearing upon decisions to be made in the future. A manager needs the qualities of a statesman to see his organization in all its relationships. He has to know his organization's objectives and policies, what resources he can call upon, and the capabilities of those who will make his decisions effective, and then he must produce plans that take all these into account. This is the leadership function of management. Every employee has a stake in leadership, because the manager is accountable not only for the success of his organization, but also for the continued employment and the satisfaction of all those associated with it. Many business decisions are routine and repetitive to the experienced manager, but he must patiently keep in mind that particular problems may be new to his staff. Therefore, it is part of his duty to provide the necessary guidance and explanations.

Two cardinal principles of management are: (1) the decision must be adequate to solve the problem, and (2) authority must be commensurate with responsibilities. There is no use in attacking a tank with a bow and arrow, and it is wasteful to shoot sparrows with a cannon. Delegation of responsibility without giving the necessary authority to carry out the responsibility is unfair to the subordinate. It leads to frustrations and ineffective administration. A disregard for the latter principle probably is the most common failure among managers and administrators.

In his book entitled *A Philosophy of Administration,*[2] Marshall E. Dimock states that administration ought to be studied according to the scientific method, but that administration ought not to aim at being a science. Yet, any philosophy of administration must be capable of passing the acid test of science, i.e., management must be capable of empiric validation based on the results of past experience, and it must be capable of further predictions and planning of future goals.

Practicing pharmacy in an economy such as ours demands *foresight, judgment, resourcefulness, knowledge,* and *courage.* Only the person who applies all these qualities in making decisions may expect to advance his pharmacy.

Styles of Management

There are basically five distinct styles of management which have evolved from the days of classic capitalism. They are:

1. The "Captain-of-Industry" style that pre-dated and later co-existed with the establishment of scientific management in 1885.

2. The "Hard-Nose" style of the mid 1910s to the 1930s.

3. The "Human-Relations" style of the 1940s and early 1950s.

4. The "Management-by-Pressure" style of the early 1950s to mid 1960s.

5. The "Management-by-Objectives" style beginning in the mid 1960s.

The various management or leadership styles are depicted as a continuum in Figure 2-1.

CAPTAIN-OF-INDUSTRY STYLE

This style is represented by the strong individualistic person who amassed a fortune through drive, hard work, ingenuity, and good luck. Well-known examples of this type of entrepreneur of the nineteenth century include Andrew William Mellon, John Davidson Rockefeller, Andrew Carnegie, and Henry Ford, who began his industrial career in the early twentieth century. These people represent only a few of the outstanding capitalists of this era. All had different personalities and characteristics, although some type of composite personality profile might be synthesized from their major attributes. Even if a person with this composite personality profile could be found, there is no assurance he would be a successful businessman. There were, of course, common traits among these men. These included drive, a dream, and definite short-term and long-term goals.

HARD NOSE ←					→ NO NOSE	
Style	*Autocrat*	*Authoritariancrat*	*Bureaucrat*	*Democrat*	*Particicrat*	*Abdicrat*
Source	Self	Position	Rules, systems, procedures	Majority	Group	Diffused
General mode of communication	Directives and order giving		Explainer and explanation	Discusser and discussion	Joint determiner and determination	Random

Figure 2-1. *Leadership styles continuum. (Adapted from Caskey, C. C.: Developing a leadership style.* Supervision, *April, 1964. By permission of* Supervision *and the National Research Bureau, Inc.)*

This style of management gradually declined as our industrial society became more mature and institutionalized. That is, large corporations began to adapt to social pressure, largely via legal regulation, and began to operate accordingly. With the adoption of the principles of scientific management, introduced by Frederick W. Taylor around 1885, this change in the style of management was accelerated.

Scientific management was based on the principles and techniques of analyzing each job down to the smallest elements that could be identified and measured in terms of the time required to perform the task. These elements were then organized into a work cycle for each job, and standards were set for each job by the use of stopwatches and statistical procedures. Thus, the workers were reduced to an almost robot level, and the base pay scale, raises, and bonuses were based on meeting or surpassing the work standards.

HARD-NOSE STYLE

After the enactment of the Sherman Anti-Trust Act in 1890, the Clayton Anti-Trust Act, and the Federal Trade Commission Act in 1914, corporate policies became more restrained in commercial dealings. However, under the increasing competitive influence brought about by these laws, management sought newer ways to compete. Armed with the techniques of scientific management, large corporations were in a position to demand high standards of work performance, thus lowering the unit production cost. This economic and political background provided the basis for the hard-nose policy of management from about 1914 through the 1930s.

HUMAN-RELATIONS STYLE

This style of management was ushered in by two major events. First was the growth in size and strength of the unions, especially after the passage of the Wagner Act in 1935. This Act gave the unions the right to assemble, associate together, negotiate, and strike if necessary without anti-trust sanctions. More importantly, World War II brought about a scarcity of workers, and it was necessary to motivate employees through good human relations programs to increase the productivity needed for the war effort. This philosophy was enhanced by two other factors: first, price stabilization, which eased the competitive pressures, and second, the research findings of the social scientists. This also was an era when fringe benefits became important considerations in lieu of frozen pay increases.

MANAGEMENT-BY-PRESSURE STYLE

This style of management originated under the economic conditions following World War II. These conditions were characterized by increasing demand, prices, and costs. Without returning to the old hard-nose policy, except in labor negotiations, management exerted pressure to hold costs down, increase productivity, and obtain a larger share of the growing market. Pressure was exerted to produce more by gearing promotion and other economic incentives to productivity, while maintaining increased fringe benefits, but putting less reliance on the policy of good human relations. This was the era when a good manager was known as someone "who could make things happen."

Meanwhile scientific management had not been ignored by personnel and industrial engineering departments. On the contrary, the tools of scientific management had been refined, and it was augmented by the observations of such famous management authorities as Peter Drucker.[3] Scientific management was being enriched and humanized by the appreciation of research findings of the industrial psychologists, notably Joseph Tiffin.[4]

MANAGEMENT-BY-OBJECTIVES STYLE

The formulation of this style, perhaps better labeled as a method, was based on analysis of the defects of the previous styles or methods of management and a synthesis of some of the better aspects of the previous methods. Since it is goal-oriented, it obviously has some of the better characteristics, philosophy, and concepts of the pressure style. Management by objectives, frequently abbreviated as MBO, accommodates all that is best in the human relations style, and it can also accommodate and use the results of well-designed behavioral science research.

Since its premises are not based on any set of personality traits or a personality cult, it is not incompatible with the "captain-of-industry" type of manager as long as the manager follows the rules set forth. Although it can accommodate the "hard-nose" style, the effectiveness of management by objectives is greatly lessened by this style and philosophy. Above all, management by objectives, like so many really useful methods, is a very simple, common sense, and logical method. One wonders why it took so long to discover it. Like many discoveries, management by objectives, though simple in content, required extraordinary insight into the various elements of the system. It was described first by Peter Drucker,[5] and later in more detail by Odiorne.[6,7]

Management by Objectives

Odiorne gave a concise *definition* of management by objectives.[8] He stated,

> In brief, the system of management by objectives can be described as a process whereby the superior and subordinate managers of an organization jointly identify its common goals, define each individual's major area of responsibility in terms of results expected of him, and use these measures as guides for operating the unit and assessing the contribution of each of its members.

Go to 30

MAJOR PREMISES

The major premises of management by objectives are as follows:[9]

1. Business management takes place within individual firms, which collectively form a major and integral component of the economic system. The economic system has undergone drastic change over the past 45 years, requiring greater social awareness and responsibility on the part of business management. The premise has a special significance for pharmacy, since health care is continuing to undergo drastic changes as a result of strong social and political pressure for improvement.

2. Management by objectives is directed toward meeting these changes and the new requirements. It presumes that the first step in management is to identify the goals of the organization, which are consistent with the goals of society. All other management methods and subsystems follow this preliminary step.

3. Once organizational goals have been identified, orderly procedures should be instituted for distributing responsibility among individuals in such a way that their combined efforts are directed toward achieving those goals.

4. Management by objectives assumes that managerial behavior is more important than manager personality, and that this behavior should be defined in terms of results, measured against the manager's goals rather than in terms of overall goals for the entire organization.

5. It also presumes that while participation is highly desirable in goal-setting and decision-making, its principal merit lies in its social and political value rather than its effects on productivity, though even here it usually has a favorable impact.

6. It regards the successful manager as a manager of defined situations, which fall within the overall purpose and scope of the firm or organization. Success is attributed to the managerial behavior best suited to achieve results with respect to defined situations and objectives. This means that there is no best pattern of management, but that management should be discriminatory, relating to specific goals, yet responsive to the larger socioeconomic system within which it operates.

PHILOSOPHY AND CONCEPTUAL FRAMEWORK

Management by objectives is essentially a system of incorporating into a more logical and effective pattern the things many people are already doing, although in a somewhat chaotic manner, or in a manner that obscures personal risk and responsibility. Management by objectives is basic and simple, yet flexible enough to incorporate subsystems such as economic order quantities and personnel development programs. Also, management by objectives does not exclude it from being a part of a larger system, especially the value system of the organization.[10]

The system of management by objectives is *not a "cookbook" approach to management* in which "cut-and-dried" procedures are followed blindly. Such an approach would render management by objectives impotent and useless. When such an approach has been used, experience has shown repeatedly that the people who are supposed to implement it never accept it. Instead they consider it as one more mechanism and an exercise in futility.[11] The system of management by objectives goes beyond a set of rules, a series of procedures, or even a set method of management. It is a *philosophy, a way of thinking,* and a *system* that incorporates objectivity, logic, and scientific management procedures. It also bridges the gap between participatory management and firm organizational control.

Odiorne described the *conceptual framework* for the implementation of the system of management by objectives:[12]

1. The system *utilizes* the basic *organizational structure* or *hierarchy* of the business and *makes it work.* This induces vitality and personal involvement of the people in the firm, and the system can be applied to a small independent pharmacy with a single proprietor, to a large drugstore chain operation, a drug wholesaler, or a pharmaceutical manufacturer.

2. Management by objectives *stimulates the growth and development* of an organization by involving all key employees, causing them to grow and develop. This is accomplished through the mutual development of statements of expectations and the necessary criteria for measuring the results.

3. The system *assigns risk* via mutual agreement and participation in the whole process. It stresses ability and achievement rather than personality and ties the employee's progress—pay raises, promotion, and even tenure—to the results achieved as measured against the objectives. Both objectives and their attainment are mutually determined by the employee and his supervisor.

4. Management by objectives is *especially applicable to professional and managerial* employees and may be extended to department supervisors, technical positions, or clerical employees with some modification in the method of setting standards and measuring results. However, at

the lower level the employees may not be as capable of identifying viable objectives as are employees at higher levels.

5. Management by objectives *helps to overcome many chronic problems* of managing professionals and store managers by negating many, if not all, of the chronic problems discussed below.

SOLUTION FOR CHRONIC PROBLEMS

The problems of management fall into two major areas: (1) problems of managing professionals and pharmacy managers and (2) problems encountered by the small business proprietor in managing employees. However, these two sets of problems are not necessarily peculiar to either category.

The solution to some of the chronic problems of managing by the application of management by objectives has been described by Odiorne[12] as follows:

1. Management by objectives provides a means of *measuring the true contribution* of managerial and professional personnel.

2. By defining the common goals of people and organizations, and measuring individual contributions toward reaching these goals, the possibility of *obtaining coordinated effort and teamwork* is enhanced without eliminating the personal risk.

3. MBO provides solutions to the key problem of *defining the major areas of responsibility* for each person in the organization, including joint or shared responsibilities.

4. MBO processes are geared to *achieving the results desired, both for the organization as a whole and for the individual contributors.*

5. It *eliminates the need for people to change their personalities,* as well as for appraising people on the basis of their personality traits.

6. It provides a means of *determining the span of control of each manager.*

7. It offers an *answer to the key question of salary administration*—"How should we allocate pay increase from available funds, if we want to pay for results?"

8. It aids in *identifying potential for advancement and in finding promotable people.*

Steinmetz et al. described the common "pitfalls" of managers of small businesses as follows:[13]

1. *Wasting time* as the most common hazard to good management.

2. *Putting fun things first, not first things first,* resulting from inability to establish appropriate priorities.

3. *Inability to delegate,* resulting from the close personal identification with the entire business enterprise.

This last problem was viewed by Steinmetz and his co-authors as one that is very difficult to overcome. Nine reasons were outlined to relate why managers and small business proprietors fail to delegate work.

1. They are little Napoleons who must satisfy their own ego by keeping all authority.
2. They feel that they can do it better themselves, and they refuse to permit others to do it in a "substandard" manner.
3. They are unable to communicate to their subordinates precisely what it is that they want done, when, where, and how much.
4. They lack confidence in their subordinates' abilities to do the work which should be delegated to them.
5. They feel that they lack feedback or other control mechanisms by which the subordinate can be "checked on."
6. They are afraid that their subordinates will "outshine" them or otherwise prove that they know as much or more about the job than the boss.
7. They are afraid to trust anyone besides themselves.
8. They suffer from a martyr complex—because they desire to have people feel sorry for them, they refuse to delegate work which logically could be done by other people.
9. They are possessed by a "guilt drive"—they feel guilty if they have nothing to do and delegating work to others leaves them in that "awkward" position.[14]

There must be an explanation for these chronic problems and "pitfalls" of management. The explanation lies in two dimensions: first, the failure to adopt an effective method of management such as management by objectives, and second, the natural tendency to put off less enjoyable tasks and concentrate on tasks that are more to our liking. An arrangement of performance priorities which depicts this dilemma is shown in Figure 2-2.

Management by objectives provides an opportunity for assigning appropriate priorities to tasks and objectives as well as a means of avoiding many of the related problems.

Installing the MBO System

There are some necessary conditions before the system can be installed properly. It must have the endorsement of the principal manager in the organizational unit.[15] This would be the proprietor of an independent pharmacy or the partners of a partnership. In a small chain of drugstores (4 to 25 units), the president and probably the board of directors should endorse the system. In a larger chain of drugstores, the system could be

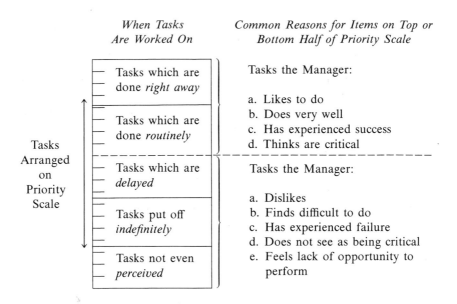

Figure 2-2. *Managerial performance priority scale. (Adapted from Caskey, C. C.: Developing a leadership style.* Supervision, *April, 1964. By permission of* Supervision *and the National Research Bureau, Inc.)*

installed in a district or regional operational unit with the endorsement of the principal manager. The manager of any functional division of a drug wholesale or manufacturing firm could endorse the system. However, it is better if the endorsement comes from top management and the system is implemented from the top down to the lowest level that is practical.

CHANGES

After obtaining the appropriate endorsement and before the actual installation of the system, the initiator of the system must involve the higher echelon of management in *four phases of changes* within the firm:

1. A *familiarization process* must be implemented, beginning with top management and proceeding down to the others involved, using the appropriate communication channels.

2. *Performance goals for the organization* as a whole must be set by the top echelon of management.

3. *Individual goal-setting methods* must be developed and extended down through the organization to the lower levels.

4. The *necessary changes* must be made in such areas as appraisal system or performance review, salary and bonus procedures, delegation of responsibility and authority, and policy clarification.

IMPLEMENTATION

There are basically *four stages of the actual implementation* of the system:

1. Establishing the goals for the firm, and then for each manager or individual involved. This is done usually at the beginning of the budget year.

2. Determining the means of measuring performance, including the necessary criteria for measuring the results for the firm and each individual involved.

3. Reviewing the results with each individual and assessing the achievement of the goals for the firm. This is done usually at the end of the budget year for the firm, but periodically for the individual.

4. Making any necessary modifications in goals or criteria that the reviews indicate. This is done usually at the end of the budget year.

Each of these stages should be broken down into *specific steps and/or elements* for efficient implementation and for good results.

1. *Setting Goals for the Firm.* Those goals should be identified which the principal manager(s) or executive(s) can reasonably expect to achieve. Some of the more common goals are given in Table 2-1.

2. *Clarifying the Organizational Chart.* The organizational chart, or

Table 2-1. *Setting Goals for the Firm*

Goal	Criteria
Profitability	$\dfrac{NP}{Sales}$; $\dfrac{NP}{Investment}$; NP (in percentages)
Competitive position	Share of the market; Market penetration
Expense control	Functional expense as % of sales; Dispensing cost/Rx
Productivity	Sales increase & Rx's increase
Employee relations	Turnover rate; Average tenure by position; Reported complaints; Suggestions
Inventory control	Turnover rate; Out-of-stock incidences; Economic order quantity, and Sources of purchasing
Public relations	Reported complaints; Returned merchandise; Compliment reports; Survey reports
Professional relations	Pharmacist avg. tenure; Prescriber complaint reports; Survey results of special projects

the informal relationship among the employees of a small firm, should be reviewed to determine the best method for assigning responsibilities in order to achieve the goals of the firm.

3. *Setting Goals for Subordinates.* Finally, implementation must be carried out on an individual basis for each employee who will assume a significant responsibility within the organization. Each employee should be asked to write down his objectives for the ensuing year. Then a date should be set to review these with him or her. The employee should be asked to organize his goals into four categories: (1) routine duties, (2) problem-solving goals, (3) creative goals, and (4) personal development goals.

Meanwhile, the immediate supervisor should construct a list of objectives before the meeting with the employee. At this meeting, the two sets of objectives should be reviewed and reconciled into one set by mutual agreement. Two copies of the new set of objectives should be typed, one for the employee and one for the supervisor. Then the supervisor should ask what he can do to help the employee to achieve his objectives, and any suggestions or requests should be documented.

4. *Measuring Results against Goals.* Some of the goals for the firm cannot be measured until the end of the year, whereas others can be reviewed monthly or quarterly. This is also true for some individual goals; however, many of the individual's goals should be reviewed frequently, depending upon the length of employment and scope of responsibility. Weekly reviews should be conducted for new employees, especially if they are not experienced in the work. Managers should review the progress of their supervisors on a monthly basis. At these meetings, goals may be altered or suggestions given, as indicated by the progress to date.

5. *Annual Review of Results.* At the end of the budget year, each employee should have an annual review of the results he achieved as measured against his goals. And, the employee should participate in this assessment. New goals should be set based on the past year's performance, keeping in mind that the employee should be challenged to do even better during the next year. The principal manager should also review the performance of his unit or area of responsibility with his superior. The review of the achievements of the firm should be performed by the proprietor or the chief executive officer, with the assistance of the appropriate staff. New sets of goals are established and the cycle is repeated each year.

RESULTS OF MANAGEMENT BY OBJECTIVES

The *primary effects* of management by objectives are tangible results in the form of profit, increased sales, growth, and lower costs. The *secondary effects* are less tangible, but very valuable in that management itself becomes more efficient, more responsive to the needs of the firm, its employees, and society. MBO reduces the stifling effects of bureaucracy. *Tertiary effects* of MBO are seen in improved employee morale, improved service, improved delegation, and a happier business family.

Improving Decision-Making

As indicated previously, decision-making is the essence of management, although it doesn't represent all that is management. The process of decision-making follows closely the scientific method of investigation. The major difference is that, in using the scientific method in research, most of the facts are known and most of the variables are controlled, whereas in making decisions, many factors and variables are unknown. This is known as making decisions under the condition of uncertainty.

This handicap is reduced considerably when the decision-maker can ascertain more of the facts through surveys of samples. New data being derived from a sample of the universe of data can be relied upon only with a degree of probability. By following a procedure of revising probabilities based on Bayes' Theorem, the degree of uncertainty can be reduced. Although discussion of this technique is beyond the scope of this text, additional information on its use can be found in *Statistical Analysis for Business Decisions.*[16] Let us now consider some of the basic principles of decision-making that every manager can use.

PRINCIPLES OF DECISION-MAKING

It is necessary in the convulsive scene of business life to assign values to our problems and to set priorities. Clearing up simple mechanical difficulties is different from reaching a decision on a course of action which involves people, budgets, and markets. It would be helpful if we had some general principles to guide us in this effort.

The *first principle* is that one needs to give patience, time, and thought to decision-making, especially when one is on unfamiliar ground. Decisions come easily to the sales manager who has been on the job twenty years, as long as they involve only the factors to which he is accustomed. When a new factor is introduced, or the manager moves into an area where he is a stranger, he must take time for orientation.

The *second principle* is the compensation principle. The power of deciding involves the danger of going astray, and that is the essence of deciding. Going astray involves some kind of penalty, and that is the essence of error. The consequences of a decision are part of the total problem, and should be considered as factors in it. We must balance risk against gain, and be neither deterred by the one nor dazzled by the other.

The *third principle* of decision-making involves forethought and anticipation. The manager is subject to one trial not common to the worker: he has the continual feeling of incompletion. His job is never done. His energy drives him to the consideration of the next job while the present job is still in the works, and he needs to keep his balance in both.

The *fourth principle* is that decisions are best made when there is a master plan to guide the manager. There is no necessary virtue in "planning" itself. Its value depends upon what the plan is for, what ends it will serve, what difficulties it is designed to overcome—difficulties arising from the caprices of fate, the actions of competitors, and the quirks of human nature. Without a plan, fluid though it may be, decisions cannot be reached intelligently. Management by objectives is a method that provides the necessary stability for solid decision-making.

The *fifth principle* is to balance the urgency of the decision against deliberation. Mere speed in coming to decisions may have small relevance at the top business management level where a man's contributions to the enterprise may be the making of two or three significant decisions a month. This is not to say that we should debate or stew over every problem. We are probably too much given to sending out a man with a red flag in front of every new idea, as they used to do with steam locomotives. On the whole, it is wiser, after giving the matter adequate thought, to make a decision promptly and crisply than to linger over it and lose momentum and drive.

To make a sound decision, it is not necessary to have all the facts, but it is necessary to know what facts are missing so that we may make allowances for same and decide the degree of rigidity to give to our decision. Some managers, in trying to avoid off-the-cuff masterminding, make it a practice to take time to sleep on a problem. This can be useful if a tentative decision has been reached or workable alternatives outlined so that the subconscious has something tangible to push around.

Very little that is good can be said about procrastinating. Any business will become paralyzed if there are persistently long delays in the making of managerial decisions. They cause waste of time among personnel, loss of teamwork, and forfeiture of faith in management.

There are, of course, times for postponement, when a resolute determination to take no action until more facts are available is a constructive contribution to a wise decision. The warning is against unwise or frivolous procrastination. We must keep in mind that to make no decision is itself a decision, and as such must be justified.

PREPARATION FOR DECISIONS

Decisions appropriate to the situation cannot be made unless there is adequate knowledge of facts and the forces acting upon them. There must be available a large store of memories of previous experiences and things learned which can be linked with the current problem.

The reasoning process requires frames of references or units of comparison gathered through experience and study. When we have sufficient data in our minds, our recall mechanism ranges over them, assesses them, takes a little of this and a little of that, relates them significantly, and produces a decision. What we call "good judgment" is the ability to bring together new facts and relate them to the archives of our memory to arrive at a decision.

The pharmacist must never stop adding to his stock of knowledge and understanding, but this need not be a burdensome task. If pressure is inherent in his daily routine, he will find it relaxing as well as useful to spend his leisure hours deliberately engaged with new ideas and new theories which will enlarge his horizons.

It is not profitable to think of the capable decision-maker in terms of a cartoon stereotype—as a table pounder, a window gazer, a pacer of the office, an aspirin user, or a man with a wet towel around his head. One general belief may be given credence in some measure: the person who makes important decisions may not be sweet tempered. He is under pressure, he takes risks, he wrestles with the task of getting his ideas carried out, he has little patience with incompetency.

Some firms make no provision for the stress of management. Their managers are loaded with detail instead of being relieved of all trivia, so that they may devote their special talents to important things.

STEPS IN MAKING A DECISION

The manager who wishes to develop the habit of making decisions with wisdom and effectiveness might do well to consider the following steps:

1. Have an objective in mind before attempting a decision.
2. Look at the situation generally, and from it extract the problem.
3. Put the problem into words.
4. Remove all of the irrelevant substance from the problem and separate it into its component parts; in other words, "tidy up" the problem.
5. Do the preparatory research thoroughly, and brush aside preconceived ideas.
6. Consider all the facts and develop alternate solutions or options and predict the effects of each option.
7. Think through to a solution and set up some controls to ensure that the decision works.

The first job is to find the real problem, divesting the situation of all irrelevant details. Masses of data may look impressive, but only those facts that apply to the problem are worth considering. It is quite right to see the pattern of the total situation and how the parts fit together, but successful managers have the capacity to reduce the whole picture to simple terms.

A problem only becomes intelligible when it is put into words. There simply is no magic formula for decision-making, but the man who approaches the point of decision by setting out his problem in an orderly way stands a better chance of reaching the right outcome than one who relies on snap judgments.

A problem can be solved if the person responsible grasps its nature, gauges its true dimension, decides what to do about it, and takes immediate steps to cope with it. He breaks a big problem down into small, easily tackled units, changing a vague difficulty into a specific concrete form. He may go so far as to answer one "yes or no" question and then ask others until the major problem is solved. One method advocated by some experts is "take it apart." The problem is first put in writing. Beneath this, in two columns, are written the arguments "for" and "against." When this is done seriously and honestly, the "pros" and "cons" can be counted.

Managers may smooth their way by having all proposals and problems in order before moving toward decisions. Almost every problem needs to be explored through such questions as these: (1) Why is this necessary or desirable? (2) What can it be expected to accomplish? (3) How can it be worked out? (4) Who will do it? (5) Who will be affected by it? (6) What harmful situations might result?

Superiority in decision-making rests on a solid basis of preparation, with a grasp of all the possibilities. When you reach a tentative conclusion, try to knock it down with dispassionate energy. Ask: "What will happen if . . . ? Does this decision take care of A, B, and C possibilities?" By proceeding in this way, the business executive borrows a bit of the value of the scientific method and spirit, the resolute asking of the questions: "What else?" "What if?"

You need to pay attention to detail in the preliminary stages, while keeping in mind the end purpose. Toscanini, the great conductor, is quoted as having said "In rehearsing a musical work, the important passages can frequently take care of themselves; it is the supposedly unimportant phrase or line that demands careful consideration."

The manager needs suppleness of mind. He should display enthusiasm, but not the sort of zeal that blinds him to facts. He should recognize that his opinion on a matter is only something that falls between ignorance and understanding. It is knowledge in the making. To change an opinion in the face of new facts is a sign of vitality and progress.

In the course of his deliberation he will have taken advantage of subconscious thought. All creative thinking, including scientific research, emerges from the subconscious. The "passed to you for action" memo which consciousness receives may be couched in vague terms, and may have to be worked into shape. But this is no mystical process; it goes on hour after hour throughout our lives. It is, however, an advantage to recognize it so that fullest use may be made of it.

Last in this group of seven suggestions is the "thinking through" of the proposed decision to its conclusion. This involves testing every step leading to the decision as well as anticipating what may follow from it.

When you have reached the point where you have gathered the facts and tested them, thought about them, and weighed the consequences, then make your decision. Here are two illustrations on the folly of hesitating. Buridan, a French philosopher of the twelfth century, told us about the ass which was placed midway between two equally attractive bales of hay, and died of starvation because he couldn't choose which one to eat. Robert Browning's poem reminds us that Saul, crowned king at a time when one swift blow would have scattered his foes and united his friends, stood midway between his duty and his task, and indecision slew him.

"FOLLOW THROUGH"

We have located and defined our problems, collected facts, and weighed the favorable against the unfavorable; we have listened to what can be said by experts, friends, and enemies; we have checked the accuracy of our information and of our thinking; we have various solutions; and we have arrived at a decision. What do we do next?

The fatal thing to do is to put the decision in a "pigeon-hole." The only place to put a good decision is into action. An idea has been born, it has evolved, and has been transformed into a decision. Now the manager must direct and participate in the execution of the decision.

It would be a mistake at this point to spend time looking back to see if you are too far from shore. You are obligated, having made the decision, to develop a certain amount of blindness to the possibility of failure. By that act you give confidence to those who must do the work of implementing the decision. However, it would be wrong to cling to a course if some vital new facts in its disfavor become known, but don't change your mind merely because you are running into obstacles. The road may be strewn with rocks, but that merely means that it is a rough road, not that it is going in the wrong direction.

Be sure that your decision is promulgated clearly. Unless you organize and clarify for your people the unrelated ideas and facts with which you have wrestled, they cannot be expected to respond with effective action. They must know what change in behavior is expected of them, what change to expect in the behavior of others with whom they work, and what change will be made in the working conditions. This is the manager's directional guidance. Together the manager and the employees establish the goals and determine the methods to achieve them.

Mechanical problems associated with your decision are relatively simple compared with the human problems. For example, your decision may change the apparent status of workers, and it is astonishing how surely a man will be annoyed and deeply pained by any wrong done to his feeling of self-importance. This is one reason for careful consultation of all those who are to be affected by the decision. It will give you the benefit of their experience and their ideas, and make them participants in whatever comes to pass.

Being a decisive manager doesn't mean being truculent, or living apart. To be part of the working force was emphasized as a necessity of management by speakers at the Duke of Edinburgh's Study Conference in Oxford. The manager must make the time to keep in touch with subordinates. Only thus can he appraise the spirit of his people, tap their interest, and ensure their cooperation in carrying out plans upon which he decides. Human motivations and human emotions are involved as factors in the solution of every problem.

Of this one can be sure: no decision can be better than the people who are assigned to implement it. Their enthusiasm, competence, and understanding determine what they can and will do.

Summary

The reader may be wondering why he should bother with these various styles or methods of management and the brief background surrounding each. The answer is that all of these styles or methods of management, except management by objectives, can be found in the various pharmacy practices—independent proprietorships, chain drugstores, or institutional pharmacies. If we include the pharmaceutical industry, we probably could find some fairly good examples of management by objectives. The young pharmacist will encounter one or more of these management styles, or perhaps some combination of them. An understanding of the nature of the various management styles and the boss's personality will aid a pharmacist to develop a better rapport and working relationship with his supervisor.

The various principles, techniques, procedures, and methods of management have been presented. Major emphasis was given to management by objectives and the importance of good decision-making. Management by objectives improves all aspects of management, but its greatest impact is on communication. It enables the manager to communicate with a subordinate without causing the subordinate to become defensive. While every technique and procedure may not be applicable to every small independent pharmacy, most of the procedures and *all the principles,* especially those related to management by objectives and decision-making, *apply* to any type of pharmacy or pharmaceutical enterprise. Indeed most of the principles and techniques can be applied to an individual in managing his time and his own personal affairs.

Most young pharmacists intend to either own their own pharmacy or become a manager of a chain drugstore or a chief pharmacist in a hospital. A word of caution is in order. Management by objectives is not a panacea, and there still is room for improvement, which is reflected by the title of the book *Beyond Management by Objectives.*[17]

REFERENCES

1. Odiorne, G. S.: *Management by Objectives—A System of Managerial Leadership.* New York: Pitman Publishing Corp., 1965, p. 39.
2. Dimock, M. E.: *A Philosophy of Administration.* New York: Harper and Row, 1958.
3. Drucker, P. F.: *The Practice of Management.* New York: Harper and Brothers, 1954, p. 280.
4. Tiffin, J.: *Industrial Psychology.* 3rd ed., New York: Prentice-Hall, Inc., 1952.
5. Drucker, P. F.: *op. cit.,* Chapter 11, pp. 121-136.
6. Odiorne, G. S.: *op. cit.,* (the entire book).
7. Odiorne, G. S.: *Management Decisions by Objectives.* New York: Prentice-Hall, Inc., 1969.
8. Odiorne, G. S.: *Management by Objectives. op. cit.,* p. 55.
9. Adapted from Odiorne, *ibid.,* pp. vii and viii of Preface.
10. *Ibid.,* p. 66.
11. *Ibid.,* p. 67.
12. *Ibid.,* pp. 54, 55.
11. Steinmetz, L. L., Kline, J. B., and Stegall, D. P.: *Managing the Small Business.* Homewood, Ill.: Richard D. Irwin, Inc., 1968, pp. 146-148.
14. *Ibid.,* p. 148.
15. Odiorne, G. S.: *Management by Objectives. op. cit.,* p. 68.
16. Spurr, W. A., and Bonini, C. P.: *Statistical Analysis for Business Decisions.* Homewood, Ill.: Richard D. Irwin, Inc., 1967, Chapters 15-17.
17. Batten, J. D.: *Beyond Management by Objectives.* New York: American Management Association, 1966.

REVIEW

1. Define management in classical terms.

2. What is the essence of management?

3. What are the two cardinal principles of management and the consequences of the failure to follow these two principles?

4. Discuss in philosophical and practical terms the differences between managers and administrators.

5. Name and describe the five historic management styles or methods, including the approximate time frame and the socioeconomic changes taking place during each era.

6. Associate the source of power and the general mode of communication with the six "styles" of management that can be identified today.

7. Define management by objectives, and discuss its six major premises, its basic philosophy and conceptual framework.

8. Explain the proper manner and sequence of implementing management by objectives and the consequence of poor implementation.

9. Explain how management by objectives accommodates the value systems of society and the special techniques and sub-systems of management.

10. Discuss how management by objectives can be used in overcoming chronic problems of both professional managers and small business entrepreneurs.

11. What are nine reasons given for failing to delegate work?

12. Explain the priority scale for arranging tasks used by some managers.

13. Discuss the entire process of setting objectives for the firm, managers, supervisors, and individual employees, including the criteria for measuring the achievement of the objectives.

14. What are the four categories of individual objectives?

15. Explain the purpose and procedure of the annual review.

16. Briefly describe the primary, secondary and tertiary effects of management by objectives.

17. Discuss the five principles of decision-making, including the related factors and implications of each.

18. Discuss the preparation and the follow-through of decision-making.

19. Outline the seven steps in decision-making and briefly explain the purpose of each.

20. Explain how management by objectives relates to the statement: "Of this be sure: no decision can be better than the people you have to carry it out."

3. *Organizational Structures*

There are three levels or kinds of organization patterns that every business or profession must consider and apply in a manner appropriate to the size and nature of the enterprise. The first level is the social organization within which a firm, including a pharmacy, can be established and operated. The second level is the legal organization of the ownership of the pharmacy. The third level is the organizational structure, usually depicted by organizational charts, which defines the lines of authority and responsibility, and the lines of communication.

Social Organization

In the past, too little attention has been given to social organization. This has resulted in a lack of understanding of the relationship between society and the business or professional enterprise. Many of the conflicts between both businesses and professions on the one hand, and especially pharmacy with its unique ambivalent characteristics, and society on the other hand can be traced to a lack of a clear understanding of this relationship. It has presented legislative problems and public relations challenges for many organizations to an unnecessary degree. The complex relationship between society and the establishment, organization, and operation of an enterprise has been depicted in Figure 3-1.

If one looks at the top echelon of the diagram, it is apparent that in a democratic society, the ultimate authority for any type of professional

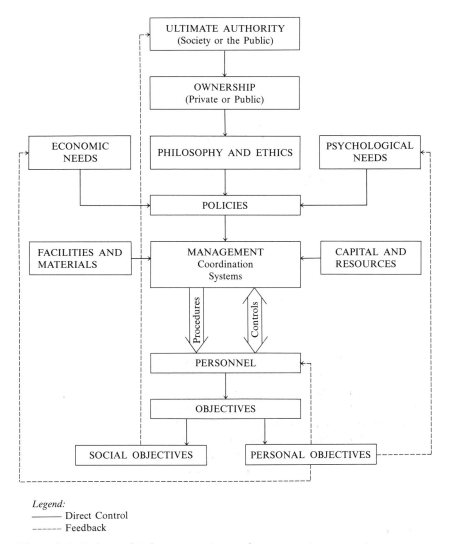

Figure 3-1. *Relationship between society and an enterprise.*

or business enterprise rests with the public or society. Property rights and professional privileges are derived from and controlled by this authority through two mechanisms, laws and the marketing process. In most enterprises, and this is especially true of pharmacy, both mechanisms function in a very real way. A cursory study of pharmaceutical law confirms the degree to which laws and regulations control the practice of pharmacy, and indeed the entire pharmaceutical industry as well. The number of pharmacies that have discontinued business in recent years is indicative of the operation of a competitive free market. Thus a pharmacist-proprietor must comply with the statutory laws and regulations, and he also must conform to a large degree with the "laws" of the marketplace.

The ownership—whether an individual, a partnership, or a corporation—will espouse a set of ethical principles and a philosophy of conduct. When these are combined with the economic and psychologic needs of the owner(s), they provide the basis for the formulation of the policies under which the firm will operate. The necessity of meeting both economic and psychologic needs is probably obvious to both pharmacists and pharmacy students. That these needs permeate throughout the organization, including the lowest level of employment, may not be as well recognized. This principle is a basic premise of management of objectives, as previously indicated in Chapter 2.

Beginning with policies as a foundation, a management system is organized to achieve the perceived objectives of the firm. This involves the coordination of capital and other resources and personnel. Procedures and control mechanisms are developed in a systematic way, such as the system of management by objectives. The philosophy of the top echelon of the firm, ranging from a proprietor to a board of directors, is important in determining the style of management and management system that will be implemented. At this point it should be noted that the objectives of all the personnel from the proprietor or chief executive to the clerk and janitor must be met, including both the economic and psychologic components of these objectives. Of course the social objectives must be met if the enterprise expects to thrive or even to continue. The pharmacy must meet the perceived needs of the people in the market. The market includes the range of merchandise and services at prices consistent with the type of pharmacy, the affluence of the people, and the perceived needs of the people within that market. The pharmacy must also conform to the laws and regulations applicable to the pharmacy.

Legal Organizations

Any time a person decides to go into business, he is faced with the decision of doing so alone or of joining with one or more other people in this venture. A second and equally important decision is the form of business enterprise which will be utilized.

There are three forms of legal organizations which are available to the owner(s) of a pharmaceutical firm, including a community pharmacy. These are the sole proprietorship or single ownership, the partnership or co-partnership, and the corporation. Each of these has advantages and limitations which the individual(s) should consider in choosing a particular form for his/their pharmacy. Certainly the nature of the business, the number and philosophy of the people involved, capital, and other factors will determine the type of organization required. In most situations, the basic factors of the operations are known or can be anticipated, and thus will provide the basis for deciding on the legal form that best meets the requirements of the firm.

Sole Proprietorship

ADVANTAGES

As the sole owner of a pharmacy there are no formal requirements for establishing the business other than obtaining the facility in which it will be housed and the various licenses and permits which are required for the pharmacy.

The owner has complete freedom, within the limits of the law, in determining the operating policies, methods, and controls. There is no one with whom the profits or decisions must be shared. As a consequence, personal incentive is strong and the responsibility is definitely established. Regulations by governmental agencies are less than for the corporate form, resulting in fewer and simpler reports which have to be submitted. Income taxes are only those required of the pharmacy owner as an individual. This is an advantage over a corporation up to a certain income level because corporations must pay income taxes on earnings, and the stockholders must pay income tax on the dividends.

DISADVANTAGES

Probably the main disadvantage of the single proprietorship is the unlimited personal liability of the owner for the debts and obligations of his practice. In the event of failure of the pharmacy, all of the owner's personal property outside of the pharmacy may be required to satisfy an indebtedness against the pharmacy. Another limitation is that the owner alone must spread his attention, time, and efforts over the many activities of his business, with none of the benefits of specialization available to a large organization. The owner is responsible for supplying all of the capital required to start and maintain the business, and often the amount of available capital is limited. Unlike a corporation, the sole proprietorship usually terminates with the death of the owner.

General Partnership

DEFINITION AND FORMATION OF PARTNERSHIPS

When a voluntary agreement between two or more individuals forms an association to carry on a business together and to share in its profits or losses, they have formed a partnership. This agreement, known as articles of co-partnership, should be in writing and should specify the name and address of the partnership or firm and the names and legal addresses of the partners. It should also identify the contributors' interests, and the duties and responsibilities of each partner. If the partnership selects a trade name for the pharmacy, a certificate indicating the trade name and the articles of co-partnership should be filed with the County Court Clerk in most states. Salaries to be paid to partners should be documented as well as expenses in connection with business functions, drawing accounts, sharing of profits, and withdrawal of the firm's merchandise for personal or family use. There should be clear-cut provisions established for dissolving the partnership, partitioning the assets and dividing the profits.

ADVANTAGES

There are two or more owners, usually one of whom is a qualified pharmacist, who can combine their respective skills, capital, knowledge, time, and efforts in establishing and operating a pharmacy under the partnership form. Several partners should obviously possess among themselves *more capital, greater knowledge and competence,* and *more diversified interests* than one person. This will allow for a degree of *specialization of functions.* For instance, one partner could be primarily responsible for the professional aspects of the pharmacy; another could handle the buying, selling, and inventory control; and a third could assume chiefly the financial, accounting, reporting, legal, and equipment responsibilities. Certainly all of the partners would be interested in, and legally responsible for, all phases of the operation. Like the sole proprietorship, the partnership has *less regulation* and *taxation* than the corporation and has fewer reports to make to governmental agencies.

LIMITATIONS

The partnership has a serious disadvantage in the unlimited liability of each of the partners. The personal property of each of the several partners is subject to be used to meet any obligations of the partnership which exceed the ability of the business to pay from its own assets and income. The personal property of a partner may be liable for the indebtedness of the partnership up to six months after assignment of his personal property to another person. Since each partner has the capacity to bind the other partners by his actions within the scope of the partnership business, any partner is at risk through foolish moves or bad judgment of another. This disadvantage is derived from the legal concept of unlimited agency. Because of this, it is very important that formal articles of co-partnership should be drawn by a competent attorney.

As with the sole proprietorship, the partnership usually terminates in the event of death, insanity, or certain other circumstances of withdrawal by a partner. It is possible to establish a new partnership, however, and the business need not be liquidated. This is normally accomplished with a purchase agreement between the partners. Business life insurance on members of the partnerships will make funds available, so that surviving partners can purchase the interests of the survivor's heirs or his estate, thus permitting continuity of the business without interruption.

RIGHTS OF PARTNERS

A general partner *may*: (1) obligate his firm by all his transactions carried out in the apparent course of the business of the partnership; (2) make the firm responsible for all commercial paper signed or endorsed by him in the course of partnership business, unless restricted; (3) buy and sell goods, hire representatives, and give warranties; and (4) share in profits.

A general partner *may not,* without the consent of all partners: (1) submit a partnership claim to arbitration; (2) dispose of the good will of the partnership; (3) transfer all or a major portion of partnership property; and (4) confess judgment against the partnership.

DISSOLUTION OF PARTNERSHIP

A partnership is considered dissolved: (1) when a partner dies; (2) when the time for which the partnership was formed has expired; (3) upon notice of termination of the partnership given by a partner if the partnership was not formed for a specified time; (4) by court decree; and (5) by the bankruptcy of any partner.

A general partner may request the court that a partnership be dissolved: (1) when due to constant disagreement between the partners the business cannot be carried on profitably; (2) when one of the partners is judged legally incompetent; and (3) when any partner has persistently breached the partnership agreement.

Upon dissolution of a partnership, due notice should be given through newspapers and by the mail, to those with whom the partnership has done business, in order to protect the interests of partners, creditors, and others concerned.

Partnership assets on dissolution are applied: (1) to partnership creditors other than partners; (2) to partners for debts due them, except for capital investment; (3) to partners for capital investments; and (4) to partners for profits.

If partnership assets are not sufficient to meet all of the above, then distribution is made as follows: (1) partnership assets to partnership creditors; (2) the deficiency is contributed by the solvent partners from their personal assets in the proportion of sharing of profits.

Specialized Types of Partnership

Various safeguards toward reducing the responsibility and liability of any partner for the conduct of the other partners' financial activities may be placed in the agreement, as well as stipulations for certain limitations in the partnership related to such matters as incurring additional indebtedness, the giving of bonds or securities, and prohibition of various unilateral actions. These, of course, must be specified in the articles of partnership.

INACTIVE PARTNER

Sometimes a person is willing to furnish part of the required capital but does not wish to take an active part in the management of the pharmacy. The articles of partnership should indicate clearly all parts of the agreement including contribution of the inactive partner, percentage of profits to the inactive partner, and a provision for the active partner(s) to purchase the interest of the inactive partner in the event of his death or withdrawal. An inactive partner, often referred to as a silent partner, is subject to unlimited liability to the same degree as an active partner.

LIMITED PARTNERSHIP

There may be one or more limited partners and one or more general partners in an organization of this type. The liability to creditors by the limited partners is confined to their investment of capital, and they cannot have a part in the management of the business. There must be a formal affiliation agreement prepared indicating the limited and the regular partners, and the length of the life of the agreement. The contributions of each partner must be indicated along with specification of the distribution of profits. The other usual details of the articles of partnership, such as names and addresses, must be included. This formal agreement of partnerships must be registered with proper authorities in the county where the firm is located and published weekly for six successive weeks in two newspapers in order for the limited liability to be effected.

PARTNERSHIP BY ESTOPPEL

Partnership may exist even when parties do not intend partnership or where the agreement between them is otherwise. When persons conduct themselves in a manner from which it may reasonably be inferred that they are partners, and a third party, relying thereon, extends credit, they may be held to be partners as to such third party. This is called partnership by estoppel.

The Corporation

DEFINITION AND FORMATION

A corporation is an association of three or more individuals chartered under the laws of the state to conduct business as an entity, separate from its members. There are various kinds of corporations such as municipal, membership, and business corporations. We shall deal only with private business corporations.

When a corporation is formed, it must file articles of incorporation with the Secretary of State. The articles must state: (1) the name of the corporation, which must not be too similar to the name of another corporation or be deceptive; (2) the duration of the corporation; (3) the names and addresses of the incorporators; (4) the location of the principal office of the corporation; (5) the business or purpose of the corporation; (6) the amount of capital stock and the value assigned to each share having par value or the number of shares of stock without par value; and (7) the names and addresses of the directors for the first year or until the first meeting of the stockholders.

After the certificate of incorporation is issued, the corporation is organized. The stockholders then proceed to elect their Board of Directors and adopt bylaws to govern the corporation during its existence. However, these rules cannot contravene State or Federal law. Bylaws may be modified or amended only by the stockholders and are binding upon the directors.

The Board of Directors then meet and elect the officers of the corporation. The officers of a corporation include the president, secretary, treasurer, and chairman of the Board of Directors. A corporation, being an artificial person, can act only through its agents. The corporation is liable for all its own lawful debts and the acts of all its agents done in the performance of their duties. It must sue and be sued in its own name.

POWERS

Every corporation has the following powers: (1) to admit stockholders; (2) to elect officers and to determine their remuneration; (3) to adopt bylaws; (4) to buy and sell real property, if granted by its charter; and (5) to make such contracts and agreements as are necessary for the transaction of the business stated in the articles of incorporation and to carry on business.

BOARD OF DIRECTORS

The Board of Directors are the agents who manage the corporation. They in turn elect the officers who are removable at the pleasure of the Board. There must be at least three directors. The Board of Directors are responsible only to the stockholders, who elect them by a plurality vote of those present at a meeting called for such purpose. If three directors are to be elected, a stockholder is voting on three questions and casts his full vote for *each* director to be elected.

The Board of Directors must act as a board and not individually. They must act by a majority vote, and any other provision of the bylaws in this respect is illegal. The directors must act faithfully in performing their duties and display a high degree of fidelity to the stockholders.

The Board of Directors, without the consent of two-thirds of the stockholders, cannot mortgage or sell real estate, dissolve the corporation, vote to merge or consolidate it, or sell its machinery or property. The Board of Directors has the sole discretion to declare dividends, including the amount per share.

STOCKHOLDERS

A stockholder is a person, partnership, or another corporation that owns one or more shares of stock in a corporation. A stockholder may vote on any major question or decision affecting the corporation and he may vote in person or by proxy.

A stockholder also has the right of preemption. When a corporation increases the number of shares of authorized stock, the stockholders have a prior right to purchase the increased shares. This is called the right of preemption. The ratio of new shares, which any stockholder has the right to purchase, is proportional to the number of shares currently held.

These rights are valuable and may be sold by the stockholder, and his vendee may acquire them and all the privileges incidental to them. In cases of stock listed and sold on a security exchange, these rights are also dealt in.

Stockholders may sue directors to account for negligent acts or acts done in bad faith or for the appropriation of any assets to their individual uses, but not for errors in judgment committed in good faith.

Stockholders are only liable for the amount of the par value of their stock, if fully paid, or the amount of the purchase price of no par value stock.

If a stockholder has not paid the full par value of his stock or the purchase price of the no par value shares, he is liable to the corporation's creditors for the difference between the amount paid in and the par value or purchase price in the event of insolvency of the corporation.

STOCKS AND DIVIDENDS

Stocks are one of two classes, common or preferred. A *common stock* is the usual class issued in the formation of a corporation. The owner of a common stock has one vote for each share, and he receives a dividend on the basis of the number of shares he owns. Dividends can be paid only from the surplus or earnings and to do otherwise is a crime.

A *preferred stock* has unique features. First, the owner of a preferred stock does not have the right to vote. The dividend for a preferred stock is predetermined as a percentage of its par value, and such dividends are paid before dividends may be declared for common stock—hence the term, preferred stock.

DISSOLUTION OF A CORPORATION

A corporation can be dissolved: (1) when it voluntarily applies for dissolution; (2) when it fails to abide by its charter, and the Attorney General of the State applies to the court for its dissolution; (3) when two years have elapsed and it has not conducted the business for which it was organized; (4) when it reaches the time limit for which it was organized; (5) when it fails to pay State Franchise Taxes for three years. Except in voluntary dissolution by consent of stockholders, a legal action for a dissolution must be instituted.

ADVANTAGES OF A CORPORATION

A corporation is preferred to a proprietorship or partnership for the following reasons: (1) the duration is perpetual unless the articles of incorporation specify otherwise; (2) inasmuch as the corporation is an entity separate and distinct from its members, the death of any or all of its members does not affect its existence or its operation; (3) it permits the attraction of capital in small or large amounts from innumerable sources and without regard to geographic location; and (4) liability of investors is limited to the amount of their investment and, therefore, one does not risk any more than he desires to invest, whereas in a partnership or individual form of conducting business, one's entire assets may be lost.

LIMITATIONS OF A CORPORATION

A corporation incurs considerable legal expense in connection with the procuring of its charter, issuing stock, and paying filing fees and capital stock taxes. The corporation must employ a brokerage firm if the Board of Directors decide to "go public," that is, make the stock available to the general public. It is subject to more governmental regulation than the proprietorship or partnership. It must submit more complex and detailed reports and is subject to higher tax rates up to a certain level of income. The corporation must also pay income tax on its earnings, and then the shareholder is taxed again on the corporation income he receives as dividends, thus incurring double taxation.

The "Subchapter S" Corporation

In 1958, Congress enacted a law giving businessmen the opportunity to do business as a corporation and allowing them the right to elect to be taxed as a partnership or sole proprietorship, thus bypassing the Federal corporate income tax. This type of corporation has the following advantages: (1) it may secure tax advantages from the fringe benefits that are available to the employees of the corporation; (2) the stockholders of a young corporation have the right to deduct on their personal income tax returns the early losses incurred while the business is getting under way; and (3) the stockholders may use a corporate fiscal year different from the stockholder's tax year, resulting in income deferment for the stockholder and controlling within limits the time when corporate income is counted as the stockholders income.

The following rules must be followed to gain the privilege of not paying a corporate Federal income tax: (1) there cannot be more than ten stockholders; (2) the decision to seek this status must be unanimous; (3) there can be only one class of stock outstanding; (4) the corporation must be organized in the United States of America, and all of the stockholders must be United States citizens or resident aliens; (5) none of the stockholders can be another corporation or trust, but an estate may be a stockholder; (6) the corporation must not be one of an affiliated group of corporations tied to a parent or holding company; and (7) eighty percent of the gross income must be from sources other than rent, dividends, interest, royalties, or capital gains from the sale of securities, and must come from sources within the United States.

Stockholders can elect to become a corporation under Subchapter S regulations one year and cancel the next. But if there is a cancellation, another election cannot be held until the fifth year starting after the year of cancellation, unless the Commissioner of Internal Revenue consents to a shorter waiting period. It is not necessary to re-elect Subchapter S treatment every year; it continues until revoked or cancelled for failure to follow the rules.

Organizational Structure

The purpose of an organizational chart is to illustrate the lines of authority, responsibility, and communication throughout an organization, beginning with the final authority at the top. There is limited application of a highly structured organization and complex organizational charts for a small sole proprietorship pharmacy employing only a few people and doing less than $250,000 annual sales volume. However, many of the principles and concepts embodied in an organizational structure as depicted by organizational charts are useful even to smaller pharmacies. The four types of organizational structures are as follows: straight line or scalar, line and staff, functional, and some combination and/or modification of these.

LINE OR SCALAR ORGANIZATIONS

This is the least complicated organizational structure, and it is most useful in organizations with fairly simple, repetitive, and uniform functions and operations. The structure allows for the direct flow of authority, responsibility, and communication from the top authority to the lowest level of work. It was the structure used in most firms during the early days of the industrial revolution and in the military services. The straight line organization is not used as much today, but it is still used with some modification in the military.

An illustration of this simple organizational structure is shown in Figure 3-2. In the pure line organization, each of the clerks or workers would have the same range of work responsibilities and tasks.

MODIFIED DEPARTMENTAL LINE ORGANIZATIONS

A modification of the above structure, which we will call the "Departmental Modified Line Organization," is adaptable to medium and large pharmacies and to other types of organizations or firms. For example, a pharmacy with self-selection layout and annual sales of $400,000 or more,

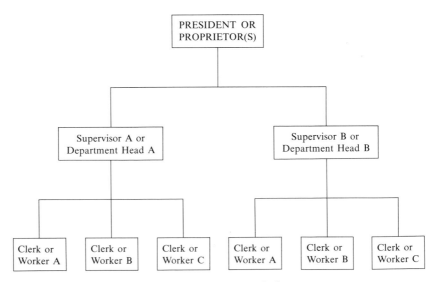

Figure 3-2. *Straight line or scalar organizational chart.*

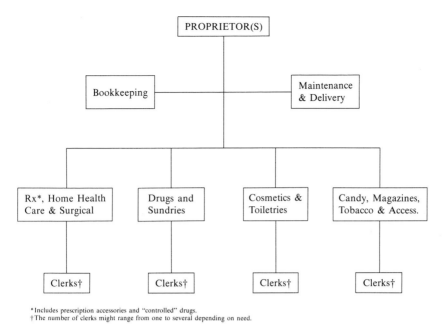

* Includes prescription accessories and "controlled" drugs.
† The number of clerks might range from one to several depending on need.

Figure 3-3. *Modified departmental line organization chart.*

four or five major departments, and twelve or more employees could very
well adapt this modified structure. Each department would be directed
by a specialist with two to four clerks under his supervision. The department head is responsible for the activities in the department including
purchasing, personnel, merchandising, and/or professional services appropriate to his department. Of course, the pharmacist-proprietor(s)
should direct and coordinate the activities of the department heads. A
system of management by objectives would be applicable to this type
of organizational structure. Some writers include this modified departmental line organization as a simple extension of the pure line organization (Fig. 3-3). The responsibilities and duties of each department
manager and employee are determined by the system of management
by objectives.

LINE AND STAFF ORGANIZATIONS

The line and staff organization was developed as the various management specialists evolved and were employed to advise management
without assuming any direct line authority within the organization. The
staff organization supplements the line organization, which has the primary responsibility for the operation of the firm. The staff organization
and functions include comptroller (treasurer), purchasing department, real

estate, personnel department, legal department, public and professional relations department, operational analysis, and market research.

This type of organizational structure is better adapted to larger firms, such as a chain of drugstores (25 units or more), large drug wholesale company, or pharmaceutical manufacturers. The number and type of staff departments vary with the type of operation, but a typical organizational chart for a corporate drugstore chain with 50 units is illustrated in Figure 3-4.

Authority, responsibility, communication, and functions flow downward through the line, to the operational division. The staff serves in an advisory position only. In certain instances, the staff may set guidelines and standards for the entire organization, but communication and enforcement normally proceed through the line organization. Although this form of organization is rather complicated, it provides some of the advantages of the functional organization in specialization in management, with the simplicity of the pure line organization in communication and transmission of authority, responsibility, and duties.

FUNCTIONAL ORGANIZATIONS

The functional form of organization shown in Figure 3-5 is an extremely old concept, albeit not very popular today. It dates back to the time of Frederick Taylor and the beginning of scientific management. However, a pharmacist or small businessman must understand the principle of the functional organization, because most small businesses start as functional organizations, formally or informally, and then grow into organizations that are either line or line and staff. What is meant by the functional organization, at least in the traditional sense, is that each supervisor is in charge of his specific function, rather than in charge of specific workers. For example, assuming there are six or eight areas of function in a pharmacy, six or eight supervisors would be needed, one in charge of each function. You would then find a supervisor who is in charge of all operations having to do with purchasing, another in charge of finances, another in charge of prescription dispensing, and so on. Each supervisor would have the last word with respect to the function he directs.

Normally a pharmacist who is just starting a business has only a few people working for him and he is in charge of all functions. However, when the organization grows—perhaps into a group practice—its character changes to that of a functional organization. Each pharmacist then is in charge of one or more specific functions of the pharmacy. Obviously, this means that as an employee moves from function to function, he works under a different pharmacist each time. And this is the source of trouble with the functional form of organization. Men become confused when they work on more than one function and therefore must work for more

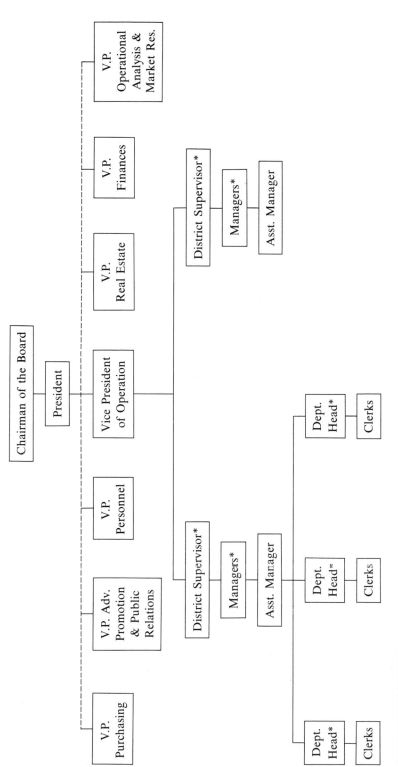

*Positions replicated as necessary.

Figure 3-4. *Line staff organization chart:* ———— *represents line operation and departments;* – – – – *represents staff functions and departments.*

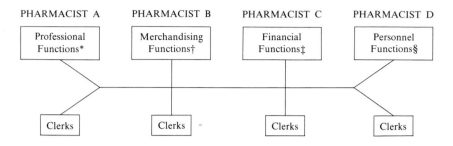

*Professional functions would include prescription dispensing, patient drug record systems, patient consultations, home health aids and surgical supplies, and professional relations.
†Merchandising functions would include purchasing, inventory control, displays, advertising, and personal selling, except prescription and professional goods.
‡Financial functions would include the general financing, budgeting, accounting, operational analysis and control.
§Personnel functions would include recruiting, selecting, firing, training, employee performance evaluation, wage determination and other employee relations including fringe benefits.

Figure 3-5. *Functional organizational chart.*

than one boss. Not only do job responsibilities get extremely confusing, but it becomes difficult for a supervisor to observe the performance of the employee. Therefore, the functional form of organization is only amenable to the small organization. However, because pharmacies tend to start small, pharmacists anticipating a group practice should be aware that in all likelihood, the first kind of organization they will utilize is the functional organization.

INFORMAL ORGANIZATIONS

A discussion of the organizations of business would be incomplete without at least passing mention of the phenomenon called the informal organization. The informal organization cannot be seen, but it certainly can be felt by the pharmacist. Unfortunately, the pharmacist can do little or nothing about the informal organization other than recognize the fact that he, and everyone else, is a part of it, that he might possibly be able to use the informal organization to his advantage, and that it can work to his disadvantage.

The informal organization is nothing more than the informal "system" of employees and employee interactions which develop in any work environment. Whereas the formal organization is something that can be charted on a graph showing direct lines of authority and responsibility between superiors and subordinates, the informal organization cannot be charted nor can any direct lines of authority be established. Rather, the informal organization is a myriad of interpersonal relationships arising as a result of friendships and other associations that develop both on and off the job, and represent the fact that employees affect each other informally as well as formally. The pharmacist also should recognize the fact that the informal organization does exist, that natural leaders will emerge in any situation, and that a leader in the informal organization can work either to the small businessman's advantage or to his detriment, depending on the attitude and aspirations of the individual informal leader. Therefore, a pharmacist should not ignore the existence of the informal organization, but rather should recognize that it does exist, try to identify the leaders, and use their abilities to positively orient his employees' efforts.

REVIEW

1. Explain what is meant by the social organization and how this is related to the management of a pharmacy.

2. Explain how the social organization correlates with the philosophy of management by objectives.

3. Describe the formation and characteristics of a sole proprietorship.

4. List five advantages and four disadvantages of a sole proprietorship.

5. Describe four types of partnerships. Compare their formation and the different characteristics.

6. List four advantages and three limitations of a general partnership.

7. Explain the purpose of an inactive partner and a limited partner.

8. What are the five bases for dissolution of a partnership?

9. Define a corporation and discuss the steps in the formation of a corporation.

10. List four advantages and four limitations of a corporation.

11. What are the five powers of a corporation?

12. Give the distinguishing features of the two classes of corporate stock.

13. What are the functions of the Board of Directors of a corporation?

14. Discuss the "Subchapter S" corporation, its purpose and advantages, and the seven requirements for its legal formation.

15. Discuss the four types of structural organization, including the functions and purposes, the strengths and weaknesses of each type, and the pattern of adaptation to the various forms with the growth of the firm.

4. Alternatives in the Practice of Pharmacy

Professions as a special type of occupational role or institution have been the object of a great many sociologic studies. Goode reduced the differentiating traits of a profession to two basic characteristics, a prolonged specialized training of abstract knowledge and a collectivity or service orientation.[1]

From these basic criteria, the following specific traits were derived: (1) the profession determines its own standards of education and training; (2) the student professional goes through a more far-reaching adult socialization experience than the learner in other occupations; (3) professional practice is often legally recognized in some form of licensure; (4) licensing and admission boards are manned by members of the profession; (5) most legislation concerned with the profession is shaped by that profession; (6) the occupation gains in income, power, and prestige ranking, and can demand higher caliber students; (7) the practitioner is relatively free of lay evaluation and control; (8) the norms of practice enforced by the profession are more stringent than legal controls; (9) members are more strongly identified and affiliated with the profession than are members of other occupations with theirs; and (10) the profession is more likely to be a terminal occupation. Members do not care to leave it, and a higher proportion assert that if they had it to do over again, they would again choose that type of work.[1]

Pharmacy: a Profession or a Business

When community pharmacy practice has been the object of sociologic research, the investigations generally have been directed toward the dual roles in pharmacy practice, viz., professional vs. business. Weinlein,[2] Thorner,[3] and McCormack[4] all drew similar conclusions from different perspectives about these dual roles. McCormack described pharmacy as a marginal occupation because of the conflict between the professional and business roles. Marginality in this context referred to the borderline or central position of pharmacy along a professional-business continuum.

Goode described a profession as a "community within a community,"[5] and even though one generation does not produce the next biologically, it does so socially. In the case of pharmacy, there still is a degree of biologic progeny, as indicated by Smith's finding that approximately 10 percent of pharmacy students were children of pharmacists, and approximately 15 percent were related to pharmacists.[6] This is supported by Caplow's research, which indicated that the most directly inherited urban occupations are those that have a proprietorial element.[7] Parsons has pointed out that there are several elements shared by both business and the professions.[8] He noted that the self-interestedness and acquisitiveness of business and the disinterestedness and altruism of the professions may not be due to motivational differences but to institutional differences. This is consistent with Caplow's view that places the occupational roles of retail business and the professions in two different occupational institutions.[9]

Whether the role conflict is one of degree, as McCormack states, or one of institutionalization, as concluded by Caplow, makes little difference to the pharmacist who, after choosing pharmacy as a career, must choose a particular type of pharmacy practice and make role adjustments. This role conflict is of equal importance to executives and managers who must recruit, select, and supervise the activities of pharmacists in their employment.

Using a questionnaire designed to measure the profession-business orientation, Quinney demonstrated that pharmacists adjusted to the role conflict in one of four patterns: (1) Professional Pharmacists (high professional and low business scores); (2) Professional-Business Pharmacists (high professional and high business scores); (3) Indifferent Pharmacists (low professional and low business scores); and (4) Business Pharmacists (low professional and high business score). The 80 pharmacists in the study responded to two questions designed to measure the existence of subjective role conflict and one question which indicated the pharmacist's satisfaction with his occupational career. The responses of the 80 pharmacists to these questions have been tabulated and classified into the four adaptive role conflict patterns and presented in Table 4-1.[10]

Table 4-1. *Objective Adaptation to Role Conflict Compared to Subjective Role Conflict and Career Satisfaction*

Item	Responses of Pharmacists By Adaptive Role Conflict Patterns			
	I	*II*	*III*	*IV*
No. in each adaptive class	13	36	15	16
% with subjective role conflict	77	64	60	25
% with career satisfaction	76	70	40	30

Source: Quinney, E. R.: *Southwestern Social Science Quarterly, 44:*373–75, 1964.

There appears to be ample evidence from both casual observation and sociologic research that pharmacy is both a profession and a business, with definite divergent roles. The pattern of adaptation to the resulting role conflict measured objectively is skewed toward the professional-business orientation, which seems consistent with a recognition of reality. Both the professional and the business-professional pharmacists indicated a high degree of awareness of the conflict, yet a high percentage of each group expressed career satisfaction. Only 40 percent of the "apathetic" pharmacists (low professional-low business orientation) expressed satisfaction with their careers. The most inconsistent finding was that only 25 percent of the business oriented pharmacists were subjectively aware of a role conflict, and yet only 30 percent were satisfied with their careers. The lesson that these data seem to indicate is that if pharmacists are aware of the divergent roles and make a concerted effort to adapt to either a strongly professional role organization pattern or to a combined professional and business role organization pattern, they can attain satisfaction within their chosen career.

Social Background and Personal Attributes

When a young pharmacist is considering a particular career choice, or when an older pharmacist considers a change in his career, he must weigh all the advantages and disadvantages of the various forms of practice as well as his personal inclination to adapt to a role conflict organization that is most compatible with the type of practice he has chosen.

In comparing large businesses with small businesses, the distinctions between the business and the professional roles become less clear with an increase in the size of the business. This is true of any organization, not only business organizations. Large organizations, either business or professional, are organized into a bureaucratic structure which subordinates individual goals to those of the organization. Thus pharmacists, attorneys, physicians, and others are employed by organizations to carry out specific functions in obtaining the organization's goals. The organization also employs professional managers or administrators with specific talents and education for the same general purpose. Bureaucracies have the type of social structure that causes role conflicts between the individual's goals and orientation and that of the organization.

Most chain drug organizations select well-schooled and motivated pharmacists for managerial and executive positions. This practice provides a wide range of role organization patterns, which has been less prevalent in the pharmaceutical manufacturing industry.

Although less than 43 percent of community pharmacists actually are owners, according to a study by M. C. Smith,[6] over 67 percent of students indicated a desire to become pharmacy owners. Figure 4-1 shows the career plans of almost 900 students from all social classes. The relationship between social class and career plans is shown in Table 4-2.

If such a large percentage of pharmacy students desire to become pharmacy owners, they undoubtedly could profit from research findings relative to success in small business generally. However, much of the research on successful small businessmen does not apply to pharmacists.

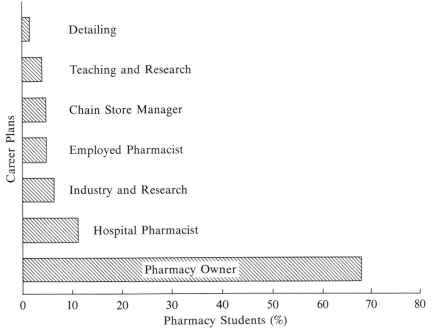

Figure 4-1. *Career plans of pharmacy students. (Adapted from Smith, M.C.:* Am. J. Phar. Educ., 32:*601, 1968.)*

Table 4-2. *Career Plans of Pharmacy Students by Social Class*

Career Plans	Social Class In %					Total Respondents*
	1	*2*	*3*	*4*	*5*	
Pharmacy owner	5	35	37	18	4	603
Hospital pharmacist	4	24	49	21	2	98
Chain store manager	3	15	44	33	5	39
Employed pharmacist	3	20	55	18	5	40
Teaching and research	6	26	49	11	9	35
Industry and research	8	27	45	15	5	60
Detailing	7	29	36	21	7	14

*Does not include all respondents; e.g., some with other types of career plans or with unidentifiable social class.
Source: Adapted from Smith, M. C.: *Am. J. Pharm. Educ., 32*:601, 1968.

For example, the family background of pharmacists is upper-middle and middle class,[6] whereas successful small businessmen in general come from lower and lower-middle classes predominantly.[11] The study of Collins and Moore also indicates that the level of education had little relationship to success as a small businessman.[11] This finding has support from other research. Also of interest is the fact that a degree in pharmacy is necessary to enter the practice, but not to own a pharmacy.

With regard to the educational background of pharmacists, a study by Braucher and Evanson indicated a positive relationship between academic grades in pharmacy administration courses and management ratings by supervisors in the Walgreen Drug Company, as indicated by the Pearson r correlation coefficient and the chi square statistical test.[12] Pharmacy courses also had a positive relationship as indicated by the chi square test only, and general education courses had a positive relationship as indicated by the Pearson r correlation coefficient. No other subject area indicated any significant relationship with management ratings.

While age per se is not a differentiating criterion of success in business or pharmacy, experience, which comes only after several years of work, is a decisive factor. Repeatedly, reports of Dun and Bradstreet indicate that lack of experience in one form or another is the major underlying cause of business failures in all types of business. In recent years they have reported the combination of lack of experience and incompetency as the leading cause of business failures. In 1971, 92.6 percent of failures in retailing were attributed to these two underlying causes.[13]

The sociopsychologic attitudes of entrepreneurs are definitely related to their affinity for proprietorship. A set of seven personality traits was identified by Collins and Moore. These traits indicated a middle class social value system; lack of social mobility—"not wanting to climb the social ladder"; unremitting pursuit of a task; lack of problem resolution;

a paternal type of relationship with subordinates; an unwillingness to submit to authority; and a perception of male authoritative figures as remote, not sought out for assistance nor models to emulate.

In another study more directly related to the success model,[14] five personality factors were identified as most relevant to success as a small business manager. These characteristics were drive, thinking ability, human relations ability, communication skills, and technical knowledge. Each of these characteristics is best evaluated by a disinterested party, preferably two or more, or by special psychologic tests.

Drive is an inherent trait that cannot be readily acquired. It may be further characterized by initiative, persistence, vigor, and willingness to accept responsibility. One should not attempt to evaluate himself on this trait or on any of the other four traits of the success model.

Thinking ability can be developed, but of course it is limited by the person's innate capacity. Thinking ability can take several forms— creative, original, critical, and analytical—all of which are important. Perhaps the most important in pharmacy management is analytical thinking. That is why problem-solving and case study should be incorporated into the pharmaceutical curriculm.

Human relations ability can be cultivated, but again the innate personality of the individual plays an important role. Good human relations ability is composed of several elements including ascendency, emotional stability, cooperation, consideration, cheerfulness, and tactfulness.

Communication ability is a trait that definitely can be cultivated and improved. A college education should provide both written and verbal skills to all graduates; however, this facet of education, along with problem-solving, is one of the greatest weaknesses in pharmaceutical education.

Technical ability can be acquired and is the one characteristic that all recent pharmacy graduates should have in abundance. Indeed, it has been stated that pharmacists are overtrained or overeducated, especially in the sciences. Of course, this point is subject to debate. However, it is doubtful whether pharmaceutical curricula provide all the necessary educational tools for the managerial or administrative challenges of managing a successful pharmacy in the highly competitive market of today.

According to authorities in the field of management and administration, there is not a unique set of characteristics that will identify a successful executive in a large firm. However, this fact does not negate the success model concept for small business entrepreneurs.

The Small Business Administration has developed a "Checklist for Going into Business" under the general title of *Small Marketers Aids No. 71*. It is available free from any of the field offices or the headquarters in Washington, D.C.

Profile of Practice Opportunities

The opportunities available to young pharmacists are varied and numerous. These may be classified in several different ways: (1) by type of practice; (2) by type of legal form of ownership; (3) by the number of units operated by a single firm (independent vs. chain); and (4) by the sales volume.

Among the types of practice there are pharmaceutical centers, other prescription shops or apothecaries, traditional pharmacies (sometimes referred to as conventional, neighborhood, or corner drugstores), large super-merchandising drugstores, hospital pharmacies, and nursing home pharmacies. The latter two types of practice are frequently referred to as institutional pharmacy and as specialty practices. These, in turn, can be classified according to size and type of ownership. Nursing home pharmacies can be further categorized with regard to the scope of pharmaceutical services involved. In 1970, 11,001 pharmacists were employed in hospitals.[15] Hospital pharmacy represents one of the fastest growing types of practice. The number of hospitals employing pharmacists in 1970 is reported in Table 4-3. An additional 553 hospitals did not report data on the services provided. In 1969, there were 13,047 licensed nursing homes with 762,465 beds and 9,966 related facilities with 262,045 beds. Together, there were 23,000 long-term facilities supplying more than 1,000,000 beds.[16]

Some pharmacists consider the pharmaceutical center, which was first introduced in 1960, to provide the ideal environment for a highly professional practice. It is estimated that there are now approximately 300 pharmaceutical centers in the United States. To be designated as such,

Table 4-3. *Hospital Employment*

		Pharmacies With Registered Pharmacist			
	No. of	Full-Time		Part-Time	
Size (*No. of Beds*)	Hospitals Reporting	Number	Percent	Number	Percent
6–24	356	24	6.7	106	29.8
25–49	1,258	173	13.8	567	45.1
50–99	1,566	569	36.3	685	43.7
100–199	1,419	1,137	80.1	224	15.8
200–299	683	644	94.3	43	6.3
300–399	424	400	94.3	30	7.1
400–499	255	242	94.9	20	7.8
500 and over	609	576	94.6	42	6.9
Total	6,570	3,765	57.3	1,717	26.1

Source: *Hospitals, 45*; Part 2, Table 4, Aug. 1, 1971.

the pharmaceutical centers must meet high standards, including the following criteria: (1) no drugs or other products on open display; (2) ample reception area for patients; (3) a patient medication profile system; and (4) the use of a professional fee, either fixed or variable, with appropriate exceptions permissible. The decor of the center is a basic feature also, which causes the center to look more like an office than a traditional pharmacy.

There is another elite group of prescription pharmacies, the owners of which form the membership of the American College of Apothecaries (ACA). There are approximately 750 members operating approximately 1000 pharmacies. The standards for membership are high, and while they do not include all the criteria of the pharmaceutical center, they do include additional criteria such as a designated amount of participation in the national or regional meetings. In addition, no merchandise that detracts from pharmaceutical practice may be stocked by ACA members.

There is a larger group of unorganized prescription-oriented pharmacies, or apothecary shops as they were called in earlier times, which emphasize prescription services and health-related products. Sometimes these shops stock cosmetics, toiletries, and a few traditional non-drug products, primarily for the convenience of their patrons. *The Lilly Digest* uses only two criteria for gathering and reporting data for this type of pharmacy, viz., floor space of 1,200 square feet or less and prescription revenue accounting for more than 50 percent of sales. Approximately 14 percent of the total *Lilly Digest* sample for 1971 was made up of prescription-oriented pharmacies.[17] It is estimated that at least 6,000 pharmacies fall into this category. Both pharmaceutical centers and ACA pharmacies make up a part of this total.

The traditional independent community pharmacies employ the greatest number of pharmacists and other employees. However, the number of chain or multi-unit drugstores has increased in terms of number of units and, more particularly, sales over the past decade. The growth in chain drugstores at the expense of the independents is illustrated in Table 4-4.

There has been a shift in the size of independent pharmacies, with the larger pharmacies increasing in number and sales volume at the expense of the smaller pharmacies. The A.C. Nielsen Company has tabulated this trend and projected it to 1980.[18] The trend in numbers of establishments is depicted in Figure 4-2, and the trend in the sales volume as shown in Figure 4-3 is even more dramatic.

The *Chain Store Age for Drug Executives* reports figures for the chain drug industry which are quite different from the Census of Business data. *Chain Store Age* reports a much higher figure in terms of both units and sales volume. This discrepancy arises from different interpretations of the definition of a chain. For example, *Chain Store Age for Drug Executives*

Table 4-4. *Comparison of Chain and Independent Pharmacies*

Year	Independents No.	Independents Sales in $1,000	Chains* No.	Chains* Sales in $1,000	% Chain of Total No.	% Chain of Total Sales
1929†	58,258	1,690,399	NA‡	NA	NA	NA
1935	52,899	914,316	3,798	318,277	6.7	25.8
1939	53,723	1,160,520	4,180	401,982	7.2	25.7
1948	43,553	2,846,065	3,402	832,398	7.2	22.6
1954	44,551	4,857,325	NA	NA	NA	NA
1958	47,697	5,095,065	3,751	1,436,084	7.3	22.0
1963	45,853	6,039,245	4,465	2,131,459	8.9	26.1
1967	40,902	6,823,235	5,342	3,464,895	11.6	33.7

*Four or more units under a single ownership.
†Data available only on total drug sales for 1929.
‡NA means data not available.
Source: *Census of Business,* several editions, 1940–1967

reported more than twice as many chain units as the Census of Business did in 1967.[19] According to *Chain Store Age,* the 15 largest drug chains operated 3,996 units, and the top 31 drug chains operated 5,513 units in 1972.[20] It should be noted that not all chains, by legal definition, are large super drugstores. Some chain firms operate all types of pharmacies and some specialize in prescription shops.

The newest development in pharmaceutical practice is the franchise system involving the entire pharmacy. The idea of a franchise merchandise line is very old, but the concept of a franchise system has developed within the past decade. It has some of the characteristics of cooperatives, but requires much more stringent controls by the system. There are several organizations offering these systems throughout the country. These franchise systems usually concentrate on prescription services, convalescent or home health care aids, orthopedic appliances, and physicians' supplies.

A typical franchise agreement would include an exclusive use of the franchise name, logo, and trademarks within a specified area. The franchisee cannot use any other signs or advertisements except those developed by the franchiser. The total package investment may range from $35,000 to $85,000 and includes approximately 10 percent for launching a promotional program and 20 percent for the franchise license and service fee. The investment is usually financed.

The franchise license and service fee includes assistance in a location evaluation, lease arrangement, setting up the fixtures, equipment and merchandise, and the initial promotional cost. The fee usually includes a management training program to instruct the pharmacist in the management and operating procedures of the system. It may include training in the fitting, servicing, and promotion of the health care equipment and devices.

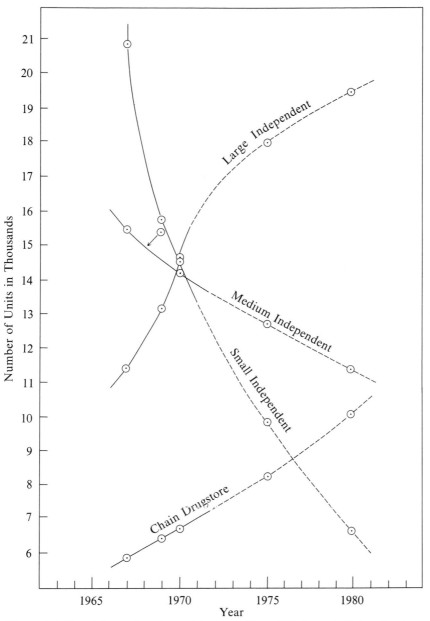

Figure 4-2. *Trends in number of establishments.* (*From* 38th Annual Nielsen Review of Retail Drug Store Trends. *Chicago: A. C. Nielsen Co., Chart 2.*)

In some cases, all designated merchandise must be purchased through the system. Usually a computerized accounting system and management assistance are provided routinely. The franchisee-pharmacist usually pays

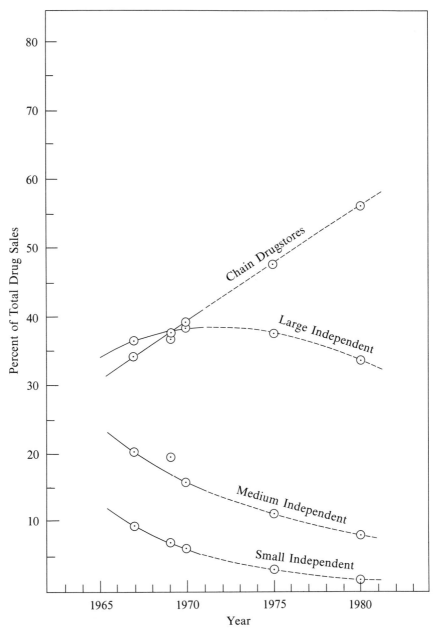

Figure 4-3. *Trends in sales volume.* (*From* 38th Annual Nielsen Review of Retail Drug Store Trends, *Chicago: A. C. Nielsen Co., Chart 1.*)

a monthly service fee of 2 to 4 percent of sales for the computerized and managerial assistance. Also, regular promotional and advertising campaigns are furnished, and the franchisee must agree to use a designated percentage of sales for advertising. The pharmacist must participate in a specified percentage of the regional promotional programs. This type of system obviously has inherent strengths, but the question to be answered by a pharmacist contemplating such a venture is whether the cost of the franchise is worth the service received. Additionally, the pharmacist must be willing to forego a large degree of independence.

In addition to the various types of practice already described, the young pharmacist may choose to work in government, industry (manufacturing, research, marketing, sales, or administration), pharmaceutical associations and journalism, law enforcement, or teaching and academic research.

According to a report of the National Association of Boards of Pharmacy,[15] most pharmacists practiced in community pharmacies—independents and chains. The major types of pharmacy employment are summarized in Table 4-5.

Practice Alternatives

Of the several employment alternatives open to the young pharmacist, basically all may be classified under two headings: *entrepreneurship,* or self-employment, and *employee* status. However, each of these major alternatives provides several variations worthy of further discussion.

As an *employee,* the pharmacist may contract to receive (1) straight salary, (2) salary plus profit sharing, or (3) salary with option to purchase an interest in the pharmacy with or without interim profit sharing. His other options are (1) to *purchase* an established pharmacy, either outright or as a partner, or (2) to *establish* a new pharmacy.

It has been noted that any of the various forms of practices may be either a chain operation or an independent operation. It should be obvious that pharmacists may seek employment in any type of pharmaceutical practice or any form of ownership, or he may seek entrepreneurship of

Table 4-5. *Distribution of Pharmacists by Employment*

Type of Employment	Number	Percent
Proprietors	45,497	35.3
Employee Pharmacists*	61,304	47.6
Hospitals	11,001	8.6
Industry	4,954	3.3
Teaching, Government, Others	6,087	4.7
Total	128,843	100.0

*Includes employment in both chain and independent pharmacies.
Source: *Licensure Statistics and Census of Pharmacy,* Chicago: National Association of Boards of Pharmacy, 1970.

any of the several forms of practice or ownership. In addition, he may seek employment in institutional pharmacy, government service, teaching, association work, or industry.

It should also be apparent that varying degrees of managerial responsibility may be delegated to an employee pharmacist, depending on his position. He may be given the responsibility of managing a chain drugstore, which requires all of the managerial skills of a pharmacy proprietor, except for financing, capital management, and the commensurate risk involved. On the other hand, the manager of a large chain drugstore may have more employees and a larger inventory to manage than a proprietor of an independent pharmacy. However, the manager of a large chain drugstore has guidelines and manuals to assist him in his overall managerial responsibility.

In contrast, a staff pharmacist has only those managerial responsibilities delegated to him by the manager. The assistant manager normally is delegated a considerable amount of managerial responsibility, and he is fully responsible in the absence of the manager.

A similar situation exists in the larger hospitals. The chief pharmacist or director of pharmaceutical services has a wide range of managerial responsibility, again excluding only capital and risk management. The assistant director and staff pharmacists have responsibilities paralleling their counterparts in a chain drugstore, recognizing, of course, the differences in the two types of practices.

The pharmacist employed in an independent pharmacy as the second pharmacist has considerable managerial responsibilities delegated to him. When he is the only pharmacist present, the law requires that he assume full responsibility for professional functions. The law also provides the necessary authority to carry out the professional responsibilities. Normally, he will be delegated the responsibility for the administrative functions as well, and this is the common practice in all types of pharmaceutical practices. Therefore, every pharmacist should be educated and trained in a wide range of managerial skills; the depth of such education and training depends on the type of practice the pharmacist chooses.

SMALL INDEPENDENT PHARMACIES

Advantages. If the typical independent pharmacy proprietor were asked why he elected to undertake the ownership of his pharmacy, he would probably give the following typical answers: "to be independent," "to be my own boss," or "to make more money." Clearly, the desire to be one's own boss is a striving for independence, which is one of America's greatest heritages. Whether or not the typical independent pharmacy owner has a true insight into his basic motivations, it is a fact that he elected the course of action as a way of life because of the perceived advantages that appealed to him, such as: (1) being your own boss; (2) doing things the way you like to do them, or self-fulfillment; (3) being secure and independent of the dictates of others; (4) being recognized in the community and playing an important role in its life; and (5) achieving the ego reinforcement motivations of personal pride, status, and profit. It is noteworthy to indicate that these appeals are primarily emotional in nature, reflecting a basic attitude acquired from the cultural and social background and personal experiences.

The young pharmacist or potential pharmacy owner should be aware of the true nature of these five advantages. Being one's own boss is not complete freedom. In fact, each patron or patient is "boss" in a very real sense. The pharmacist must satisfy his needs and desires, first to attract his patronage, and second to merit his continuing patronage. Also, "to be the boss" requires a great deal of responsibility and concern, not only with respect to the public, but especially for employees.

If, in fact, a young pharmacist, as a potential pharmacy proprietor, is properly motivated in his desire to "do things the way he thinks they should be done," this is one of the most laudable reasons for undertaking the independent proprietorship of a pharmacy. Certainly pharmacists should not be encumbered by overpowering commercial interest in making professional decisions. This is one of the fundamental ways pharmacy, with its professional considerations, differs from ordinary small businesses. Similarly, the same thing applies to being independent from the dictates of others. Security in the professional context is a combination of independent discretion and economic and psychologic security. A professional pharmacist feels the need for all three.

The fourth advantage is not restricted to independent pharmacy proprietors, but can be attained by a manager of a chain pharmacy, provided he remains in one community for a sufficient length of time. Also, he must be motivated to seek a significant role in the community. This advantage accrues to an independent pharmacist more readily because of his greater visibility usually, and the fact that the community benefits from the local retention of the profits.

The fifth advantage or appeal is probably the most powerful for most pharmacists. Historically, status and prestige are inherent characteristics reserved primarily for the pharmacist-proprietor in the American pharmacy tradition. This is particularly true in the smaller cities and rural towns. In recent years there has been a considerable reduction in the prestige and status of the pharmacist-owner, particularly in the metropolitan areas. This has come about primarily because of the dominance of commercial activity in pharmacy in these areas. Also, the profit and salary of the independent pharmacy proprietor are not much more, on the average, than the salary plus the bonus of the manager of a chain drugstore, who has very little invested.

Disadvantages. The very first disadvantage encountered by the independent pharmacy proprietor is the fact that he is not so independent after all. In fact, he will discover that everyone, in a sense, is his "boss." In other words, some of his ideas may have to be subordinated to those of others. This extends not only to his patrons, but also to his banker, his suppliers, the physicians, and others. For example, if a note is due at the bank, the banker may well offer some suggestions, or even make demands, before the renewal of the note, which may affect the manner in which the owner operates the pharmacy. This could also apply to suppliers who may have sold him the opening inventory on credit. It is obvious that the pharmacist and the physician must have professional working relations to function for the maximum benefit to society and each other, and this need not require a simple "yes man" attitude by the pharmacist.

The second disadvantage of ownership is the inherent responsibility and liability. The pharmacist-proprietor must be willing to assume full financial, professional, and legal responsibilities for the entire operation of the pharmacy. This particularly is true of the sole proprietorship. In this regard, the new pharmacy proprietor may have to deprive himself, and his family, during the formative years of the practice until he can develop the practice into a profitable one. This may require several years, depending on the location, type of pharmacy, and managerial ability of the pharmacist-proprietor.

Another obvious disadvantage consists in the long hours and work week during the formative years of the practice. This can be avoided in two basic ways. First, if the pharmacist selects an excellent location and has sufficient capital to begin a going practice, he may be able to employ the second pharmacist soon after beginning his practice. Second, he may form a group practice with other pharmacist(s) with the understanding that each may supplement his income by part-time practice in another pharmacy in another location.

Another disadvantage of independent ownership, and one about which pharmacists frequently complain, is the amount of paper work required. This complaint is exaggerated in the opinion of some. The reasons for the seemingly great burden of paper work is the failure to formalize business and professional procedures, develop good routines, and delegate as much as is feasible and consistent with good professional practice. Adequate records are required to chart the course of an enterprise and analyze its progress, and executed properly, the paper work is an advantage, not a disadvantage.

LARGE CHAIN PHARMACIES

Advantages. Some advantages associated with employment in a large organization are: (1) stability of employment and less susceptibility to economic change; (2) fixed hours, salary, vacations, and fringe benefits; (3) financial strength to carry out the organization's plans; (4) the opportunity to identify and associate with a group; (5) opportunity for advancement in the company with the accompanying status and titles; and (6) opportunity to have anonymity and avoidance of social or community responsibility to a degree.

Little explanation of these advantages is required because they largely are self-explanatory. Some of these advantages may be partially realized in an independent pharmacy. One of the more recent organizational advancements among "traditional" pharmacists is the establishment of a package of fringe benefits for their employees through an association. These benefits are transferable as long as the employee remains employed by a member of the group. The philosophy has also been extended to group buying and cooperative promotion. These cooperative efforts provide economic strength to the members of the group along with a measure of the large-chain type of security, both psychologic and economic, to the proprietors and their employees.

Disadvantages. The primary disadvantages of employment in a large chain organization are: (1) job insecurity brought about by frequent transfer, and the resulting lack of sense of permanent local associations and job commitment; (2) receiving blame for certain uncontrollable events; (3) less flexibility in scheduling regular hours and "time off" when necessary or desirable; (4) the policies associated with any large organization; and (5) the highly competitive nature of the operation with emphasis on commercialism.

A brief comment on the first disadvantage is necessary because it may appear to be contradictory. Job security per se should be contrasted with the economic stability of the overall organization. Although the organization can withstand economic changes, even crises, the individual may not feel secure in his job. During an economic recession, a new employee is expendable, but this is not the primary point. The basic point is that the employee must adapt himself to the organization's goals and be productive. Failure to perform as expected is sufficient reason for dismissal. This should be true in small organizations, but more leniency is practiced in the smaller organizations. Management by objectives is the technique designed to avoid this hazard for the benefit of both employee and employer.

Uncontrollable events for which an employee, or especially an employee-manager, may be held accountable are numerous. One example is pilferage by both customers and employees. This can be controlled to a degree, but complete eradication of this costly practice is not possible with today's methods of merchandise displays and controls. The automatic shipment of goods that will not sell in certain markets is another example. Transfer and re-assignment of personnel are further examples.

Frequency of transfer of personnel, especially management, within a chain organization is a real weakness in establishing loyal patronage on a professional and lasting personal basis. This can, and often does, distract from a complete commitment to the community by pharmacists in a large chain organization. The feeling of anonymity, one among so many others, is a common complaint of our modern-day society. If pharmacists have this feeling themselves, they can hardly transfer a warm, personal, and helpful feeling to the patients and patrons with whom they come in contact. That is why there is so little patient consultation among *some* chain pharmacists; however, this fault is found much too frequently among traditional independent pharmacists as well.

Scheduling flexibility need not be a major problem in chain pharmacies, and often it is not. Pharmacists should be aware of company policies and operations in chain pharmacies before accepting a position with a company. Individual needs can be accommodated in most instances with a little effort and ample patience.

It is axiomatic that whenever a sizable group is involved in any activity you will have politics. Conventionally, the term is applied to the activities of government. However, the term is derived from the same root word as "policies" and "polite." Thus, politics will evolve any time a group is formed in which policies are developed and a hierarchy is present. As a general rule, the larger the group, the more likely it is that politics will become a part of the group's activities.

A business firm with a well-defined structure and set of policies has a formal method of controlling activities, making decisions, and achieving goals, which presumably minimizes politics. When efforts are expended to influence decisions, activities, or goals outside the formal procedures, these efforts are labeled as "politics" in business. Unwarranted influences on decisions through regular communication channels, for example by a special group within the organization, should be labeled political as well. Seldom is a business organization of any size free of political activities. This is probably best described by the cliché, "It is not what you know, but who you know." One of the reasons for adopting management by objectives is to minimize undesirable politics in business.

The highly competitive posture of many chain pharmacies is well known. As a consequence, many independent pharmacies are failing in business.[21] The degree of competition varies among chains as well as between chain and independent pharmacies. Some of the newcomers in the chain drug business have advertised prescriptions as low as the average wholesale cost plus $.49 in order to break into a market. Older, established chain drugstores are forced to engage in competitive pricing in order to maintain their market position.

INSTITUTIONAL PRACTICE

A pharmacist may elect to practice in one of the several types of institutions. The hospital is the primary employer of pharmacists in institutions; however, skilled and other nursing homes, and penal institutions employ pharmacists, either full-time, part-time, or as consultants. Although the duties of the pharmacist vary considerably with the type of institutions, the basic duties are common to all. There are as many differences between hospital pharmacists employed in an acute, short-term general hospital and a long-term mental or tuberculosis hospital as there are among pharmacists employed in these other various types of institution.

Characteristics. There are certain basic distinctions between the institutional pharmacist and the general, community pharmacist:

1. The institutional pharmacist primarily serves patients confined to the institution, with the exception of those outpatients having prescriptions dispensed at the institutional pharmacy.
2. The institutional pharmacist's professional relationship involves primarily the physician and the nurse, his involvement with the patient being only an indirect one through the nurse. Again, the exceptions are the outpatients and certain large teaching hospitals in which skilled pharmacists serve patients directly on the floor, taking drug histories, and providing information in certain instances.
3. The institutional pharmacist operates on a nonprofit basis, but in a revenue/expenditure budget context. This distinction should not be overemphasized because hospital administrators often expect the director of pharmaceutical services to generate revenues in excess of expenditures to offset deficits in other departments. Thus the director of pharmaceutical services, or chief pharmacist, is expected to be a good administrator.
4. A final distinction is that an institutional pharmacist must be knowledgeable and feel comfortable in a bureaucratic organizational structure, especially in larger institutions. He must understand the interrelationships in the organization, the lines of authority, responsibility, and communication, and be able to function efficiently within the organization.

Advantages and Disadvantages. The *advantages* of institutional practice include: (1) insulation from severe economic, competitive pressures; (2) opportunity to relate to and consult more frequently with other health professionals; (3) opportunity to influence prescribing patterns through the Pharmacy and Therapeutics Committee; (4) opportunity to teach other health professionals and assist in research, especially in the large, teaching hospitals; (5) opportunity to engage in limited manufacturing of pharmaceuticals in larger institutions; and (6) opportunity for advancement in the larger institutions.

The *disadvantages* include: (1) limited direct contact with the patient and the resulting absence of patient consultation concerning prescriptions (with the exception noted above); (2) almost complete absence of direct contact with patrons (customers) and the opportunity to assist in the primary care of simple ailments; (3) less opportunity to function independently in several facets of practice—especially in comparing the independent proprietor with the institutional practitioner; and (4) absence of the opportunity to be self-employed and the advantages inherent in proprietorship.

PURCHASING AN ESTABLISHED PHARMACY

Advantages. In general, the purchase of an established pharmacy entails less risk than does the establishing of a new pharmacy. Because the financial records are available for study, the buyer is dealing with a known quantity to a large degree. If all other economic factors remain equal, the purchase of an established pharmacy has the advantage of not increasing the number of competing pharmacies in a given market. If the location is a good one, this fact supports the general proposition of less risk and better chance of success. Related to these two concepts is still a third advantage, namely, no lag time before attaining a profitable status, barring some unusual economic or market upheaval.

An established pharmacy has an established clientele with entrenched shopping habits or patterns. Habits are not easily changed; therefore, one can expect to retain most of the patrons. The set of charge accounts or accounts receivable is a closely related but separate factor. If the pharmacist purchases the accounts receivable with the pharmacy, then he has the opportunity to begin a sound professional and business relationship if he meets the patrons when they pay their accounts. If the accounts are paid by mail, an appropriately composed letter can accomplish similar results, since the ledger of accounts receivable provides an excellent mailing list. The third item in this category is the prescription files. The prescription files are of definite value because an average of 55 percent of all prescriptions dispensed are refills. Frequently, prescription files are sold to another pharmacist when a pharmacy discontinues its operations.

Collectively the aforementioned make up the concrete aspects of goodwill. Goodwill is an illusive asset and can be readily overpriced. It is considered to be an *intangible* asset representing the potential earning capacity of the pharmacy. As already indicated, this intangible asset can have, and should have, some of the tangible items in support of its valuation. "Goodwill," if overpriced, can be a disadvantage.

Disadvantages. As previously indicated, one disadvantage in purchasing an established pharmacy is the possibility of paying too much for goodwill. This factor should be studied critically before reaching an agreement on its value. A more detailed discussion of evaluating goodwill will be given in the chapter on capital requirements.

Other specific disadvantages include used fixtures and equipment, which may require replacement in the near future. Although the old fixtures and equipment may have served the purposes of the former proprietor, they may simply be inadequate for the style of pharmaceutical practice you envision. This, of course, will require additional capital outlay. Also, the inventory of merchandise may be too large in relation to sales; it may contain items that will not sell; or it may be unbalanced generally, meaning quantities of various goods out of proportion to their sales potential. This problem can be avoided by having a third party take the inventory and make corrections for unsaleable or deteriorated merchandise. He can identify certain merchandise which may be eligible for return to the supplier for credit.

Two other disadvantages, which are interrelated, are inadequate policies and procedures and undesirable personnel. The former owner may not have been diligent in formulating and implementing good policies and procedures or in the hiring and training of employees. Like bad habits, bad precedents are difficult to rectify. Dismissal of an old employee can have repercussions in the community, creating ill will among the friends and family of the dismissed employee, and it may have an unfavorable effect on employee morale, although in some instances the reverse may be true.

There is yet one other potential disadvantage in purchasing an established pharmacy—and this can be critical—namely, the lease for the building. The lease may be near its termination and the former owner may have failed to protect himself adequately with appropriate renewal options. The landlord may have ideas of increasing the rent substantially, or even leasing the building for some other purpose. Related to this problem are such other considerations relative to the building as meeting the fire and sanitation codes and appropriate insurance coverage, which could affect the operation.

ESTABLISHING A NEW PHARMACY

Advantages. In considering both the advantages and disadvantages of establishing a new pharmacy, one is confronted to a large degree with a "mirror image" of the advantages and disadvantages of purchasing an established pharmacy. The advantages of one are the disadvantages of the other, with certain exceptions. For example, in a new pharmacy one can purchase new fixtures and equipment and a model inventory; develop sound policies and procedures; employ and train personnel of his choosing; check the terms of the lease carefully; and avoid the problem of purchasing goodwill. One other advantage is the potential for finding a superior location with greater potential earnings for the new pharmacy in view of expanding suburbia, the development of shopping centers, and the relocating of many physicians.

Disadvantages. As a general rule, establishing a new pharmacy involves greater risk, basically because (1) the entrepreneur is dealing with unknown quantities, such as shopping habits and possible new competition, and (2) new pharmacies, as a rule, are larger, requiring more capital. It may be more difficult for a young independent pharmacist to borrow the necessary capital for a new pharmacy in a new location. In fact, it is virtually impossible for an individual pharmacist to obtain a lease in a large shopping center because the developers of the center rely upon lessees with large amounts of capital and a superior credit rating to finance the cost of developing the center.

The most obvious disadvantage is the lag time before the practice reaches a profitable level of operation. This lag period can range from approximately one year to three or four years. If it requires more than four years to reach a profitable status, the cause is either poor management or a poor location in a competitive market. If the location is not a good one, relocating should be considered.

JUNIOR PARTNERSHIPS

As indicated previously, a pharmacist has a choice of seeking employment in a pharmacy or owning his own pharmacy. As an employee, he may receive a straight salary, a salary plus a share of the profits, or either of the above two arrangements with an option to purchase an interest in the pharmacy. Under this latter arrangement, a preliminary period of one or two years is stipulated to determine mutual compatibility. Following the preliminary period, a purchase agreement is drawn, usually specifying a percentage of the pharmacy's valuation to be sold to the junior partner annually up to a designated percentage. Frequently, this is accomplished over a period of time when the senior pharmacist is phasing into semi-retirement and finally into full retirement. He may retain an interest in the pharmacy after his retirement for a retirement income, or he may sell the entire pharmacy and invest the proceeds along with other savings to provide a retirement income. Payments may be spread over a longer period of time for tax advantages.

Advantages. First, there is little risk involved in this method of becoming a proprietor. The pharmacist has ample opportunity to evaluate the potential and the risk of investing in a pharmacy with which he has been associated for a year or more. Generally, the initial capital is relatively small, and part of the increments of the investment over time can be derived from the pharmacist's share of the earnings. This type of arrangement provides for immediate profit in addition to the salary in almost every case.

In addition, there are non-monetary advantages in this arrangement. These include incentive, professional pride, self-esteem, and self-fulfillment. The profession and society as well are benefited from the stabilizing influence this arrangement has on pharmacists' employment. There is greater likelihood that a pharmacist will remain in a permanent location. This saves money in retraining pharmacists in new operations, and the pharmacist can better serve patients whom he has known over a period of years. In summary, there are less risk, less initial capital required, a profit in addition to a salary usually, greater incentive and self-fulfillment for the pharmacist, and greater stability in pharmacists' employment with this type of arrangement.

Disadvantages. Some critics have stated that this arrangement has many disadvantages. They include investment without any real authority in the decisions, the potential of personality incompatibility, the difficulty of disposing of the minor interest without assuming at least some financial loss, and finally, the potential legal entanglements in a partnership. This latter criticism is very real and was discussed in more detail in the chapter on legal organizations. The other criticisms are potential disadvantages, but only if appropriate steps have not been taken to prevent or mitigate these disadvantages. Compatibility should be determined in advance of the purchase agreement. Participation in decisions can be expected to be at least proportionate to the interest owned and will probably exceed this level since the intent is for the junior partner to assume an equal or senior status in the future. Disposing of the minor interest can be prearranged under specified conditions in the purchase agreement.

REFERENCES

1. Goode, W. J.: Encroachment, charlatanism, and the emerging profession: psychology, sociology, and medicine. *Am. Soc. Review, 25*:902-914, 1960.
2. Weinlen, A.: Pharmacy as a profession with special reference to the state of Wisconsin. Master's Thesis, University of Chicago, 1943.
3. Thorner, I.: Pharmacy: the Functional Significance of an institutional pattern. *Social Forces, 20*:321-28, 1942.
4. McCormack, T. H.: The druggists' dilemma: problems of a marginal occupation. *Am. J. of Sociology, 61*:308-15, 1956.
5. Goode, W. J.: Community within a community: the professions. *Am. Soc. Review, 22*:194-200, 1957.
6. Smith, M. C.: Social background of pharmacy students. *Am. J. Pharm. Educ., 32*:596-609, 1968.
7. Caplow, T.: *The Sociology of Work.* Minneapolis: University of Minnesota Press, 1954, p. 76.
8. Parsons, T.: The professions and social structure. The motivation of economic activities. *Essays in Sociological Theory,* Glencoe, Illinois: The Free Press, 1949, pp. 185-217.

9. Caplow, T.: *op. cit.,* pp. 100-123.
10. Quinney, E. R.: Adjustment to occupational role strain: the case of retail pharmacy. *The Southwestern Social Science Quarterly, 44*:367-76, 1964.
11. Collins, O. F., Moore, D. G., and Unwalla, D. B.: *The Enterprising Man.* East Lansing, Michigan: Bureau of Business and Economic Research, 1964.
12. Braucher, C. L., and Evanson, R. V.: Academic factors related to success in community pharmacy management. *Am. J. Pharm. Educ., 28*:56-66, 1964.
13. Wyatt, R.: Business failures. *Dun's Review, 99*:97, 1972.
14. Pickle, H. B.: *Personality and Success.* Washington, D.C.: Small Business Administration, 1964.
15. *Licensure Statistics and Census of Pharmacy.* Chicago: National Association of Boards of Pharmacy, 1970, Table 2.
16. *Pharmaceutical Services in the Nursing Home,* Washington: APhA, ANHA and ASHP, 1972.
17. Slavin, G. F.: *The Lilly Digest.* Indianapolis: Eli Lilly and Co., 1972, p. 26.
18. *38th Annual Review of Retail Drug Store Trends.* Chicago: A. C. Nielsen Co., 1972.
19. *Chain Store Age for Drug Executives. 49,* No. 5, p. 81, 1973.
20. *Ibid.,* pp. 84, 145-209.
21. *Drug Topics, Chain Edition,* April 16, 1973, pp. 25, 26.

REVIEW

1. Name the *two basic* characteristics of a profession and the ten specific traits associated with a profession according to Goode.

2. Discuss the extent that pharmacy possesses these ten specific traits.

3. Correlate the four adaptive role conflict patterns with the degree of awareness of the subjective role conflict and the percentage of pharmacists with career satisfaction.

4. In sociologic terms, what is the basis for describing pharmacy as a marginal occupation (or marginal profession)?

5. How does the reported desire of pharmacy students to own their own pharmacy compare with reality?

6. What subject matter in the pharmacy curriculum correlates best with success in a large chain drugstore as indicated by supervisors' ratings?

7. What are the seven sociopsychologic *attitudes* of entrepreneurs as reported by Collins and Moore?

8. Describe the five personality *factors* of the success model of the small business entrepreneur.

9. Discuss the profile of practice opportunities in pharmacy, including the significant trends and the relative extent of the opportunities among the various specialities.

10. Discuss the alternate means of entering the practice of pharmacy.

11. Discuss the five perceived advantages of owning a pharmacy and why each may or may not exist in real life.

12. What are six advantages and five disadvantages of employment by a large chain drugstore?

13. What are five advantages and four potential disadvantages of entering practice as a junior partner?

14. What are the six advantages and six potential disadvantages of purchasing an established pharmacy?

15. What are seven potential advantages and three potential disadvantages of establishing a new pharmacy?

5. Planning for Capital Requirements

Capital is the wealth, or tangible assets, used in a business enterprise to produce income. Its various forms include actual cash, bank deposits, notes, and property, either real or personal. Capital may be classified in several ways for various purposes. In terms of capital resources, the first classification that comes to mind is equity capital and borrowed capital. *Equity capital* is defined as tangible assets owned free of financial obligations or debts, whereas *borrowed capital* is the term applied to assets obtained from other sources such as banks, other firms, or individuals.

Classified according to the manner in which it is to be used, capital may be either working capital or fixed capital. *Working capital* consists of cash on hand or in the bank, accounts receivable, and inventory; in other words, it is the capital that is working for the firm. The capital is transformed from one form to another through the transactions of the merchandising cycle as shown in Figure 5-1.

On the other hand, when funds are committed to long-term or continuing investment for a fixed purpose, such as the purchase of equipment and fixtures, they are no longer available for other purposes. Thus, capital so committed is called *fixed capital* or *fixed assets.* In contrast, working capital may be shifted, to a degree, for alternate purposes, variation in quantity or lines of merchandise, expansion or decrease in accounts receivable, or a corresponding decrease or increase in cash. A more thorough discussion of the management of the merchandise cycle is included in later chapters.

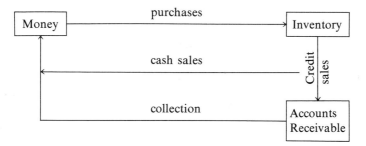

Figure 5-1. *Schematic diagram of the merchandise cycle.*

Borrowed capital may be classified further as short-term and long-term. *Short-term liabilities* are those debts that become due within one year or less; *long-term liabilities* are those debts for which payment takes longer than one year. In general, it is better to use short-term liabilities to finance working capital, if necessary, and to use long-term debts to fund fixed assets.

Sources of Capital

It should be apparent that the ideal situation exists when the pharmacist has all the capital he needs to purchase or establish a pharmacy. There would be little or no financial strain on the firm and no interest charge to decrease the profits. This situation is seldom the case. Where does a pharmacist borrow funds and how much should he borrow? The answer to the second part of the question is "as little as possible." The answer to the first part is more difficult and depends on the sources available to him and the route of entry into entrepreneurship he is taking.

If a pharmacist is purchasing an interest in a pharmacy in increments over time—a junior partner as it were—the senior partner or a bank note with a co-signature of the senior partner may be the most logical source of borrowed capital. The junior partner should have a significant amount of his own capital to invest in the pharmacy, ranging from 10 percent to 30 percent of the purchase value.

Relatives or friends are another source of borrowed funds. This source has come under severe criticism because of potential entanglements and disputes. These can be avoided with appropriate advice and arrangements. First of all, the lender should view the loan as a business proposition as well as an opportunity to assist the pharmacist to get a start in business. The lender should not offer to provide the funds unless he has confidence in the pharmacist and has reasonable expectations that the venture will succeed. A business life insurance policy should be purchased by the borrower to protect himself, his family, and the person lending the money. Appropriate interest rates should be charged. Finally, a mutual understanding and the necessary legal arrangements are a must to avoid unnecessary disputes or liabilities.

Banks and other financial institutions are the logical source of borrowed funds because this is the purpose of these institutions. There is a degree of security in using this source because a bank will investigate the potential of success of the pharmacist and the pharmacy to safeguard its loan. In general, banks are the preferred source of borrowed funds. Usually the person borrowing the capital, normally in the form of money, executes a note indicating the amount borrowed, the interest rate, and the date(s) the note or fractions thereof is/are due. Such notes or any form of borrowed capital are commonly referred to as debts, and in the language of the accountant, they are called liabilities.

Another potential source of borrowed funds is the suppliers, generally the full-service wholesaler. This source was the one most frequently used in the past. This is no longer true today. Most wholesalers would rather see the pharmacist obtain the necessary borrowed capital from a bank, and they will gladly assist through such efforts as location evaluation, layout design, and other services. These services assist the bank in making a decision on credit extension.

Suppliers will still provide restricted credit for inventory. The prevailing practice is to sell a "model" opening inventory with a down payment of 10 percent to 25 percent and the balance due in 90 days net of cash discounts. The rationale is that the "model" inventory will be turned or sold in 90 days or less, thereby generating enough cash to pay for the opening inventory and replenish the inventory stock. This rationale would have to be based on the assumption that the "model" inventory was minimal and that additional stock would be added as demand indicated it was needed.

As a general rule, it is best to purchase inventory with your own funds or from funds provided by relatives or friends. Banks are most reluctant to lend money to purchase inventory. Fixtures can be financed through banks, drug wholesalers, or the fixture company with long-term financing.

Financing an Established Pharmacy

First, the purchase price must be agreed upon before financial arrangements can be made. An owner's concept of the value of his pharmacy usually is considerably higher than that of a prospective buyer. The seller naturally wishes to recover his total investment and to retain all of the accumulated profits remaining in the business. The buyer, of course, is earnestly intent upon obtaining his money's worth in all particulars and in preserving the maximum opportunity for making future profits.

There are at least four methods used to approximate the value of an established pharmacy.

One method, which is a very realistic approach, is the *capitalization of the return on investment method.* This method is best explained by example. Assume the pharmacy's net profit or net return for the past year was $10,000 before taxes and assume further that you are willing to pay a price that will yield a 20 percent return, before taxes, on the investment or purchase price. If we let X equal the purchase price, we can express the relationship of the above assumptions as follows:

$$(0.20)\ (X) = \$10,000$$
$$X = \frac{\$10,000}{0.20}$$
$$X = \$50,000\text{—the purchase price}$$

To project further what an enterprising pharmacist may expect, let us make a few more assumptions and determine the outcome. Let us assume the proprietor's salary is $18,000, giving a total income of $28,000. Assume that the income tax and social security liability is $7,000 per year, leaving an income after taxes of $21,000. If we assume the young pharmacist can save approximately $10,000 annually, he could pay for the pharmacy in five years. Let us assume he had made a 20 percent down payment and had financed the remainder ($40,000) with a bank note at 7 percent simple interest on the unpaid balance and renewable annually for five years. The debt would have been amortized as shown in Table 5-1.

Two other methods of estimating the value of a pharmacy utilize *projections from the sales volume.* These are more arbitrary than the other methods. One method is simply taking *one-third of the annual sales,* and the other is *100 times the average daily sales.* To illustrate these two

Table 5-1. *Amortization of Bank Note, 7 Percent Interest on Unpaid Balance Computed Annually*

Year	Unpaid Balance	Payment on Principal	Interest Charge	Total Payment
1	$40,000	$ 8,000	$2,800	$10,800
2	32,000	8,000	2,240	10,240
3	24,000	8,000	1,680	9,680
4	16,000	8,000	1,120	9,120
5	8,000	8,000	560	8,560
Cumulative Value	0	$40,000	$8,400	$48,400

methods, let us use an annual sales volume of $210,000. The respective estimates of purchase prices are $70,000 and $57,534 ($210,000 ÷ 365 × 100 = $57,534.) The first of these two methods tends to overestimate the value of the pharmacy.

The fourth, and perhaps the most valid method, is the *summation of the relevant factors method.* Relevant assets can best be described by taking a typical balance sheet and selecting those assets and liabilities used in this method (Figure 5-2).

A few common-sense observations will identify those items on the balance sheet that normally would not be transferred. These include cash and notes payable. In our particular example, these two items were equal and thus cancel each other in considering the purchase price. If we total the rest of the assets and liabilities and subtract the liabilities from the assets, we get a difference of $64,000, which *coincidentally* is the same as the net worth. This is not the purchase price, because the seller will want a reasonable price, to say the least, for the goodwill associated with the pharmacy. In reviewing the profit and loss statement, we find the net profit last year was $12,800 on $256,000 sales volume. A "rule of thumb" valuation for goodwill is a year's net profit, $12,800 in this example. The estimated purchase price is $76,800. The capitalization of the net profit method, using a 15 percent return on the investment, yields a purchase price of $85,300. One-third of annual sales and 100 times the average daily sales yield purchase prices of $85,333 and $70,137, respectively. These four methods provide a range of $70,137 to $85,333 as an estimate of the value of the pharmacy. This provides ample opportunity for negotiation to arrive at a fair price near the $75,000 figure.

These four methods of estimating the value of a pharmacy can be refined by projecting the next year's sales volume or profit, depending on which method is used, to correct for the trend effect. The projection can be made by using a straight line equation and the middle year as the origin to determine the projected values for each year from the straight line equation. Data for a five-year period would be required.

After a purchase price has been agreed upon, the buyer must determine what sources of financing are available and select the one best suited to his situation. Bank financing similar to the example illustrated in Table 5-1 is probably the best choice if the buyer has a sufficient down payment and a good bank credit. It is a good idea for a young pharmacist to develop a good bank credit by dealing primarily with one bank and meeting his payments regularly on loans to purchase an automobile or other property.

ASSETS

Current Assets:

Cash	$12,000	
Accounts receivable	17,700	
Inventory	55,500	
Total Current Assets		$ 85,200

Fixed & Other Assets:

Fixtures, equipment & leasehold improvements (net after reserve for depreciation)	$12,000	
Prepaid expenses, deposits, etc.	2,800	
Total Fixed & Other Assets		14,800
Total Assets		$100,000

LIABILITIES & NET WORTH

Current Liabilities:

Accounts payable	$17,000	
Notes payable (within 1 yr.)	3,000	
Accrued expenses	7,000	
Total Current Liabilities		$ 27,000

Long-term Liabilities:

Note payable (over 1 yr.)	$ 9,000	
Total Long-term Liabilities		9,000
Total Liabilities		$ 36,000
Net Worth		64,000
Total Liabilities & Net Worth		$100,000

Figure 5-2. *Balance sheet for pharmacy X.*

Financing a New Pharmacy

Again, the cost of establishing the pharmacy must be estimated before financing arrangements can be made. The cost will be directly related to the size of the pharmacy, the estimated sales and thus inventory, and the quality and type of the fixtures, furnishings, and equipment. All of these factors, in turn, depend upon the location analysis. The type and sales potential of the location will determine the type and size of the pharmacy. The eight factors that influence the type and size of the pharmacy and the required capital outlay are discussed here.[1]

SOCIOECONOMIC CLASS SERVED

A pharmacy serving a number of persons in exclusive residential districts will require a more spacious and prestigious pharmacy, finer fixtures and equipment, broader assortments of merchandise, the offer of generous credit, delivery and various special services. Farmers, dependent upon the yield of a single crop, or workers for an industrial plant subject to seasonal or cyclical irregularity, may create the necessity for furnishing credit over long periods and to unusually large proportions of patrons.

GENERAL ECONOMIC CLIMATE

Poor or depressed conditions can reduce the volume of sales and slow the stock turnover while requiring approximately the same inventory investment, with its inherent expenses of insurance, interest, taxes, storage costs, and deterioration.

EXPECTED SALES VOLUME

Even though a larger pharmacy can make more efficient use of its personnel and buy in larger than "normal" quantities that provide quantity discounts, additional capital will be required to carry a wider range of merchandise and services.

DISTANCE FROM SUPPLIERS

A pharmacist receiving more rapid delivery from suppliers should be able to maintain the same sale volume with less investment in inventory.

PURCHASE TERMS

Special purchase terms, e.g., 2 percent cash discount or quantity discount will allow a decrease in the amount of funds required to maintain the necessary inventory level.

MANAGERIAL EXPERTISE

The pharmacist trained to analyze financial reports and utilize other managerial tools should be able to make more effective use of his capital.

COMPETITION

The competitive situation may create the need for additional funds to finance a high level of advertising and other promotional activity, selling numerous products at low margins, maintenance of a larger sales force in order to provide prompt service, including prompt and frequent delivery service.

PROFESSIONAL RELATIONS

In a pharmacy dispensing prescriptions written by a large number of prescribers, expanded capital will be required to maintain a wider variety of products necessary to meet the demand, including duplicate lines from many manufacturers.

Capital Requirements

There are three major categories of capital requirements: (1) inventory; (2) fixtures, equipment, and furnishings; and (3) necessary working capital to sustain the operation until the pharmacy generates enough sales to meet these needs.

Let us take an example of a typical traditional pharmacy and estimate the capital requirements. The pharmacy is in a moderately competitive market. The dimensions are 100 feet long and 30 feet wide, providing an area of 3000 square feet. The estimated sales volumes for the first five years, based on the location analysis, are $100,000, $135,000, $165,000, $185,000, and $200,000, respectively.

CAPITAL FOR INVENTORY

Since prescription sales are slower in developing, a lower than average percent gross margin should be estimated for the first year—probably $33^1/_3$ percent. Thus the estimated cost of goods sold (CGS) for the first year is $66,666 ($100,000 × .66$^2/_3$). The *initial inventory* may be estimated by dividing the CGS by the turnover rate (TOR). There are two schools of thought relative to this step, but both reach approximately the same estimate. One school assumes a TOR of at least four because the pharmacy is carefully stocked with saleable merchandise. Thus, $66,666 ÷ 4 = $16,667, which would be the initial inventory.

The other school states that sales volume will reach a modest figure the first year, yet a sufficient assortment of merchandise must be offered the public. The result is a lower TOR, about 3. Dividing $66,666 by 3 gives an *average* inventory of $22,222. However, the proponents of this school assert that the initial inventory can be carefully selected, and by restricting initial quantities of many product lines, only three-fourths of the *average* inventory or $16,667 will be necessary for the *initial* or model inventory. This rationale is probably more realistic, but the results are the same.

CAPITAL FOR FIXTURES

The cost of the fixtures, equipment, and furnishings can vary considerably, depending on the quality and source of supply. For example, the cost of the fixtures may vary from $3.00 to $6.00 per square foot, the average being $4.00 to $5.00. Carpeting cost may range from $10.00 to $20.00 per square yard, with $13.00 being a typical figure. A medium-sized fountain, if one is to be installed, will cost about $15,000. These and other costs have been summarized in Table 5-2.

The fixtures, equipment, and furnishings may be financed through a bank or through the various suppliers. In either case the method of financing most likely to be available is known as the "add-on" interest charge, which is considerably more than simple interest. The interest rate will normally be $1/4$ percent to $1/2$ percent above the prime interest rate—the rate banks charge preferential customers, those with large amounts of assets and high credit ratings. The prime interest rate, in turn, ranges from $1/4$ to $1/2$ percent above the discount rate set by the Federal Reserve Bank System. The discount rate is used by the Federal government to regulate the availability of money and set monetary policy consistent with the needs of the economy.

A pharmacist can expect to pay an interest rate of 7 to 8 percent, or even more, during an inflationary period. The computation below illustrates how the add-on interest works. Using 8 percent interest rate and a five-year repayment period, the interest rate is multiplied by the number of years $(.08 \times 5 = .40)$, this percentage is multiplied by the principal ($14,500 \times .40 = $5,800), and the product is added to the principal, making a total obligation of $20,300. This sum is paid in 60 equal installments of $338.33 per month.

WORKING CAPITAL

The enterprising pharmacist should have sufficient *working capital* to cover the expenses for two to three months in addition to the installment

Table 5-2. *Capital Requirements for Fixed Assets*

Item	Total Cost	Down Payment	Balance
Fixtures	$12,000	$3,000	$ 9,000
Carpeting	4,150	1,150	3,000
Sign	600	300	300
Cash registers	3,000	800	2,200
Card racks	No charge	—	—
Rx equip. & references	250	250	—
Totals	$20,000	$5,500	$14,500

payments. Figure 5-3 provides a projected cash flow account for the first three months, which indicates the necessary extra working capital.

Table 5-3 summarizes the initial capital requirements and the monthly payments.

Sales		$21,000
Cost of Goods		14,000
Gross Margin		$ 7,000
Expenses:		
Proprietor's Salary	$3,000	
Employee Wages	2,500	
Rent	1,200	
Heat, Light & Power	250	
Licenses & Permits	100	
Insurance	200	
Fees, Legal & Accounting	300	
Delivery	150	
Advertising (Grand Opening)	500	
Depreciation	non-cash	
Bad Debts	none	
Telephone	100	
Miscellaneous	200	
Total Expenses		8,500
Deficit		$ 1,500
Add Estimated Accounts Receivable Accumulation		500
Total Required Working Capital		$ 2,000

Figure 5-3. *Projected cash flow for first 3 months.*

Table 5-3. *Summary of Capital Requirements*

Item	Initial Capital	3 Monthly Payments
Inventory*	$ 8,333.50	$ 8,333.50
Fixtures, etc.	5,500.00	1,015.00
Working capital	2,000.00	—
Totals	$15,833.50	$ 9,348.50
Total capital requirements for 3 months: $25,182		

*One-half down payment required on the inventory with remainder due in 3 months.

The sales estimate for the first three months was conservative, which is a realistic approach. Assuming a normal or average sales growth pattern, the break-even point may be reached about the fifth month of operations. Some additional working capital may be required, perhaps as much as $2,000 to $3,000. If better credit terms can be obtained for the inventory purchases, this will reduce the initial capital requirements substantially and perhaps the monthly payment as well.

REFERENCE

1. Adapted from Swafford, W. R., Huffman, D. C., Ryan, M. R., and Watkins, J. R.: *Community Pharmacy Management, Planning and Development,* Memphis, Tennessee: University of Tennessee, 1973, pp. 112, 113.

REVIEW

1. Define each of the following: equity capital, borrowed capital, working capital, and fixed capital.

2. What are the various sources of capital?

3. Liabilities are classified as short-term and long-term. Which of these is more appropriate for financing working capital and fixed capital, respectively?

4. Use the four methods of estimating the purchase price (value) of an established pharmacy.

5. What are the methods for estimating the value of goodwill?

6. Discuss the eight factors that influence the amount of required capital to establish a new pharmacy.

7. Discuss the three major categories of capital requirements for a new pharmacy, and from appropriate data provided, be able to calculate the initial capital requirements in each category.

8. Given the appropriate data, calculate the annual payment on principal and interest on a bank note with simple interest on the unpaid balance.

9. Given the appropriate data, solve a problem involving the "add-on" interest rate concept, including total obligation and monthly payments.

10. Given appropriate data and other necessary information, estimate via a cash flow chart the amount of working capital necessary to sustain a new pharmacy for three months, including payments on principal and interest.

6. *Location Analysis and Evaluation*

The importance of a good location to the success of a pharmacy practice can hardly be overemphasized. This point is readily understood if one considers the extreme case, for example, of the so-called "ghost town." Many small rural communities that once thrived and supported a physician and pharmacy can no longer do so because of the migration from rural to urban and then to the suburban areas. This migration has been brought about by technologic and sociologic changes, the mechanization of farming, the deterioration of the quality of life in the inner core of the cities, and the appeal of suburbia to the more affluent taxpayers. Migration has reduced the market value of some locations while increasing the value of others. These changes have been enhanced by the increasing reliance on the automobile and the development of planned shopping centers.

Another way to view the importance of the location is to recognize the frequency that locations are evaluated and revaluated. At first, one might think that the typical pharmacist will evaluate one location once in his entire practice. This is a myopic and static view of the subject. A more dynamic and practical view of location evaluation is to consider that a pharmacist revaluates his location each time he renews his lease, and although more subtly, he revaluates the location each morning when he turns the key to unlock the door. Even the newly graduated pharmacist evaluates a location when he accepts his first position and each new position. After all, it could be the pharmacy where he will practice the remainder of his lifetime.

One should also consider location analysis in the light of the significance of a poor location with regard to business failures. Although the selection of a poor location is considered by experts, such as Dunn and Bradstreet, as a symptom of the underlying deficiencies of inexperience or incompetence, it is one of the major apparent causes of business failures. Good management and aggressive promotions cannot overcome a weak location.

The basic principle, therefore, is very simple. Locate in or near high population density, and where competition is not too severe. This does not mean that one should avoid all rural towns and the inner core of the cities. There are people in these places who need health care services, including pharmaceutical services. Several government programs, such as urban renewal, Medicaid, and others are available to assist the people in these areas. Also, it has been shown that people in these areas relate favorably to the community pharmacist. For these, the pharmacist is often their first medical care contact and resource. The pharmacist can function effectively as a medium of entry into the medical care system for the underprivileged people in these locations.

Classification and Definitions

Locations may be classified in two general ways—*geographic* and *functional.* The geographic classification is further classified broadly into either *rural* or *urban* areas. Urban areas constitute a much smaller proportion of the geographic area, but a much larger proportion of the population. According to the definitions used by the United States Census Bureau and other government agencies, "urban places" comprise all incorporated and unincorporated places having 2,500 inhabitants or more, and certain other towns, townships, and counties classified as urban in the *1970 Census of Population.*[1] A complete definition of urban places may be found in the *1970 Census of Population.*[1] All other areas, of course, are designated as rural areas.

GEOGRAPHIC AND DEMOGRAPHIC CLASSES

Size. The term urban places is used for all the urban classifications including the smallest classification unit, towns with a population of 2,500 or a density of 1,000 persons per square mile, and the largest classification unit, the standard metropolitan statistical area. Urban places are further classified as follows: (1) standard metropolitan statistical areas (SMSA), (2) urbanized areas (UA), (3) cities (C), and (4) other urban places (OUP).

A definition of each of the above classifications will provide the basis for understanding the nature of the various types of urban locations. The definition of an individual SMSA involves two components: (1) the central city and the corresponding central county, and (2) a social and economic relationship and integration of contiguous counties which are metropolitan in character. A standard metropolitan statistical area must include a city with 50,000 inhabitants or more, or two cities with contiguous boundaries and a combined population of 50,000, the smaller of which must have a population of at least 15,000.

The population of the contiguous counties must be primarily non-agricultural in nature as indicated by 75 percent of the labor force. This criterion may be met if a minimum of 10 percent of the nonagricultural population in the central county or counties either work or live in the contiguous counties, or a minimum of 10,000 nonagricultural people either work or live in each contiguous county. In addition, 50 percent of the population in the contiguous counties must have a population density of 150 persons per square mile in an unbroken pattern radiating from the central city.

The criteria of economic integration are fundamental to the concept of SMSA. Either 15 percent of the workers living in each of the contiguous counties must work in the central county (or counties), or 25 percent of the people working in a contiguous county must live in the central county or counties. If the above two criteria are not met, other information may be used to demonstrate social and economic integration. These include newspaper circulation, telephone listings, analysis of charge accounts of retail stores in the central cities, the extent of delivery service, official traffic counts, public transportation, and local planning, which demonstrate a social and economic interrelationship of the central city (or cities) with the outlying contiguous counties.

An *urbanized area* is similar to the SMSA, but the emphasis is placed on population density in a defined geographic area rather than social and economic integration. An urbanized area is defined as a city of 50,000 inhabitants or more, or twin cities of 50,000 people or more, the smaller of which must have a population of at least 15,000. In addition it includes the surrounding area that meets the following criteria: (1) contiguous incorporated places with 2,500 inhabitants or more, (2) contiguous incorporated or unincorporated places with less than 2,500 inhabitants, but having 100 housing units or more in a closely settled area, (3) contiguous unincorporated census districts with a population density of 1,000 inhabitants or more per square mile, and (4) any other census district within one and a half miles of the main city of the urbanized area meeting the population density criterion to eliminate enclaves or indentation of one mile or less in the circumference of the total urbanized area.

The designation "city," in general, refers to a political subdivision of a state which is incorporated and has a population of 25,000 inhabitants or more. The Bureau of Census recognizes unincorporated cities with 25,000 population or greater, but since this classification has the same general characteristics as incorporated cities, we have chosen not to differentiate between the two. Finally, there are all of the other urban places that do not fall into one or the other classifications. The above classifications have been tabulated and given common names in Table 6-1.

Location. In addition to the above general geographic classifications, locations may be classified more precisely according to their characteristics and scope of commercial services and functions provided. These locations may be classified as (1) central business district (CBD); (2) major outlying retail districts (MORD); (3) neighborhood or suburban residential locations (NSR); and (4) shopping centers (SC).

The first two classifications are recognized by the Census Bureau and defined in the *County and City Data Book, 1967.* The *central business district* is described as an area of high concentration of retail businesses, offices, theaters, hotels, and other services, and an area of high traffic flow. Central business districts have been delineated officially only in cities with a population of 100,000 or more; however, a central downtown shopping district can be presumed to exist in all cities of 25,000 population or greater.

The *major outlying retail center* has been defined by the Bureau of Census as a concentration of retail stores located inside a standard metropolitan statistical area in which the central business district is located, but outside the central business district itself, which includes, among other stores, a major general merchandise store, usually a department store. Major outlying retail centers normally do not include the larger planned suburban shopping centers, but rather the older neighborhood developments which meet the above requisites. There is a major distinction between shopping centers and other major retail centers. Shopping centers are planned and well designed for efficient shopping and off-street parking, while the older type of major retail centers grew in a haphazard and unplanned manner.

The *residential neighborhood* or *suburban location* is just what is implied by the words. The term "neighborhood" is used most frequently

Table 6-1. *Modified Classification of Geographic Locations*

Bureau of Census Designation	Approx. Population	Common Name
Standard metropolitan statistical areas	100,000 or more	Metropolitan area
Urbanized areas	50,000 or more	Large cities
Cities	25,000–49,999	Small cities
Other urban places	2,500–24,999	Large towns
Towns in rural areas	less than 2,500	Rural towns

to denote a location in the older residential part of a city, whereas the term "suburban" is used to denote a similar location in the newer, sprawling residential developments in the cities. This type of location is characterized by a few convenience stores and service establishments without a particular design. Generally, they have been established to serve the residents within an immediate area of approximately a mile radius. A pharmacy located in an older neighborhood section traditionally has been referred to as the "neighborhood pharmacy." The term "corner pharmacy" is sometimes used to refer to the same type of pharmacy located on the corner; however, the term "corner pharmacy" (or drugstore) is more frequently used to designate a traditional pharmacy in the smaller cities and rural towns.

The neighborhood or convenience shopping center differs from the older neighborhood or suburban location in that the shopping center must have been planned and designed in such a way that each establishment compliments the others and attracts patrons to the center. Accessibility to the center is a prime requisite. Also, the neighborhood or convenience shopping center normally will have a greater variety of stores and services than the older neighborhood location.

A new type of pharmacy location found in the newer suburban section of our cities has been described as an "island" location in the *American Druggist*. The *island location* may be described as a single, free-standing building in a residential area. It houses the pharmacy and is surrounded by a parking area—thus the label, "island" location. Infrequently, a second commercial or service establishment will be located in the building. The island location was born of economic necessity. It provides the independent pharmacist a location with adequate off-street parking at a cost he can afford. Rental charges in the better shopping centers are prohibitive for many independent pharmacists. In addition, the independent pharmacist can hardly obtain a lease in the larger centers because the developers prefer lessees with greater assets and a higher credit rating, the reason being that the developer will use the credit strength of the larger lessee as leverage in obtaining funds from financial institutions for developing the center. One usually will find a modern conventional pharmacy in the island location; on occasion, a prescription speciality shop may be located in an island location. It is apparent that the island location is a special case of the neighborhood or suburban residential location. Figure 6-1 shows a view of a typical island location.

SHOPPING CENTERS

Shopping centers are further classified and defined according to the size of the trading area and the classes of goods that are prevalent in the center. These are summarized in Table 6-2.

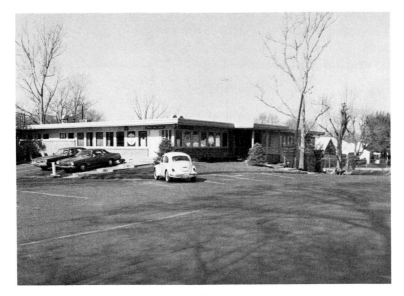

Figure 6-1. *View of a typical island location.*

Neighborhood Centers. This type of shopping center is frequently designated as a *convenience* center. It consists of a few stores that purvey primarily convenience goods such as food, drugs, some hardware goods, liquor, and variety store items. It serves a district approximately the size of a grade school district, normally a radius of two to three miles. These centers are usually of the "strip design" along one side of a street.

Community Centers. Community centers are sometimes referred to as *suburban* centers. They are larger than the neighborhood centers, consisting of a dozen or more stores that carry convenience goods, some shopping goods, and limited specialty goods. These centers approximate the size of a city high school district with the usual radius being three to five miles. They sometimes draw patrons from distances up to ten miles. Nearly all types of stores and goods may be found in these centers including a junior-size department store, frequently a branch super-

Table 6-2. *Classification of Shopping Centers*

Common Name	Radius of Drawing Area	Dominant Class of Goods
Neighborhood	Up to 2–3 miles	Convenience goods
Community	Up to 3–5 miles	Convenience and shopping goods
Regional	Up to 50 miles or more	Convenience, shopping & specialty goods

variety store, or a full-size department store. These centers are usually of the "strip" or "mall" design.

Regional Shopping Centers. This type of center is the largest of shopping centers, characterized by a large department store—more frequently, two department stores—and one or more general line stores such as pharmacies, groceries, hardware stores, and variety stores. These centers draw trade for shopping goods, such as clothing and appliances, from as far as 50 miles away and occasionally farther. Several designs may be found among these centers. The regional center designation is often misused. Very few shopping centers are actually regional in their characteristics.

FUNCTIONAL LOCATIONS

So far we have discussed five general classes and four specific geographic types of location that are generally familiar to most students and pharmacists. In addition, locations may be classified functionally as suscipient, interceptive, or generative. These terms are less familiar. This classification is distinct and any of the geographic classes of location may be further classified in this manner.

A *suscipient* location is one to which patrons are coincidentally or impulsively attracted while away from their place of residence for any primary purpose other than shopping. Thus, a pharmacy located in a hotel, an airport, a resort area, and similar places is a suscipient location. Pharmacies located in clinics and hospitals are special cases of this class of location. Although these latter examples must be considered prime locations, care should be exercised not to overestimate their value. This is especially true of the pharmacies located in clinics with a large number of low prescribing specialists.

The *interceptive* location receives its label from the fact that the strategy of such a location is to intercept patrons on their way to a shopping district, whether the shopping district be a central downtown business district, a major outlying retailing center, or a shopping center. This strategy is most effective among convenience and specialty shops located, for example, between a large office building and the central downtown business district. A pharmacy located near but not within a clinic is an example of this type of location.

The *generative* location is the most common among this classification. It derives its name from the fact that patrons are attracted to it for the purpose of shopping—thus it generates business. Obviously, the central downtown business districts, the major outlying retail centers, and the shopping centers are examples of the generative class. Most pharmacies in the small cities, rural towns, and neighborhood locations fall within this class. In many instances, one would have to investigate the particular situation surrounding the pharmacy to classify its functional location accurately.

In summary, a location may be one of the general geographic locations (SMSA, urbanized city, smaller city, other urban place or large town, or a rural town). Additionally, a location site may be in a central downtown business district, a major outlying retail center, a shopping center, a neighborhood or suburban area, or an island location. Any of these locations may be classified further as suscipient, interceptive, or generative. Each particular type of location has its advantages and disadvantages, but in the final analysis each individual location must be analyzed and evaluated for its market potential.

Variables Affecting Choice of Location

Demographic factors are the primary variables in the selecting of a location. These factors are important because they determine to a large degree the need of, if not the demand for, health care services. The aged and infants use more medication than other age groups. Ethnic groups sometimes require special consideration in their specific needs and demands. Other variables include the *economic activity,* the *social and cultural institutions of the community,* the *type of pharmacy,* and the *pharmacist's inclinations and desires.*

The primary measures of economic activity are the *per capita income* and the *median family income.* The underlying factors of economic activity include *economic input factors* and *economic organization.* To investigate these, the following questions should be raised. Is the economy of the community primarily agricultural or industrial, or does it include both? If it is primarily agricultural, does the community rely mostly on one or two crops, or is the agriculture diversified? If it is an industrial community, does it rely primarily on one or two basic (heavy) industries such as steel, or is the industry of the community diversified? The implications of the questions should be obvious. Reliance on one major crop involves heavy risk from drought, floods, and other disasters. The same is true with a single industry since risks inherent from strikes, riots, or failure of the company to obtain a government contract are very great.

Supportive social and cultural institutions are important to the growth and development of a community. These institutions include the economic institutions, such as banks, and the proper number and types of shops and stores. Adequate transportation, utilities, professionals, services, good educational and health institutions, and religious and cultural institutions are also important parts of the social and cultural institutional milieu. Of course, natural resources are vital, but human resources are the most important of all. Often a community has a dearth of skilled artisans and professionals, and these people are essential to the growth of a community.

Another variable to be considered is the type of pharmacy practice to be established. For example, a large super drugstore is hardly feasible in a rural town with a population of a thousand or less. At one time it was thought that the strictly prescription shop was not feasible in a small community with less than 10,000 population. This theory has proved to be erroneous, since several pharmacists have successfully established this type of practice in some of our smaller communities. *Pharmaceutical centers* have also been successful in smaller communities. The pharmacist's inclinations and desires are important considerations in the selecting of a location and constitutes yet another variable.

Analysis of the Market Potential

IDENTIFYING THE TRADE AREA

Once a pharmacist has identified tentatively a location, or perhaps several locations, he must delineate more precisely the trade area of each. There are several methods of accomplishing this task.

The *interview* technique, which is the most accurate and the most costly method, is also time consuming. The primary requisite is that an appropriate sample of the people in the projected trade area be selected. The object is to determine where the people purchase, or would prefer to purchase, the particular goods and/or services in question—in our case drugs and pharmaceutical services. The projected trade area is then divided into smaller units, and each unit is sampled and studied individually. This method has the following advantages:

1. The researcher can better analyze the smaller units and more readily perceive and make sounder judgments concerning the various factors requiring judgment.

2. The multiplicity of many discrete judgments tends to prevent accumulative error, since the chances are greater that errors in judgment will cancel each other.

3. Unusual situations—including demographic, economic, and social variables—can be uncovered through the interviews.

A modification of the interview technique may be used to evaluate central business districts, major retailing centers, or large shopping centers. The object is to interview a sample of the foot traffic passing a particular site during appropriate time intervals and identify the addresses of those passing the site. A plot of the addresses on a map will identify the boundary of the trade area. Based on the distribution of the sample, a percentage value can be assigned to each discrete population unit surrounding the site under consideration. These percentages are then multiplied by the population in each population unit to estimate the potential more precisely. Questions pertaining to the reasons the people are in the area are included in the interview. Thus, the percent of people making pharmaceutical purchases can be used to estimate the potential for a pharmacy.

Of course, the accuracy of the interview technique varies with the type or class of location and pharmacy, as well as the sampling procedure used. For example, this technique is usually successful for drugstores located in central business districts, major retail centers, and the large regional shopping centers of a metropolitan area. However, since pharmacies primarily sell convenience goods and services, they do not attract many patrons from the outer fringes of the metropolitan area to the same degree as stores handling many shopping goods, and this must be taken into consideration in evaluating these locations for a pharmacy. Yet, the entire trading area must be considered as the base when this method is used.

The second technique of delineating the potential trade area of a location is *Reilly's Law of Retail Gravitation.* The usefulness of Reilly's Law is restricted primarily to rural and small city locations. Reilly's Law is represented by the following formula:

$$D_{a \to b} = \frac{d}{1 + \sqrt{\dfrac{P_b}{P_a}}}$$

where:

$D_{a \to b}$ = Outer limit of the trading area of community A, expressed in miles, along each major paved road between community A and community B.

d = Distance in miles between community A and community B.

P_a = Population of community A.

P_b = Population of community B.

The assumption underlying this equation is that patrons normally travel to the larger and more accessible community. A modification of this equation substitutes, in the case of two shopping centers, the square feet of space in the respective shopping centers for the population of the communities and the driving time for the distance between the communities, respectively. However, the application of the modified formula for estimating the trade area of a shopping center is less valid than the original formula for estimating the trade area of rural towns and small cities.

It is rather obvious that Reilly's Law can be employed with a minimum expenditure of time, money and effort. It is a reasonably accurate technique for a rural setting, but it must be used with caution in an urban situation. In an urban setting the situation is more complex, and factors other than distance and population must be considered to be equally and sometimes more important.

A technique for estimating the trade area of an existing pharmacy is to *sample the prescription file* and/or *charge accounts* and plot the addresses of the customers on a map. The sample should be sufficiently large, about 400 prescriptions or accounts, and selected randomly. The area represented by the plot of the addresses represents the trade area of the pharmacy. This technique is discussed in more detail in the section on relocating a pharmacy.

Another technique is the *"vacuum" calculation* technique. This technique is best utilized when the geographic boundaries of the trade area are fairly well defined, such as rural areas, small urban towns, most neighborhood districts in cities, and small convenient shopping centers. The vacuum technique has been applied, however, to nearly all classes and types of locations and pharmacies.

The first step in the vacuum technique is to delineate geographically the trade area. The county boundary is most frequently used for rural areas and smaller urban towns when the populations of neighboring towns are approximately equal. For neighborhood or residential locations in cities, the trade area for the site is determined using one or more of the following criteria and applying it to each major street leading to the site: (1) the distance to the nearest pharmacy; (2) two miles or ten minutes driving time from the site; and (3) any natural traffic barrier or busy railroad crossing. The geographic limits of the trade area for central business district, major retail center, and large regional shopping centers cannot be determined by this technique.

ESTIMATING THE MARKET POTENTIAL

After the trade area has been identified geographically, one can proceed to estimate its sales potential. Two demographic units and economic measures are available for this purpose: (1) the number of families and the median family income, and (2) the population and the per capita income. The latter criteria are preferred since they provide for inclusion of individuals not living in family households.

The *first step* in estimating the market potential is to ascertain the population of the trade area. This may be accomplished in one of two ways: (1) get the information from a reliable source, such as government publications, postal lists, Chambers of Commerce, or tax rolls for adults and school rolls for children, or (2) count the number of households and multiply this by the mean number of persons per household. (In the United States, 3.67 persons per family.)

The *second step* is to multiply the population by the per capita income for the area. An alternate method is to multiply the number of families by the median family income for the area. This calculation gives the total personal income for the entire area, which is reduced to the amount of disposable income by multiplying by the ratio of disposable income to personal income. (This ratio for the United States was 87.6 percent in 1965.) The disposable income is then used to estimate the potential for the trade area by applying the appropriate percentages from Table 6-3. The appropriate percentage is based on the contemplated departments in the pharmacy, e.g., prescriptions, over-the-counter drugs, health aids,

Table 6-3. *U.S. Expenditures for Drugstore Products in 1971*

Category	U.S. Expenditure (in thousands)	% of Disp.[a] Income	% Spent in[b] Pharmacies Range (Mean)	Per Capita[c] Expenditures
Prescriptions	$ 5,652,700	0.81	80–100 (90)	$24.90
Packaged medication	2,874,140	0.41	50– 80 (65)	9.15
Sickroom & convalescent aids	321,830	0.04	30– 50 (39)	0.62
First aid	254,080	0.03	35– 75 (53)	0.66
Foot products[d]	107,190	0.01	50– 90 (61)	0.32
Baby needs	722,220	0.10	30– 50 (40)	1.41
Feminine needs[e]	505,930	0.07	30– 50 (40)	1.01
Duplication for fem. needs	− 75,170	–	–	–
Veterinary	339,710	0.04	10– 45 (28)	0.47
Dieting aids	140,460	0.02	25– 50 (34)	0.23
Subtotal	$10,843,090	1.57	–	$38.61
Duplication[f]	− 757,570	–	–	–
TOTAL FOR DRUGS, OTHER HEALTH AIDS	$10,085,520	1.46	60– 90 (73)	$36.15
Toiletries[g]	7,454,510	1.08	20– 30 (25)	9.18
TOTAL FOR DRUGS, OTHER HEALTH AIDS, TOILETRIES	$17,540,030	2.54	45– 65 (53)	$45.33
Other sundry products	$15,764,660	2.29	10– 20 (16)	$12.26
Fountain & luncheonette	3,621,630	0.52	– (10)	1.85
Packaged ice cream	1,033,180	0.15	– (6)	0.32
Candy, tobacco, & accessories	13,247,170	1.92	– (10)	6.21
Unclassified	nd	–	–	2.58
GRAND TOTAL	$51,206,670	7.44	20– 40 (27)	$68.55

Adapted from *Drug Topics,* Sept. 25, 1972, pp. 21–23, 36, 37.

[a] Estimation based on data from *U.S. Statistical Abstracts,*[2] 1972, and *Drug Topics,*[3] Sept. 25, 1972.

[b] The ranges were estimated, based on national averages reported in *Drug Topics,* Sept. 25, 1972, taking into consideration the variations due to different types of locations, e.g., rural areas, central downtown business districts, etc. The means are those reported in *Drug Topics.*[3]

[c] In pharmacies only.

[d] Athlete's foot medication under "Packaged medication."

[e] Feminine bulb syringes are in "Sickroom & convalescent aids."

[f] This is the estimated amount received when packaged medications and other health aids of the types listed above are supplied as prescriptions.

[g] Includes oral hygiene, hair preparations, shaving products, hand products, cosmetics, and other toiletries.

and toiletries could expect a potential sales volume of 2.54 percent of the disposable income, provided there was *no* competition. An alternate method to obtain this figure is to multiply the per capita expenditures for various drugstore products by the population of the trade area to determine its potential. This is the most accurate and the preferred method in most instances, especially when the population is known or can be determined accurately.

If the percent of disposable income is used, a correction should be made for non-drugstore competition. The upper limits of ranges of percentages spent in pharmacies apply to locations with little or no non-drug competition, for example, rural areas. The lower limits may be used in highly competitive markets; the mean percentages apply to the typical location with moderate competition. If the per capita drugstore expenditures column is used, non-drug expenditures are already taken into account. Simply multiply the population by the per capita expenditures corresponding to the departments and product lines contemplated for the pharmacy.

The *third step* is to estimate the sales volume for the competing pharmacies located in the trade area. After allowing for non-drug competition, the remainder of the expenditures is available to all the drug outlets, including chain drugstores and discount stores with prescription departments. The sales volume of each pharmacy within the trade area can be estimated by multiplying the estimated payroll, including the proprietor's salary, by a factor of five. This procedure is based on the statistics reported in *The Lilly Digest*[4] and is valid for most pharmacies with sales volumes over $100,000 a year. The total of the estimated drug competition is then subtracted from the estimate of the expenditures for pharmaceutical products, after allowing for non-drug competition. This is the "potential" available for a new pharmacy, which is called the "vacuum" potential. Of course, these people currently are obtaining their drugs and pharmaceutical services from some source, but the significance of the vacuum potential is that a new pharmacy, properly located, should have a better chance of attracting and holding these patrons than any other pharmacy. In addition, the pharmacy may attract some patrons from existing pharmacies and non-drug outlets. The ability to do this will be determined by the relative strength of the several location sites and management.

ESTIMATING RELATIVE STRENGTH

The relative strength of pharmacies should be estimated from several points of view, some of which are more significant than others. For example, proximity to physicians' offices should be a consideration for prescription shops, whereas foot traffic should be a determining factor in the location of a conventional pharmacy, especially for a super drugstore in a shopping center or a downtown location. To arrive at these estimates, percentage weight should be assigned to the following factors:

Size. For maximum volume, conventional pharmacies with fountains need approximately 3,500 square feet; traditional pharmacies without fountains need at least 3,000 square feet. Both figures are exclusive of storage area. Super drugstores need a minimum of 5,000 square feet and preferably 10,000 square feet or more. Prescription pharmacies require approximately 1,000 to 1,500 square feet.

Shape. Traditional pharmacies are most efficient when customers are readily drawn throughout the pharmacy. Thus, the most efficient design is a rectangular shape with the short side facing the street. An ideal ratio between the length and width of the front is three to one. The percentage of efficiency of the pharmacy should be decreased only slightly for less than an ideal ratio. However, the percent efficiency should be decreased greatly if "L" shapes or hidden alcoves exist within the store. These configurations tend to make it difficult to activate all of the selling area. Super drugstores may be either square or slightly rectangular. Decrease the percent efficiency slightly for a super drugstore as the space departs from the square or near-square configuration. Shape is not as crucial in the prescription pharmacy, but clumsy alcoves make the store difficult to lay out.

Front. Except for a few downtown locations, the fully open or nearly fully open front should be rated 100 percent efficiency. As the front departs from this ideal, the percentage should be reduced. In heavily traveled or downtown districts, a display window front is desirable, but some vision into the pharmacy is also desirable because "people go to people." An entrance above or below street level may reduce volume potential, and an allowance for this should be made in the efficiency rating.

Parking. In modern shopping centers, a ratio of three square feet of parking area to one square foot of selling area is considered the *bare minimum.* In the better centers, a ratio of at least four and one-half to one is maintained. If the ratio of parking area to selling area falls below this value in a shopping center, the efficiency percentage is decreased. In older existing shopping districts, where no such ratio can be established, it would be wise to make an observation at peak selling periods. Parking spaces should always be available near enough to the location under consideration so that it will be more convenient to stop and shop there than to go to another pharmacy. In downtown shopping locations, parking is quite a different matter. Most shoppers usually park in some commercial facility and shop several stores on foot. However, if commercial parking facilities in a downtown shopping area are distant from the location, the percentage is decreased. Finally, if all parking spaces in the shopping district or area are filled during peak periods the percentage is decreased.

Traffic. Passing foot and car traffic are of promotional value and should also be considered. Minimums or ideals depend on whether the site being considered is in a central business district, a major retailing center, or a shopping center. They also depend on the type of pharmacy being considered. Passing traffic is qualitative and traffic going to and from work is much less valuable than shopping traffic. A foot and car traffic count, showing the number of passersby in a given period, should be made during several periods selected at random. Surveys should be made both at the proposed location site and at the competing pharmacies in the same trading area. The site with the greatest traffic count is rated 100 percent efficient. Other sites are rated as a ratio of their traffic count to the count of the 100 percent site. Efficiency ratings should be adjusted in relation to the 100 percent site. If the pharmacy is in a shopping center, it should be located in the active end. Also, it should be easily accessible to the main thruway and from nearby residential areas.

Proximity to Merchants. Pharmacies, particularly those without fountains or other strong traffic-building facilities, need to be located either very near the population center or very near strong traffic-building stores. A spot adjacent to an aggressive supermarket or department store is considered to be 100 percent efficient and the efficiency percentage should be adjusted accordingly for those not adjacent to such stores.

Proximity to Physicians. This factor is important for prescription pharmacies, less essential for traditional pharmacies, and still less essential for super drugstores. One can check with pharmaceutical detail men or make his own estimates of the number of prescriptions written by physicians in the area. At least twice the number of prescriptions expected for the new pharmacy should be written by prescribers in the area. This is especially true of clinic pharmacies. The efficiency rating should be decreased accordingly if this is not the case.

Proximity to Other Health Facilities. A medical clinic near the pharmacy would constitute a location with a 100 percent efficiency rating for this factor. A hospital with active outpatient clinics should be rated rather high, but less than 100 percent. This factor, as with the one above, is important for prescription pharmacies and less essential for the other types.

Care should be exercised in attaching too much significance to some of these factors for certain types of pharmacies. On the other hand, these factors should not be ignored. If there is a problem in estimating the percentage reduction for any of the given factors, the best course is to force rank the competing pharmacies for each factor, obtain a sum, and average the scores. These values are then used to estimate the portion of the "vacuum" volume one can expect.

EVALUATING SUSCIPIENT LOCATIONS

The evaluation of suscipient locations requires special techniques. For example, the potential of a clinic pharmacy is estimated by ascertaining the number of prescribers by specialty, and multiplying this by the average daily prescriptions written by the respective specialty. Next, the total estimated number of prescriptions is multiplied by the percentage one can expect to dispense in the pharmacy. Experience indicates that on the average, the pharmacy will dispense about 50 percent of the prescriptions written in the clinic. Obviously, this percentage may vary from very low to nearly 100 percent. The basic factor determining this percentage is the ratio of the patients who are referred to the clinic by physicians from other communities. This, in turn, is related to the ratio of the number of specialists in the clinic to the number of primary care specialists, such as internists, pediatricians, and general practitioners.

Other special suscipient locations, such as airports, require still other special techniques. Basically, these consist of estimating the number of people in transit and then estimating the percent of these people making purchases of pharmaceutical products and the average transaction value. Multiplying the latter two statistics by the daily average number of people in transit provides an estimate of the average daily sales.

When to Relocate Your Pharmacy

A change of location for any firm will depend on many factors, a number of which are obscure and difficult to assess. The pharmacist should always be sensitive to changes in the marketplace that affect the potential of his present site in relation to other possible locations. All managers should periodically consider the desirability of a change in location. A formal analysis on an annual basis might be advisable. Relocation would be beneficial when: (1) growth or shift in the population within the market area, especially in older sections of a city, may not be benefitting the pharmacy at the present site; (2) recent site developments and new locations may provide opportunities not previously available; (3) upgrading of the present pharmacy by sizable capital expenditures to achieve a proper operating environment may be better accomplished at another site; (4) relocation may preclude or eliminate the possibility of increased competition in the market; and (5) change in location may be a stimulus for the improvements in business and professional operations that otherwise would be delayed or never achieved.

If a pharmacist/proprietor is considering relocating his pharmacy for any of the above reasons, he should appraise both his present location and any new proposed site along the lines indicated in the preceding sections. In addition, he should investigate the area of the community that is the source of his present trade in order that he may choose a location where he may best serve those patrons. This investigation can be accomplished by an analysis of the prescription files or charge accounts. Also, he may determine his potential trade area by obtaining names and addresses of patrons on slips deposited for a "drawing" for selected item(s) of merchandise. The following sections describe the procedures for determining both present and potential trade areas for established pharmacies.

ANALYSIS OF PRESCRIPTION FILES

A statistical analysis of a sample of new prescriptions will assist the pharmacist in determining the trade area of patients purchasing prescriptions in his pharmacy. Although a discussion of statistical methods is beyond the scope of this text, the following procedure is recommended for such an analysis.[5]

First, the pharmacist should randomly select a sample of new prescriptions purchased during the past 12 months and plot the patients' addresses on a map.* The term "randomly selected" means that each new prescription, or combination of prescriptions, dispensed during the past 12 months has an equal probability of being a part of the sample selected. For example, the eighth new prescription dispensed on the tenth day of November must have exactly the same probability of being selected as any other new prescription dispensed during the time period under study. Selecting a sample in a random manner is important because all other methods introduce a possible bias, thus limiting their usefulness or statistical validity. Also, the pharmacist must have a large enough sample to be confident that the results obtained will represent the entire population within an acceptable range of error. In our example, this means the trade area found by using the sample will be approximately the same as the trade area found if the pharmacist used all new prescriptions dispensed during the past 12 months.

The sample size will vary based on how confident we desire to be that the sample represents the population and the percent of error we are willing to tolerate. The more confident we wish to be that the sample represents the population and the less error we are willing to accept, the greater the number of prescriptions which must be included in the sample. Of course, if we would accept no error and desired to be 100 percent

---

*Stated in statistical terms, a sample is defined as a limited number of units selected from the total group. The entire group of items is called the population or universe. In our example, the population or universe would be all new prescriptions dispensed during the past 12 months.

confident, the sample would have to include all prescriptions dispensed during the time period under study. However, reviewing all new prescriptions would be a long and expensive task and should be avoided by the use of a random sampling technique.

Although statistical formulas are available to determine the proper number of prescriptions to include in the sample for various confidence limits, allowable errors, and variances, experience using these formulas indicates that reasonable results will be obtained if the pharmacists will review at least 400 prescriptions in a random manner.

A table of random numbers may be used to select the first prescription in a random sample of prescriptions. Alternatively, the following procedure may be used:

1. Determine the total number of new prescriptions dispensed during the past 12 months and number each prescription consecutively. All prescriptions, including drugs controlled by the Drug Enforcement Agency (DEA), should be included in this group and assigned a number.

2. Determine the percentage of prescriptions to be selected so that a minimum of 400 prescriptions will be included in the sample, and use this percentage to determine the number of prescriptions, consecutively numbered, that you should skip (omit) between each prescription you will review.

3. Place consecutively numbered slips of paper of equal size in a box. The number of slips to be used should be equal to the number of prescriptions you will omit between those selected, *plus* one slip for the prescription selected. After throroughly mixing all the slips of paper, select one number. Beginning with the prescription represented by the assigned number, select each assigned prescription thereafter until all chosen prescriptions have been selected.

The following example will clarify the statistical procedure used to determine a trade area:

STEP 1—Determine total number of prescriptions dispensed during the last fiscal year.

Regular R Nos. 398,621 to 408,615 = New Regular Prescriptions =   9,995
DEA Nos.   112,134 to 116,205 = New DEA Prescriptions   =   4,072
Total new prescriptions   = 14,067

STEP 2—Assign the number "1" to the first prescription dispensed during the fiscal year and number the 14,067 prescriptions consecutively. NOTE: The prescriptions need not actually be numbered, but you must be aware of the number each prescription has been assigned.

STEP 3—Divide the number of new prescriptions dispensed by 400.

$$14,067 \div 400 = 35.2$$

(For this analysis the number may be rounded to 35)

STEP 4—Choose a number between 1 and 35 using one of the procedures outlined for selecting a random starting point. For this example the number "5" was chosen.

STEP 5—Starting with the prescription assigned number "5" (actual ℞ No. 398,626), select every 35th prescription filled during the year. This will result in a total sample of 402 prescriptions.

STEP 6—Plot the address from each prescription selected on an area map.

The above procedure will ensure that each new prescription dispensed in the past 12 months will have the same probability of being selected. Also, the sample is large enough to ensure that the trade area determined represents the *true* trade area. These data also can assist greatly in the decision to relocate and in the selection of a new site that will still be convenient to current prescription patrons. It is strongly suggested that all managers, regardless of their present plans concerning relocation, complete this process on at least an annual basis to determine shifts in the patient population being served.

ANALYSIS OF CHARGE ACCOUNTS

The same sampling procedure may be used to determine the present trade area of persons maintaining charge accounts at a pharmacy. Although experience indicates the trade area for charge customers usually does not differ greatly from the patient population trade area, both groups are extremely important to the success of the enterprise, and thus, an occasional analysis should be completed for both groups and the results compared. If a major difference is found, the reasons for this difference should be determined and the proper adjustments made. Such adjustments may include a change in emphasis or method of future promotional programs.

SPECIAL EVENT TO DETERMINE POTENTIAL TRADE AREA

A manager may obtain a good indication of the potential trade area for an established pharmacy using the "special event" technique. Plan a major event, such as a weekend sale, and offer a special gift or prize. Advertise the event consistently using all feasible media to ensure excellent penetration to all parts of the potential trade area. Have all persons sign their names and addresses on special cards of equal dimensions. Thoroughly mix the cards and draw a name for the prize. Then, randomly choose at least 400 of these cards and plot the addresses on a map. If a major difference exists in this potential trade area and the present trade area, a decision to relocate or change promotional and merchandising practices may be made. The results, together with those of previous surveys of prescriptions and/or charge accounts, may indicate a shifting of the population served, which would in turn indicate relocation.

Summary

The pharmacist should screen several potential locations by comparing the basic variables affecting choice of location. After the choice has been narrowed to one, or possibly two or three locations, a more detailed analysis should be made. The method to be used depends largely on the class or type of location, the type of pharmacy, and the amount of time and money available for analysis and evaluation. More than one method should be used as a double check on the estimates. The importance of location analysis and evaluation is such that time and money should not be the major consideration in the choice of methods.

The potential pharmacy proprietor should be aware of the social and economic changes that are taking place in many of the older neighborhood or residential areas as well as the rural areas. The quality of life and standard of living are deteriorating in many of the older sections of our cities, and consequently, these locations should be evaluated carefully and periodically. Also, the commercial potential of many of the central business districts is not as lucrative as it was in former years. This trend is largely the result of the development of the shopping centers. Urban renewal, Medicaid, and other Federal programs, together with the building of "high rise" apartment houses in the central portions of cities, serve to militate against the deteriorating force of the social and economic changes.

The analysis should proceed logically as follows: (1) several locations are screened; (2) the trade area is delineated; (3) the population of the trade area is determined; and (4) the potential total sales volume for the scope of lines of goods and services to be offered is estimated by use of the appropriate expenditure percentage or the appropriate per capita expenditure; (5) allowance must be made for both non-drug and drug competition; and (6) the relative drawing power of the competing pharmacies is estimated and the potential sales allocated on this basis.

Special techniques should be used for suscipient locations and for certain types of pharmacies such as the pharmaceutical centers. Also, an evaluation of the location of established pharmacies may require other methods and techniques. Finally, it should be recognized that the procedures that have been suggested provide only estimates and not precise measurement. Judgment must be exercised in all phases of these procedures.

REFERENCES

1. *1970 Census of Population, Vol. 1, Characteristics of the Population.* Dept. of Commerce, Bureau of Census, Washington, D.C., pp. x-xv.
2. *Statistical Abstract of the United States, 1972.* Dept. of Commerce, Bureau of Census, Washington, D.C.
3. *Drug Topics,* Sept. 25, 1972, pp. 21-23, 26, 37.
4. Slavin, G. F.: *The Lilly Digest.* Indianapolis: Eli Lilly and Co., 1973.
5. Huffman, D. C., et al.: *Community Pharmacy Management and Development.* Memphis: University of Tennessee, 1973, pp. 38-45.

REVIEW

1. Discuss the importance of location evaluation in terms of changing socio-economic conditions, frequency of tacit or actual evaluation, and business failures.

2. What is the simple and basic principle of location choice?

3. Discuss the five variables or factors affecting location choice.

4. Classify locations into their various geographic and functional classifications.

5. Define and describe each type of location, including shopping centers.

6. Describe the four types of locations based on the nature of the location and scope of commercial services and functions found in the larger cities.

7. Contrast the differences among suscipient, interceptive, and generative locations.

8. Describe an "island" location.

9. Discuss the strength and weaknesses of each technique of location analysis.

10. Outline the necessary steps used in the "vacuum" calculation technique.

11. When provided with the appropriate data, evaluate the sales potential of a location using the "vacuum" calculation technique.

12. Discuss each of the following factors in the evaluation of the market strength of a pharmacy.
    (a) Size   (e) Traffic
    (b) Shape   (f) Proximity to merchants
    (c) Front   (g) Proximity to physicians
    (d) Parking   (h) Proximity to other health facilities

13. Given the appropriate data, calculate the trading area in square miles using Reilly's Law of Retail Gravitation.

14. Discuss the techniques used in analyzing and evaluating the trading area of an established pharmacy.

15. When provided the appropriate data, analyze and evaluate the trade area of an established pharmacy; outline the necessary steps to evaluate such a location.

7. Pharmacy Layout Design

The location of a pharmacy, its management, and sufficient capital are major factors contributing to a pharmacy's success. Another major factor in determining the success of a pharmacy is its general appearance, including the layout design of the pharmacy and the arrangement of the individual departments. Before a pharmacist undertakes to design a layout or modernize a pharmacy, he should consider the objectives of the various designs, the type of pharmacy, the classes of consumer goods and purchases, and the principles of layout design.

Objectives of Layout Design

The *major objective* in the design of the exterior of a pharmacy is to attract more patrons into the pharmacy. The overall *objective* of interior *layout design* is to increase the amount of the total purchases of each person who enters the pharmacy.

In addition to the above general objectives, there are *six specific objectives:* (1) to enhance the general appearance of the pharmacy and to project a professional image; (2) to control payroll expenses through convenience and efficiency of the layout; (3) to improve patrons' satisfaction and convenience; (4) to maximize the utilization of space; (5) to disperse and control the traffic pattern within the pharmacy; and (6) to provide surveillance and reduce pilferage.

One other important factor to consider is the philosophy of the pharmacist-owner. Many pharmacists prefer to practice in a specific type of setting. Thus, the design required by a service-oriented pharmacist would differ from that needed by the pharmacist interested in using mass merchandising techniques.

Types of Community Pharmacies

PHARMACEUTICAL CENTER

The pharmaceutical center, designed and developed by McKesson & Robbins and the American Pharmaceutical Association, is similar to the prescription-oriented pharmacy, but it must conform to certain standards as described in Chapter 4. The layout design of this center is not so critical as with the other types because no merchandise of any kind is displayed. The inventory is confined to legend and non-legend medication and few convenient goods. The decor, the atmosphere, and the uncluttered floor space are the hallmarks of the pharmaceutical center.

PRESCRIPTION-ORIENTED PHARMACIES

This type of pharmacy usually occupies 1,000 to 2,000 square feet and is so designed that the patrons will have a comfortable waiting area near the prescription department. Health-related items, including drugs, home health care appliances and supplies, and prescription accessories, are displayed near this vicinity. The pharmacy may have a separate room for fitting trusses and other orthopedic and surgical appliances. Cosmetics, gifts, and a limited number of other items are displayed in the other areas of the pharmacy.

TRADITIONAL PHARMACIES

The traditional or conventional pharmacy usually occupies between 2,000 and 5,000 square feet. The major objective of the layout design for this type of pharmacy is to disperse the customers and expose them to all areas in the pharmacy. These pharmacies also should have a pleasing appearance, project a professional atmosphere, be convenient for both consumers and employees, and provide the opportunity for maximum sales at minimum expense. Of course, surveillance for shoplifters must be included as one objective in the design and layout process.

Although traditional pharmacies vary in design, it is generally agreed that the best traffic flow can be achieved with a 3:1 length-to-width ratio.

THE SUPER DRUGSTORE

The super drugstore occupies more than 5,000 square feet, generally 10,000 square feet or more, with the design approximating a square. The basic objective in a super drugstore is traffic control rather than traffic dispersal, which is achieved by the merchandising techniques used. Many lines of goods are sold in this type of drugstore, and the layout design is usually of the self-service type to facilitate traffic control and to provide maximum sales at minimum cost.

Figures 7-1 through 7-4 show inside views of the four types of community pharmacies.

Consumer Goods and Purchases

CLASSIFICATION OF CONSUMER GOODS

Definitions of the classes of consumer goods are included to provide an understanding of the relationship between consumers' activity in the purchase of various goods and good layout design principles. In addition to the classification of consumer goods, the manner in which consumers purchase them is very important to the success of a layout design.

Convenience Goods. Convenience goods normally have a low unit value and are purchased frequently, with little effort on the part of the

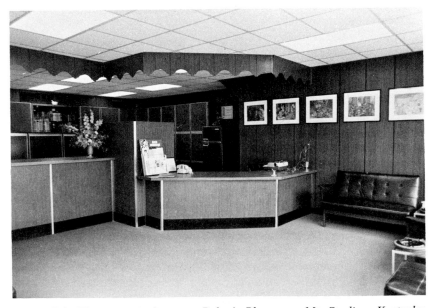

Figure 7-1. *Pharmaceutical center: Baker's Pharmacy, Mt. Sterling, Kentucky.*

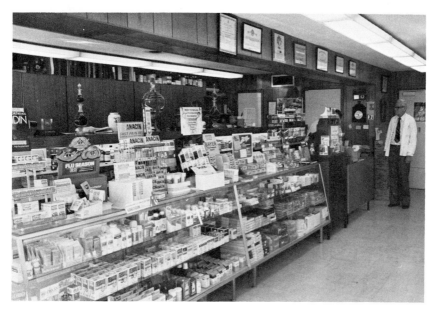

Figure 7-2. *Prescription-oriented pharmacy: Hubbard & Curry Pharmacy, Doctors Park, Lexington, Kentucky.*

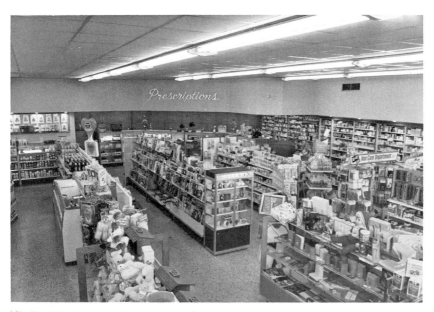

Figure 7-3. *Traditional pharmacy: Gardenside Pharmacy, Gardenside Plaza, Lexington, Kentucky.*

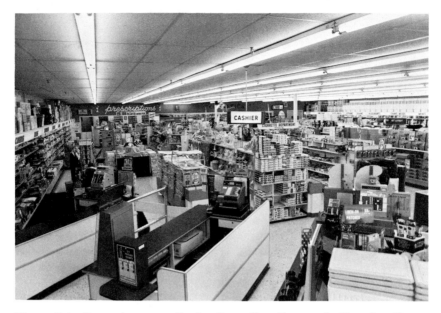

Figure 7-4. *Super drugstore: Begley Drug Co., Crossroads Shopping Center, Lexington, Kentucky.*

consumer. Convenience goods make up the large majority of the stock of grocery stores, variety stores, and pharmacies.

Shopping Goods. Goods in this class normally have a high unit value, are purchased infrequently, and require considerable effort on the part of the consumer. For such purchases the consumer will compare prices, quality, special features, and required services among other features. Shopping goods are found mostly in department, furniture, clothing, and similar stores.

Specialty Goods. Specialty goods normally have a high unit value, possess unique qualities or features and are purchased infrequently; consumers exert a great deal of effort to purchase them. Rare antiques and exclusive brands of clothing are examples of specialty goods.

It should be noted that pharmacies stock predominantly convenience goods; however, most pharmacies stock some shopping and specialty goods. The prescription is a special case; it includes attributes of all three classifications. For example, some patients shop for expensive or maintenance drugs, while other patients patronize only one pharmacist even at considerable expense and effort because of the personal and special services provided.

CLASSIFICATION OF PURCHASES

Demand Purchases. When consumers enter a pharmacy, or any other place where goods or services are sold, with the deliberate intent of purchasing a particular item and/or service, the purchase is considered to be a *demand purchase.* A prescription is a classic example.

Impulse Purchases. Impulse purchases are purchases made *after* the consumer has entered the pharmacy to purchase one or more other items, or are purchases made when the customer has entered the pharmacy for no particular purpose. This type of purchase frequently is suggested by an attractive display or price. Cosmetics, toiletries, and sundries often are purchased on impulse.

The percentage of pharmacy sales bought on impulse is not known. It can be assumed that all prescription and most nonprescription drugs, prescription accessories, surgical and orthopedic appliances and supplies, and other home health care aids are purchased on demand. A significant percentage of other types of products is bought on impulse.

It should be noted that classes of goods and purchases are not always mutually exclusive, but may be integrated in varying degrees in the mind of the purchaser.

Classes of Layout Designs

HISTORIC TYPES OF SERVICE-ORIENTED LAYOUT DESIGN

Historically, there are three basic types of layouts: (1) clerk, or personal service, (2) self-selection, and (3) self-service. Each is designed to achieve the objectives of the three basic types of pharmacies, professional, traditional, and super drugstore, respectively.

Clerk Service. The clerk service layout is the old traditional design used in most pharmacies before the trend toward self-service and mass merchandising. It consists primarily of complete clerk service with only a small part of the merchandise exposed for patrons to handle. The modern example of this layout design is the pharmaceutical center in which no merchandise is on display. Traditionally, pharmacists have used the clerk service design because it facilitates maximum interchange between pharmacy personnel and patrons, one of the major reasons many independent pharmacies have survived. Convenience and friendly service are still important factors in the patronage of a specific pharmacy.

However, the quality of clerk service has not been maintained in many instances. In addition, prices for pharmaceutical products have risen and the importance of price in relation to service has also increased. Therefore, this combination of factors has caused many managers to reduce services and seek an alternate type of layout design as a solution.

Self-Selection. In an attempt to provide adequate personal service in a more efficient manner, and thus be more competitive with the larger super drugstores, many independent pharmacists now use the self-selection layout design. This type of layout design dictates that clerk service be maintained at all service-oriented departments, such as cosmetics, photo supplies, prescription and selected nonprescription drugs, surgical and orthopedic appliances and supplies, and veterinary departments. Much of the other merchandise, however, is displayed in a manner that the patrons may see, handle, and select themselves. This layout is most frequently found in the modern conventional pharmacies.

Self-Service. The term self-service is restricted for those layouts that utilize a minimum of clerk service and expose the maximum amount of merchandise for patrons to handle. It is not possible to have 100 percent self-service in a pharmacy because of the prescription department. Central check-out of all purchases is the one criterion most commonly used to identify a truly self-service layout, although some "experts" dispute the appropriateness of this basis of distinction alone. This type of layout is most often used in the super drugstores.

STYLES OF LAYOUT DESIGNS

Styles of layout design emphasize *physical configuration* of the layout rather than the degree of service provided, although variations in services will coincide with several of the styles as shown later. Four distinct styles of layout design have been developed over the past three decades. They include: (1) *center service,* (2) *lobby check-out* or *bull pen,* (3) *off-the-wall,* and (4) *right-rear service.* The latter style is often referred to as the "self-selection" style, but we have chosen not to use this term in order to avoid confusion with the use of the term with regard to the concept of a combination of clerk service and self-service.

Center Service Style. This style features an elongated, two-sided wrapping counter and check-out "island" located in or near the center of the selling area of the pharmacy. Usually convenience goods such as tobacco, candy, and sometimes magazines and photo supplies are stocked in the island. The objective is to align the major traffic-generating departments around the perimeter and then pull all of the traffic through the check-out island in the center of the pharmacy. It has been tried in several traditional pharmacies, especially those that are rather wide or approximate a square configuration. The concept is good in theory, but it has been less than satisfactory in practice in most instances (Fig. 7-5).

Lobby Check-Out Style. This approach utilizes a square, clerk service check-out "island" near the front of the pharmacy, but there is enough space between the check-out island and the front window to form a "lobby." Again, candy, tobacco, photo supplies, and men's sundries are

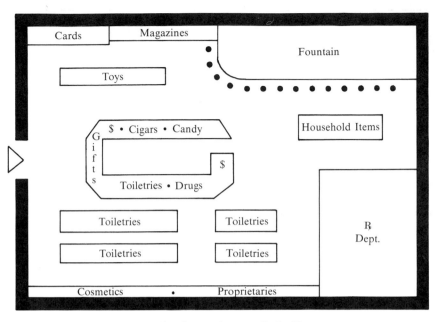

Figure 7-5. *Layout Design for Center Service Style Pharmacy*

stocked in the island, while seasonal and promotional merchandise are displayed in the lobby where the traffic is heavy. Frequently, the check-out island is supplemented by a short wrapping counter in the rear of the store in front of the prescription department.

The major traffic-generating departments are located around the walls with display counters or showcases placed in front of the wall shelves. Gondolas are aligned front-to-rear in the center portion of the pharmacy. This style is used in the larger traditional pharmacies with floor space of 5,000 square feet or more. A modification of this style, substituting several check-out lanes for the "bull pen," has been used successfully in super drugstores. The main disadvantage of this style in the traditional drugstore is the reduction of the depth penetration of the traffic flow caused by the short wrapping counter and the check-out island (Fig. 7-6).

Off-the-Wall Style. This style features open display of merchandise on the wall shelving without showcases or counters in front of the wall shelves. The main wrapping counter, short or long, is placed across the rear of the store in front of the prescription counter. One or two rows of gondolas are placed in the center of the pharmacy. This style became popular for a time because of the ease and low cost of installing fixtures. It is well adapted to a *very* narrow building, but it is not conducive to personal, clerk service. Large super drugstores utilize a modification of this style (Fig. 7-7).

Right-Rear Service Style. This style frequently is called the self-selec-

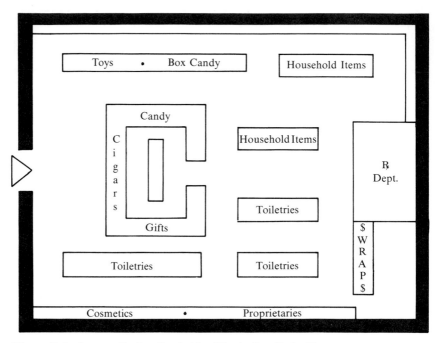

Figure 7-6. *Layout Design for Lobby Check-Out Style Pharmacy*

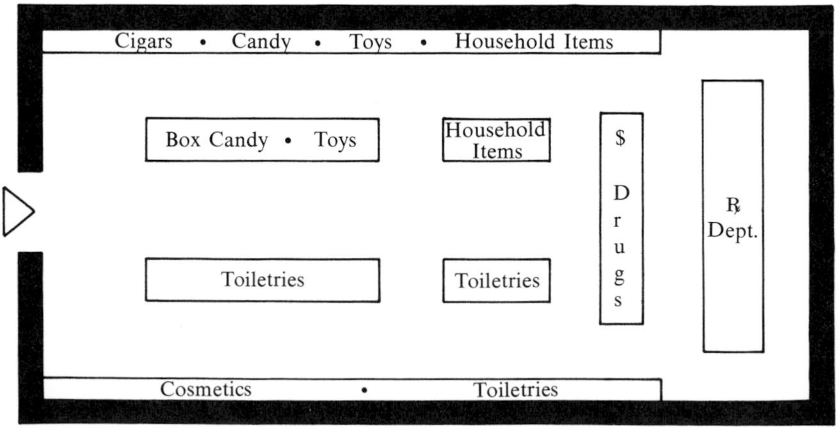

Figure 7-7. *Layout Design for Off-the-Wall Style Pharmacy*

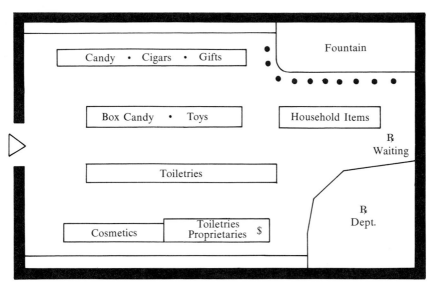

Figure 7-8. *Layout Design for Right-Rear Service Style Pharmacy*

tion style because it accommodates this concept so well. The concept permits self-service where desirable, and thus promotes efficiency and reduces costs. At the same time, it permits personal clerk or professional services as appropriate. When this style is properly designed and implemented, it has twelve characteristics of optimum design which are discussed below. The right-rear service style is well suited for most traditional pharmacies, especially those that approximate a 3:1 length-to-width configuration (Fig. 7-8).

Principles and Characteristics of Layout Design

The principles of layout design include the selection of the appropriate service-oriented design and the physical configuration best suited for the type of pharmacy and location. They also include the appropriate arrangement of departments and merchandise in order to achieve optimum design characteristics.

OPTIMUM DESIGN CHARACTERISTICS FOR THE
TRADITIONAL PHARMACY

1. All four corners of the merchandising and service area of the pharmacy should be activated. This is achieved by strategic placement of clerk-activated service or special-skills departments, plus selected

"self-selling" departments such as greeting cards, gifts, and magazines.

2. All displays are departmentalized and well identified. Related departments and merchandise are grouped adjacent or near similar departments and merchandise.

3. The main wrapping counter with a cash register is placed along the longest clear wall—right side if walls are equal length—and deep to the rear.

4. A selected assortment of the fastest selling nonprescription drugs, dental products, and toiletries are displayed on the main wrapping counter.

5. The prescription department is located in the rear and adjacent to the main wrapping counter. The prescription department is dramatized with commanding identification and a floor elevation of seven inches. There should be a minimum of 150 footcandles of light within the prescription department.

6. An adequate waiting area with comfortable chairs and health-related reading materials should be provided near the prescription department. Sickroom supplies, home health aids, and prescription accessories should be displayed near the prescription department and the waiting area.

7. The cosmetic and toiletry department is aligned with the nonprescription drug and prescription drug departments from front to rear, respectively, along the right or longest wall. Pre-sold, nationally advertised cosmetics and toiletries, such as hair care products, lotions, and creams are placed on open display on gondolas across from the cosmetic department.

8. Special skill departments such as photography, imported gifts, costume jewelry, veterinary drugs and pet supplies, and orthopedic and surgical appliances and supplies should be given special treatment and well identified. Clerk service should be provided in these departments.

9. Special care should be given to use of color and special design features so that the pharmacy is a restful, pleasant place to shop and reflects professionalism and pride of ownership.

10. The lighting layout in the pharmacy must conform with the fixture layout, highlighting the merchandise, not the fixtures. A minimum of 100 footcandles should be provided in the selling or merchandising area.

11. The fountain, if one is installed, is located across from the main wrapping counter on the opposite wall deep in the rear of the pharmacy.

12. All clerk service stations must be self-supporting, that is, the service-merchandise departments must produce gross sales at least ten times the weekly payroll.

ARRANGEMENT OF DEPARTMENTS AND MERCHANDISE

The prescription department and other high-skill or specialty departments should be located in the rear or toward the rear of the pharmacy. If the pharmacy has a fountain, it should be placed in the rear of the pharmacy across from the main wrapping counter and the prescription department. Ideally, the fountain should be separated from the prescription department and the prescription waiting area by an attractive planter, a partial partition perhaps made of pegboard on which home health care products can be displayed, health information displays, or other suitable means of separation. This type of arrangement maintains the integrity of the professional atmosphere of the prescription and drug area.

If the pharmacy has a surgical and orthopedic appliance department, a special fitting room is a must. The door of the fitting room and any intermediate door through which a patient must pass should be adequately identified. A separate toilet for men and women should be located near the fitting room because in nearly every instance, the patient will need to use the toilet after a fitting, especially the fitting of trusses.

If the pharmacy does not have a fountain, greeting cards and a gift department are the best choices to replace the fountain in the rear of the pharmacy. A photographic department or a veterinary drug department, if developed into a high-skill department by highly competent clerks, provides another option. A special room located in part of the stockroom in the rear makes an ideal veterinary drug department, provided the entrance is well identified.

The cosmetics, toiletries, and nonprescription drug departments should be arranged as described in characteristic number 7 (p. 122). The tobacco, candy, and magazine departments are usually located in the front of the pharmacy across from the cosmetic department. Smoking accessories, photo supplies, and/or men's toiletries are often included in this area to provide greater sales potential, but more importantly, greater gross margin. This is desirable in order to achieve characteristic number 12 (p. 122). Other major departments can be used to fill the remainder of the wall space opposite the cosmetic and drug side of the pharmacy. Gondolas normally are aligned lengthwise in the center portion of the pharmacy to complete the layout.

Goods and services purchased on demand, and specialty goods, should be placed in or toward the rear of the pharmacy. This arrangement draws the patrons deep into the pharmacy. Convenience goods generally are placed near the front of the pharmacy. Selected convenience goods are displayed near the cash registers. Many shopping goods and most products often purchased on impulse are displayed in the middle portion of the pharmacy. Selected products of both categories are displayed in the front part of the pharmacy and near the cash register. Household products, school supplies, and many sundries are displayed on the gondolas. Promotional merchandise frequently is displayed on gondolas, especially the ends of the gondolas.

Traffic Flow Analysis

There are two types of traffic flow analyses, qualitative and quantitative. The first is *very* simple to perform and can be done frequently, two or three times annually if desired. The second, quantitative analysis, requires more time and would be performed no more frequently than once each year.

QUALITATIVE TRAFFIC FLOW ANALYSIS

A qualitative traffic flow analysis is performed by tracing the path of each patron who enters the pharmacy. First, three layouts of the floor plan of the pharmacy are drawn on graph or grid paper. Three time intervals representing morning, afternoon, and evening traffic, of either 30 minutes or one hour, depending on the amount of traffic, should be selected randomly over a period of a week. The path of each patron is traced on the graph paper from the moment he enters the pharmacy until he leaves. Appropriate marks are made at each point of purchase. It is useful to use three colors for tracing, one representing ladies, another for men, and a third representing children under the age of eighteen (Fig. 7-9).

The three tracings are then compared. Usually, they have similar traffic patterns with some variation due to the different times of day the data were taken. The primary purpose of the qualitative traffic analysis is to identify "dead" areas in the pharmacy where few or no patrons shop. Dead areas are an indication that the pharmacy needs to be modernized with significant changes in the layout design.

The impact that remodeling has on traffic flow is vividly depicted in Figures 7-10 and 7-11.

QUANTITATIVE TRAFFIC ANALYSIS

The following procedure is used to determine quantitatively whether the present layout of the pharmacy is adequate.[1] At the end of the study you will be statistically confident that the results achieved are correct.

STEP 1—Divide the pharmacy into major departments. In a traditional pharmacy, these departments generally include: (1) the prescription department, (2) nonprescription drugs and health-related items, (3) cosmetics and toiletries, (4) baby department, (5) feminine hygiene, (6) candy, tobacco and accessories, and magazines, and (7) in some instances, veterinary supplies. Pharmacies containing less than 5,000 square feet generally can be divided into fewer than ten departments, usually six or seven. The cash register(s) should be keyed to each of the major departments to record sales and number of transactions.

STEP 2—Randomly select enough hours during a one-month period to be assured that at least 400 patrons will be observed. For example, if an average of 40 patrons entered the pharmacy each hour, ten one-hour intervals or 20 one-half hour intervals should be selected in order to conduct a complete and quantitative traffic flow analysis.

STEP 3—Record the data from the cash register at the end of each sampling period and label them with date and time of sampling.

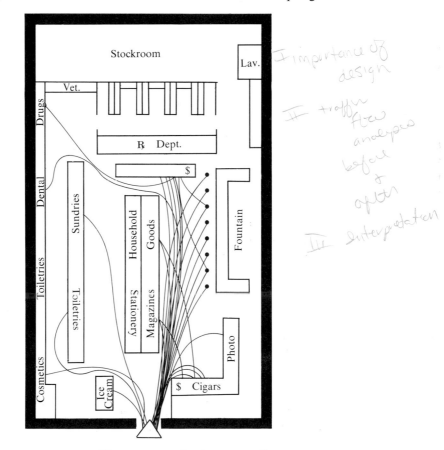

Figure 7-9A. *Illustration of Qualitative Traffic Flow Analysis to be Placed over Work Sheet in Figure 7-9B.*

Adapted from McKesson & Robbins, Inc.

WORK SHEET FOR TRAFFIC FLOW ANALYSIS

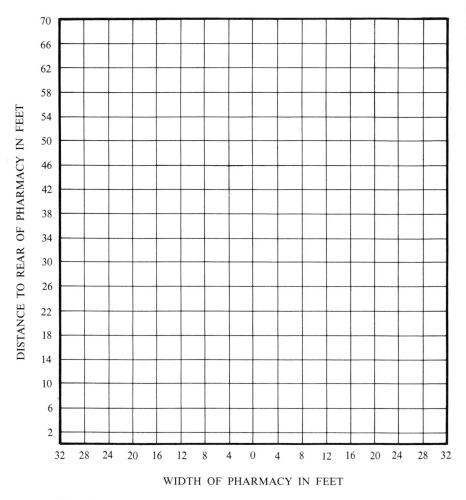

Directions:

1. Sketch floor plan on grid showing department locations.
2. Show each customer's route by colored line.
3. Terminate line at point of final purchase.

Figure 7-9B

STEP 4—Total the sales for each department for all sampling periods and calculate the average dollar value per transaction.

STEP 5—Conduct a qualitative traffic flow analysis as described previously during the same time interval used to obtain the data in Step 2.

STEP 6—Compare the sales efficiency by department and transaction

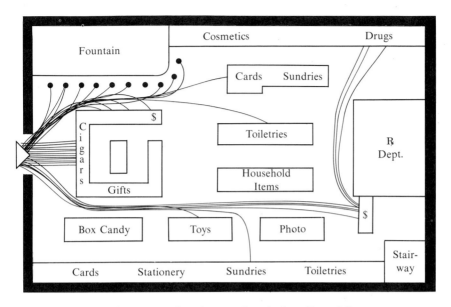

Figure 7-10. *Qualitative Traffic Flow Analysis* before *Remodeling*

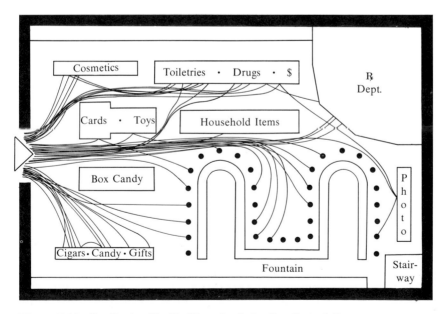

Figure 7-11. *Qualitative Traffic Flow Analysis* after *Remodeling*

with the qualitative traffic flow to locate "dead" spots within the store and redesign the layout based upon the data and space needed for each department.

The procedure for selecting the times for sampling may be demonstrated with the following example. Assume the pharmacy is open from 9:00 a.m. until 9:00 p.m., Monday through Saturday. The sampling is to be conducted during June, 1974. Since the month contains 30 days and five Sundays, the pharmacy will be open 12 hours per day for 25 days for a total of 300 hours. The number "1" is assigned to the hour beginning at 9:00 a.m. on Saturday, June 1, and each hour thereafter is numbered consecutively. This means that the hour beginning at 8:00 p.m., Saturday, June 29, is assigned the number "300." Assume an average of 40 patrons per hour and 400 observations are to be made. A total of 10 hours should be selected—one hour for each 30 hours the pharmacy is open during June, 1974 (300 hours ÷ 10 hours = 30 hours).

Next place 30 slips of paper of equal size numbered 1 through 30 into a container, mix them thoroughly, and select one. Assuming number 13 was drawn, the traffic flow analysis would begin at 9:00 a.m. on Monday, June 3, 1974. Similar analysis would be conducted each thirtieth hour the pharmacy was open in June.

At the same time a traffic flow study is being conducted, determine the average amount per sales transaction for the entire pharmacy for each time interval. Also, the sales in each major department should be segmented to determine the total sales for each department and the dollar amount per sales transaction for each department. (The average sales transaction per customer will range between $1.00 and $3.00, depending on the merchandise mix and clientele of the pharmacy.) This can easily be accomplished by means of a modern cash register, which shows the number of transactions and sales by departments. This analysis will provide a comparison of sales efficiency and the relative space needed for each department when the pharmacy is renovated.

After a complete renovation or any major change is made within the pharmacy, another traffic flow analysis should be completed and the results compared with those before renovation. In addition, it is suggested that the pharmacist complete a traffic flow analysis on an annual basis.

APPLICATION OF TRAFFIC FLOW ANALYSIS

A traffic flow analysis was conducted on traditional prescription-oriented pharmacies located in a medical building in a city of approximately 40,000 people. The pharmacy was approximately forty years old and had not been remodeled over the past fifteen years. In addition to the street entrance in the front of the pharmacy, patients could enter directly by a side door from the lobby after visiting the physicians in the building. Stock was stored in two rooms in the rear of the pharmacy and in several rooms on the balcony level. It was obvious that there was inappropriate use of all the space. The prescription department was located on the balcony level and utilized a dumbwaiter to transfer the prescription orders and the finished prescriptions between the service area and prescription department. Thus, the pharmacist had very little patient contact. The pharmacy generally was cluttered, although it was kept clean. The cosmetic department, which had several prestige lines and a large inventory for this particular size of pharmacy, was kept fairly attractive.

A qualitative description traffic flow analysis was conducted on several occasions before remodeling. These revealed that only minor parts of the pharmacy were not active because large numbers of patrons were forced to circulate throughout the store because of the small waiting area in the prescription department. However, inefficiencies did exist in several areas.

The renovation included the following changes. The prescription department was relocated on the first floor. A first-level stockroom was converted into a surgical and orthopedic fitting room. One of the second-level stockrooms was converted into a physicians' reading lounge where physicians could come to read the most popular medical journals, inspect package inserts of new drugs, and drink free coffee. (This room was entered from the second floor corridor of the building.) The ceiling of the pharmacy was lowered and modern fluorescent lighting was installed. All-weather carpeting was placed on the floors. Wood paneling was installed throughout the selling area, the prescription department, the physicians' reading room, and the fitting room. New fixtures were installed throughout the pharmacy. In addition, an individual patient medication record system was implemented and the APhA Health Education Center was installed. A professional fee for pricing prescriptions was also put into effect.

A quantitative traffic flow analysis was performed before and after the renovation and revealed the following data: Using random samples of time intervals, approximately 31 percent of the patients entered the pharmacy from the lobby through the side door before renovation. After renovation, 56 percent of the patients entered the pharmacy by this entrance. This difference was statistically significant at the 0.01 confidence level—in other words, the investigator was 99 percent confident that the difference was not a result of chance. Each patron entering the pharmacy before renovation made an average of 1.2 purchasing stops. After renovation, each made an average of 1.4 purchasing stops.

The annual sales increased by 14 percent over the previous year, taking into consideration the sales decline rate of the previous year. Prescription sales increased an effective 16 percent on an annual basis—reversing a 14 percent decline trend plus a net 2 percent absolute increase.

Most significant of all was the increase in *new* prescriptions, which reversed a downward trend of 15 percent annually plus an actual increase of 37 percent over the previous year.

REFERENCE

1. The quantitative traffic analysis was adapted from Huffman, D. C., et al.: *Community Pharmacy Management, Planning and Development,* Memphis: University of Tennessee, 1973, Section IV.

REVIEW

1. What is the major objective of the exterior design of a pharmacy?

2. What is the basic objective of the layout design of the interior of a pharmacy?

3. What are the six specific objectives of the layout design of the interior of a pharmacy?

4. Describe the four major types of pharmacies.

5. Distinguish between the three basic service-oriented layout designs.

6. Describe the four styles of layout design and include the advantages and disadvantages of each.

7. Define and distinguish the characteristics of convenience goods, shopping goods, specialty goods, and demand and impulse purchases.

8. Describe the 12 optimum design characteristics.

9. Outline the most appropriate arrangement of departments and merchandise according to classes of consumer goods, and impulse and demand purchases.

10. Perform a qualitative and a quantitative traffic flow pattern analysis of a traditional pharmacy.

8. Personnel Administration

What we frankly give, forever is our own.
George Granville

Personnel administration probably is the most important aspect of pharmacy management; yet it is the most neglected phase. Today we read and hear a great deal about pharmacy becoming people-oriented or patient-oriented. Most *successful* practitioners have always been people-oriented. Furthermore, these practitioners have used this philosophy in their relationships with their employees. Just as "charity begins at home," people-orientation begins with the employees in our pharmacies.

Importance of Personnel Administration

There are *three important reasons* why good employee relations should be emphasized and practiced in every pharmacy. The *first* involves *finances.* According to the *1973 Lilly Digest,*[1] the "average" pharmacy spent $49,408, or 20 percent of sales, for salaries and wages. This figure represents the largest single expense item in the profit and loss statement. Some pharmacists may view expenditures for salaries and wages as a type of investment, but in reality, they are not. Money expended for salaries and wages must be productive as it is spent, or at least in the near future;

otherwise the money will not be recovered or produce a net return. Therefore, payroll inherently has an immediacy which creates an urgency in its judicious use.

Another way to view the financial importance of the payroll is to contrast it with the investment in inventory. Inventory represents an *investment* on which a net profit may be earned, while the payroll is an *expense* of doing business. A pharmacist has at least two options in the use of the inventory investment: (1) he may return the goods for credit under certain conditions, and (2) he may reduce the price and enhance the sale potential. Such options are not available in respect to the payroll expense.

There is yet another financial aspect of personnel administration, namely, the high cost of personnel turnover. Normally it requires three to six months of training before a new employee becomes sufficiently productive to be profitable. If a pharmacy has a high personnel turnover rate, an unprofitable situation could easily exist because of the cost associated with the constant training of new employees who, at the beginning, are not proficient enough to be productive and profitable.

The *second reason* personnel administration is important derives from the interrelationship between the behavior of the employees and the *pharmacy's public image.* To a great extent, the attitudes and behavior of the employees will create the public image of the pharmacy. Of course, their attitudes and behavior reflect the personality of the proprietor or pharmacist-manager and the type of employee relationship he maintains. This points to *one of the basic rules* of personnel relations, that is, *good employee relations begin with the proprietor or manager* himself. His attitudes toward work, people, and the profession have a tremendous influence on those in his employ. A good personnel relations program is essential to cultivate a good public image for any organization. This is especially true of a pharmacy because a successful, professional enterprise such as a pharmacy must exhibit a warm and friendly atmosphere.

The *third reason* personnel administration is important relates to the *achievements of the objectives of the pharmacy.* From a strictly economic point of view, the proprietor, in addition to his entrepreneurship, provides a managerial function, an economic input. The economic reward is reflected in the form of the proprietor's salary before the net profit is computed. The *net profit* is the economic reward for entrepreneurship, and it is one of the basic objectives of the pharmacy. Without good employees supporting the proprietor, a healthy net profit cannot be achieved.

Principles of Personnel Administration

There are several basic principles of good employee relations. These include: (1) people-orientation begins with the proprietor and his employees; (2) good employee relations emanate from the attitudes, philosophy, and leadership of the employer; (3) the "golden rule" is an excellent principle to follow, but most people need additional guidelines and principles to assist them in making personnel decisions; (4) the techniques and methods of employee relations should not be depersonalized, although objectivity and fairness must be used judiciously; (5) a good manager will delegate authority to the lowest level consistent with the capabilities of the employee; and (6) adequate resources should be supplied and authority should be delegated to subordinates commensurate with the delegated responsibilities.

These principles apply to all types and sizes of pharmacies; however, the scope of the application of specific techniques and methods is limited by the number of employees. In this regard, trends toward fewer smaller pharmacies and more larger ones are significant considerations.[2]

Methods of Personnel Administration

PRESELECTION TECHNIQUES

Job Analysis. Before a manager begins to recruit and select employees, he should perform certain analyses and describe the jobs or functions for his pharmacy. This process is aptly called *job analysis,* and the description written from the analysis is called *job description.* This process is meticulously carried out in large organizations using time and motion, work monitoring, and work sampling techniques. It is not necessary for the usual community pharmacy; however, each job or position to be filled should be analyzed and described in sufficient detail to permit both employer and employee to know what is expected in each position. The emphasis in job analysis and job description falls upon the work elements to be performed, and by implication or explicit descriptions, the qualifications of the person who will fill the position.

Job Specification. Based on the personal qualifications extracted from the job description, a *job* or *position specification* is written. Whereas a community pharmacist may not perform a detailed job analysis or write a detailed job description, he should write a fairly complete job specification based on the requirements of each job or position to be filled. Job specification emphasizes personal qualities, while job description emphasizes work elements to be performed. The job specification provides the basis for selecting the right employee for each position in the pharmacy.

RECRUITMENT AND SELECTION

Recruitment. A pharmacy manager can launch an intelligent employee recruitment and selection program on the basis of the job specifications for unfilled positions in his pharmacy. The sources for *recruitment* will be determined by his needs at any particular time. For staff pharmacists, the colleges of pharmacy are the best source at graduation time. During the rest of the year, other pharmacies, health care institutions, government, and industry may be approached. These sources are the only ones for experienced pharmacists for managerial positions. Another good source (and perhaps an important one for the future) consists in the married female pharmacists who want to reenter the profession after their children have reached school age. Part-time employees, both professional and nonprofessional, may be a solution to the profit squeeze caused by rising costs on the one hand and increased competition on the other. Classified ads are the medium used most widely to locate experienced pharmacists, but employment agencies can be useful in large competitive markets.

Different means are used to recruit nonprofessional personnel. High schools and colleges offer possibilities for part-time personnel, as do married females. However, school "dropouts" usually do not make good pharmacy personnel. Newspaper ads and word-of-mouth advertising are the best media. "Help Wanted" signs in the windows have fallen into disuse for good reason. Such signs usually are not attractive or dignified, and they use valuable space that can be used better for professional displays.

Personnel Selection. The *selection process* is probably the most *critical phase* of personnel relations. Here the decision must be made. The question to be answered is, "Is he the kind of person I want in my organization?" Once an employee is hired, it is difficult to discharge him without some repercussions and considerable cost.

There are *four steps* in the selection process. The *first step* is the *initial interview* with the prospective employee and completion of a prepared *application form.* The initial interview serves as a means of appraising the applicant's apparent qualities—appearance, speech, mannerisms, and attitudes. The application form should provide essential personal, educational, experience, and health data as well as references to serve as a basis for preliminary selection. From a list of seven applicants, four might be eliminated on the basis of the application form and the initial interview.

Tests, although not widely used in community and hospital pharmacies, are the *second step* in the selection process. They are more common in chain pharmacies, industry, and government. Simple tests, properly constructed, can prove useful in personnel selection. Such a test may be written, oral, or practical, and it must be designed for the level of the position being filled. Although a proprietor may think it unnecessary to test a registered pharmacist on his professional knowledge, he may want to ascertain some measure of the applicant's managerial potential.

Written tests may cover problems, letter writing, or general knowledge about drugs. Oral questions may determine the applicant's ability to express himself and handle a particular situation, or again, his general knowledge about drugs. Practical or performance tests may include making change, typing speed and accuracy, preparing a prescription, especially the label, and patient consultation. Many such tests may be simulated; however, an actual test under real conditions is to be preferred.

Honesty and *ethics* are difficult to measure. A test can be made of an individual's basic honesty through a few questions, the answers to which can be validated. For example, the manager may ask the applicant about his relationship with his previous employer(s) and then check with the employer(s). Polygraph tests are widely used in many industries, including the chain drugstores. A recent survey indicated that 73 percent of the responding drugstore chains use the polygraph and 80 percent stated they favor its use. The widest use of the polygraph is reserved for theft and robbery problems; however, 40 percent of those using this technique also use it for pre-employment examination.[3]

The *third step* is to employ *references* to assess the applicant's honesty and willingness to work, the quality of his work, and any personality or disciplinary problem. References may include former employers, teachers, and friends, but former employers are preferred. Oddly enough, *oral recommendations are more reliable than written ones.* People are more inclined to "tell it like it is" about a person if they do not have to put it in writing.

The *final interview* is the *last step* in the selection process. After studying the application, the results of any tests that were used, and the recommendations of former employers, the manager is ready to make his decision. On the basis of preliminary considerations, the field may have been reduced to two or three applicants. In any case, a final interview should be conducted to check on any unanswered questions and to clarify any potential problem area. The final decision will be made at this time, and the manager will want it to be the best possible.

A pitfall to be guarded against in any interview is the "halo" (positive) or "horn" (negative) effect. This is simply a lack of objectivity on the part of the interviewer by which he allows one particular characteristic to color his judgement about other characteristics or qualities. For example, the interviewer may like or dislike a certain color of hair, accent, or manner of dress so much that his judgement of other qualities is distorted. The use of two or three interviewers serves to minimize the halo or horn effect and provides for more objectivity in the interviews.

ORIENTATION AND TRAINING

Orientation. The purpose of *orientation* is to acquaint the new employee with the organization, its history, its objectives, its policies, and other employees. Personnel psychologists have demonstrated a high degree of relationship between good orientation programs and the results of subsequent training programs. It is very important for each new employee to be properly indoctrinated and made to feel "at home" in his new work surroundings. Failure to orient and indoctrinate new employees properly is probably the most common failing of community pharmacy proprietors.

Orientation can be made more effective by the use of concise written statement of policies and by the use of the "buddy system." Written policy statements may be compiled into a booklet that functions as an employee manual. The American College of Apothecaries has compiled a prototype policies and procedures manual for its members.[4] This manual contains a statement of objectives and general policies, employee policies and procedures, including company rules, fringe benefits, information for pharmacy personnel, such as telephone technique, consulting with patients, information for typists, and use of the patient medication record system. This manual can be easily adapted for an individual pharmacy. The large chain drugstores have seen the wisdom of writing employees' manuals and developing extensive training programs for nearly all levels of employees.

Training. Training and development of employees should be distinguished from education. Whereas education has broad objectives, training has specific objectives related to proficiency on a particular job. Training objectives are either the acquisition of skills or a change in behavior. Personnel training may be either formal or informal, but most of the training in pharmacies is considered to be informal.

The most common method of conducting training for nonprofessional personnel is *on-the-job training.* This type of training consists of four basic steps:

1. Tell the trainee what the job is, how the job is done, and why it is done.
2. Show or demonstrate how the job should be done.
3. Allow the trainee to do the job.
4. Follow up by explaining what was done correctly and what was done incorrectly. Corrections always should be made as privately as possible.

The *conference* is the next most frequently used means of training pharmacy personnel. Conferences may be either formal or informal. A formal, regularly scheduled meeting is effective in maintaining the proficiency and morale of experienced personnel if it is planned and conducted well. Each conference should have an objective (or objectives) and a planned agenda covering such subjects as sales, special promotion, public relations programs, or product knowledge. Experience has shown that combining an evening meal or breakfast with a conference is a good morale booster. Advantage should also be taken of the special schools and seminars offered by cosmetic manufacturers, surgical supply houses, and veterinary drug manufacturers.

Information to be supplied in an orientation and training program should include the history, objectives, and policies of the pharmacy. Next, the pharmacy's systems and procedures, especially those for which the new employee will be responsible, should be taught. These should include the organization of the pharmacy, lines of responsibility and authority, location of departments, maintenance of inventory, handling of cash, checking registers, special controls for certain departments and products, and related restrictions. Methods of dealing with patrons, especially in unusual situations, require more time. Knowledge of new and existing products requires still more time, and teaching this is a continuous project.

The proprietor or manager of a pharmacy should realize that his personal example is a powerful teaching tool. It is especially true that poor examples have a negative effect on the learner.

Employee orientation and training are the most neglected aspect of personnel administration. There is too little—far too little—of it done. Too frequently the training that is provided is neither well planned nor often evaluated.

SUPERVISION

Supervision is necessary even in a small pharmacy in which only two or three people are employed; it cannot be avoided if the employees are to perform satisfactorily and achieve their objectives and those of the pharmacy. There is the danger, however, of oversupervision. Oversupervision reduces the self-confidence of the employees and creates a morale problem.

Supervision is simply a process of open communications between the supervisor, the manager in most small pharmacies, and the employees, and a general overview of the work performance by the supervisor. Communications always should be conducted on a two-way basis to be effective. Being a good listener is inherent in good communication. Understanding is important, but listening and understanding must be genuine. This is especially true in performance review and evaluation.

It is a well-known fact that there are good and bad supervisors. Since good supervision is so important to the success of any organization, there must be an explanation why there are many poor supervisors. Laurence

Peter offers a plausible explanation in his book entitled *The Peter Principle.*[5] According to Peter, our modern society has the inherent tendency toward developing hierarchies in all organizations. In these structures, every person tends to rise to his first level of incompetence. The phenomenon is universal and inevitable because of the characteristics of our social system. These characteristics include: (1) social mobility which rewards competent people in a specific area of endeavor with a promotion to a higher position for which the person is not trained or qualified; (2) the tendency to preserve the hierarchy which produces conformity of action for the security it provides; and (3) the absence of a method or system of identifying and distinguishing the necessary qualities for good supervision.

The reasons for, and the methods used, in promoting people to their level of incompetency are beyond the scope of this book. However, *The Peter Principle* and its companion, *The Peter Prescription,*[6] are recommended reading. The books not only provide a good insight into organizational hierarchy; they permit a better understanding of society in general and more specifically how one can cope with the difficulties encountered in many organizations.

EVALUATION AND COMPENSATION

A manager should realize that he is evaluating himself and his personnel relations program when he evaluates his employees. This procedure is even more personal than a teacher's evaluation of his students. After all, the manager selects and trains his employees, whereas the teacher normally does not select his pupils.

Principles of Personnel Evaluation. There are some general principles of employee evaluation which should be observed.

1. The manager must have a genuine desire to be fair and honest. Personal bias must be avoided if at all possible.

2. Allowance must be made for nonproductive (nonselling) duties. This is one of the purposes of a rating system.

3. The pay scale must be competitive within the market. Parsimony is unprofitable in personnel relations.

4. Incentive and opportunity for advancement must be incorporated into the pay scale. Insufficient incentive and opportunity for advancement are the most common faults in current pay scales for pharmacists. This may be overcome if the starting salaries are lowered and a profit-sharing plan and/or an opportunity to purchase an interest in the pharmacy is provided as a strong incentive for achievement.

5. The method of calculating wages or salary should be simple enough to be easily understood by the employee involved.

6. Clerks' wages should be approximately 10 percent of their sales,

but this rule should not be applied to managers or pharmacists.

7. Wages should be fairly uniform from week to week, especially for young married people with tight budgets.

8. Finally, compensation alone cannot replace proper supervision and good human relations.

Personnel Evaluation. Achievement measurements and rating scales are the two primary means of evaluating employees. The former are more objective, easier to devise, and easier to use. Examples of such measurements include sales per employee, number of transactions or patrons served per day, dollar value per transaction, and incidents of out-of-stock situations in an assigned department of the pharmacy.

Rating scales are more difficult to design, use, and interpret. One such instrument, the graphic rating of employees on various qualities, as illustrated in Figure 8-1, is sufficiently simple to be used by the typical pharmacy proprietor or manager. However, rating of employees on a scale used alone is inferior to a system of management by objectives.

Compensation. Methods of compensation were implicit in the discussion of principles of evaluation. Although straight salary is commonly found, it offers the least in incentive. It does provide wage stability, it is simple and easily understood, and it can provide compensation for nonselling duties. Selling on commission provides a strong incentive, but it may create overly aggressive attitudes. It also lacks wage stability. Salary plus PM ("push merchandise") techniques are to be discouraged for the same reasons. In addition, PMs may divide employee loyalty between the proprietor and the manufacturer of the product. Salary plus profit sharing and/or opportunity to own an interest in the pharmacy seems to have most of the advantages and none of the disadvantages of other methods.

Proprietors and managers should be aware of the Federal and their respective State minimum wage and hours laws. The Federal law exempts an independent pharmacy (one unit only) if the sales are less than $250,000 annually. Both independent and chain pharmacies (two or more units) with annual sales of $250,000 are covered by the Federal minimum wage law; but individual units of either chains or independents with less sales volume are exempted. However, the 1974 Amendments will reduce the exemption for chains to $225,000 in gross annual sales per unit by January 1, 1975, to $200,000 by January 1, 1976, and will repeal the exemption altogether January 1, 1977.

The increases in the minimum wage are scheduled to become effective in stages, and the minimum wage schedules are different for the large chains with a million dollar annual volume and for those pharmacies with $250,000 annual gross sales per unit. For the large chain, the new minimum wage schedule is $2.00 per hour, May 1, 1974, increasing to $2.10 per hour January 1, 1975, and $2.30 by January 1, 1976. For the

Characteristic	Scale

Dependability

Loyal attitude
toward the firm

Awareness of
assigned respon-
sibilities

Knowledge of the
stock in assigned
departments

Order and clean-
liness of assigned
sections

Courtesy and co-
operativeness with
fellow employees

Courtesy and gen-
uine interest in
dealing with
patrons

Alertness and
promptness in
dealing with
patrons

Warm and pleas-
ing personality

Appearance

Poor	Fair	Average	Good	Excellent

Figure 8-1. *Rating Scale for Evaluating Employees*

smaller pharmacies, the increases are $1.90 May 1, 1974, $2.00 January 1, 1975, $2.10 January 1, 1976, and $2.30 by January 1, 1977. Small independent pharmacies with less than $250,000 annual gross sales are still exempted from the law.

Motivation

Motivation is perhaps the most difficult aspect of employee relations. Every individual is different and reacts to a given situation differently. Sometimes people, or at least a portion of them, can be predicted to react to a well-defined stimulus under controlled conditions. But these conditions seldom exist, and therefore, prediction of their reactions is extremely difficult.

Several theories of motivation have been formulated. One of the better known theories is expounded by Maslow and can be described as an *integrated hierarchy of needs* theory.[7] Maslow has labeled his motivational theory a synthesis of holistic-dynamic theories. He borrowed concepts from the functionalist tradition of James and Dewey, fused these with the holistic approach of Wertheimer, Goldstein, and Gestalt psychology, and the dynamics of psychoanalysis of Freud, Jung, and others. Maslow prefaced his theory on sixteen propositions, many of which were self-evident. The essence of these propositions may be abridged and summarized in a few well-chosen statements.

1. An individual functions as an integrated whole and not in parts, and thus his motivations are integrated and not isolated.

2. Hunger is not the paradigm or base for all other motivations even though hunger and the sequential behavior can be readily observed and subjected to experimentation. On closer analysis, hunger is seen as more of a special case of motivation than a general one because it is more isolated.

3. The observed, everyday desires and drives may be only a means to an end, which may not be apparent at all. Underlying motivations may actually exist in the subconscience.

4. There is sufficient evidence to indicate that desires or motivations are conditioned by cultural and environmental factors.

5. There are so many specific desires or motivations which are not of equal force that they cannot be enumerated and placed into mutually exclusive classes or atomistic lists. There are indeed multiple motivations operating sometimes synergistically and sometimes antagonistically.

6. Motivations are interrelated and may be loosely subsumed into categories forming a hierarchy of *needs,* but they cannot be formed into classes of discrete drives. This interrelationship is manifested by the fact that man rarely, if ever, reaches a state of complete satisfaction, except for a very short period of time. At any given time, the need that is manifested depends upon those needs already satisfied. Because some needs are more basic to survival than others, a hierarchy of needs or basic goals may be constructed, keeping in mind that even these goals are perceived in an integrated fashion by an integrated, whole person. This is the holistic approach to psychology and motivation.

7. People's expectation, motivation, and behavior are influenced, and generally limited, by reality and the possibility of attainment of goals. People may behave in a manner that demonstrates maturity and various expressions of self-actualization without any apparent motivation in the conventional sense.

Maslow's theory may be expressed simply as an integrated hierarchy

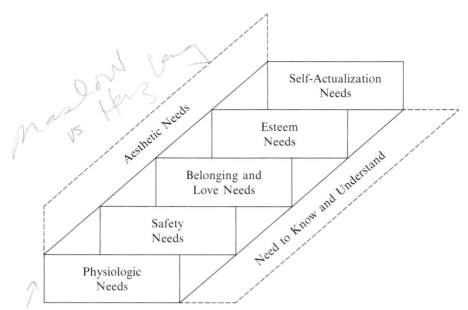

Adapted from Maslow, A., *Motivation and Personality,* 2nd, ed., New York: Harper and Row, 1970.

Figure 8-2. *Motivational Drive Based on a Hierarchy of Needs*

of five basic needs, the satisfaction of which is preconditioned by cognitive impulses, the need to know and understand, and aesthetic needs. This hierarchy is depicted in Figure 8-2.

Physiologic needs form the first order of motivational drives. Satisfaction of the physiologic needs may dominate, but only with total deprivation. When this is the case, hunger is the most prepotent of all, followed by thirst, sexual drive, and other basic physiologic needs.

When the basic physiologic needs are met, higher needs emerge as motivators, and these, rather than physiologic needs, dominate the organism. When these in turn are satisfied, again new and still higher needs emerge, and so on upwardly through the hierarchy of needs. Thus, basic human needs are organized into a hierarchy of relative prepotency.

An implication of this concept is that *gratification* becomes as important as *deprivation* in motivational theory. In a society such as ours, most people are released from the domination of satisfying the relatively-more-basic physiologic needs, permitting thereby the emergence of other goals. A need that is satisfied is no longer a "need" in respect to motivational theory. The organism is dominated and its behavior organized only by unsatisfied needs.

Safety needs may be characterized by security, stability, dependency, protection, freedom from fear, anxiety, and chaos, and the need for structure, order, law, and limits. Under certain conditions, people are dominated by this set of needs, and this may be easily seen in the case of infants. One influence of culture on motivation is that adults are taught to inhibit reactions to the deprivation of safety, that is, to be brave and self-reliant. A broader aspect of seeking safety and security is the common preference for the familiar rather than the unfamiliar and the tendency to fear change and innovations. A highly mature person can cope with and accept change more readily than one less mature.

Third in the hierarchy is the *belonging* and *love needs*. These encompass, in addition to belonging and love, the need to be accepted, to have friends, to have "roots" in a particular location, to belong to the "in-crowd" or class, and comradeship. All of these needs are fulfilled on a two-way basis; you must give to receive. This fact is especially true of love.

Esteem needs consist of two subsidiary sets, namely, *self-esteem* and *esteem of others*. The first includes the desire for strength, for achievement, competency, confidence, independence, and freedom. The second set includes reputation, prestige, respect, recognition, status, attention, importance, dignity, and appreciation. These are powerful motivators, and the thwarting of these needs produces feelings of inferiority, of weakness, and of helplessness. These feelings, in turn, give rise to either basic discouragement or else compensatory or neurotic tendencies.

Self-actualization is the pinnacle of the hierarchy of motivational needs; it is the desire for self-fulfillment. A person *must* do what he *can best* do if he is to fulfill himself and be true to his real nature. Putting square pegs in round holes, as it were, is a weakness of our bureaucratic society, as described in *The Peter Principle*.[5] The emergence of these needs and their fulfillment usually proceeds after satisfying the other basic needs. However, a good administrator or manager must always strive to provide this means of motivation. Herein lies the real payoff in productivity and efficiency. To do less is to cheat the manager, his organization, and most of all, his subordinates.

Maslow sees the *noble concepts,* which might better be called precepts, such as freedom to seek knowledge and express oneself, freedom to do what one wishes to do as long as it does not bring harm to others, justice, honesty, and orderliness in the group as preconditions for satisfying the basic needs. Thwarting these freedoms is a threat to a person and will produce emergency reactions. These freedoms are defended because, without them, the basic needs satisfaction is quite impossible, or at least, severely endangered. These conditions are not ends in themselves, but they are almost so, since they are so closely related to the basic needs.

In addition to the prerequisite, functional role of the desire to know and understand, Maslow postulates a positive, inherent impulse to behave in this manner. He bases his case on observations of the behavior of lower animals which cannot be explained by normal animal instinct patterns, by historic facts, and by many clinical cases of psychopathology. He strongly suggests that one must guard against the tendency to separate the desires to know, to be curious, and to understand from the basic needs. The same caution is given for dichotomizing cognitive and conative needs. It seems more logical to assign the need to know and understand as a simple extension of the need for self-actualization. The same is true of the aesthetics needs. To pursue these needs is to fulfill oneself more completely, to become a whole person.

The model adopted from Maslow's original five basic needs theory has been criticized by some as being too simplistic on the one hand and too complex on the other, especially the highest level of self-actualization. Some of the criticism arose before the publication of the second edition of his book.[7] For example, McFarland states the "first level needs are satisfied before going to the next level."[8] This is an oversimplification based on Maslow's first edition of *Motivation and Personality,*[9] rather than an appropriate interpretation of either edition. Maslow's theory has much support from the research of Argyris,[10] McGregor,[11] Whyte,[12] and Porter.[13] Maslow's theory provides a much deeper understanding of personality and motivation, and his model (Fig. 8-2) provides a tool for supervisors in personnel relations, especially for motivation.

The skeptics of Maslow's theory include Sayles,[14] Herzberg,[15] and Vroom.[16] Sayles views the concept of self-actualization permeated with too much value judgment, reflecting a moral judgment as to how people ought to behave, and not directly connected with organizational life. Herzberg, in his motivation-hygiene theory, divides all motivating factors into two categories as shown in Figure 8-3. One category is job-related, which he calls hygienic factors or dissatisfiers, and the second category contains the job-content factors, which he labels motivators or satisfiers. Further elaboration on the theory and supporting research is given in *Work and the Nature of Man.*[17]

Herzberg's basic work,[15] which consisted of in-depth interview of 200 engineers and accountants, produced the data from which he derived his *motivation-hygiene* model. The subjects were asked first about specific events on the job that produced job satisfaction and positive feelings, and then about those events that produced job dissatisfaction or negative feelings. All events had to meet five objective criteria to be used. The responses were analyzed and coded, and from the coded data, five motivating factors (satisfiers) and five hygienic factors (dissatisfiers) emerged. The length of each bar in Figure 8-3 represents the relative frequency with which the factor was identified among the events as presented in the interviews. Herzberg included another dimension, which is not represented in Figure 8-3, namely the duration of the good or bad feeling representing the motivators and hygienic factors, respectively. *Short duration* was defined as two weeks or less: *long duration* was defined in

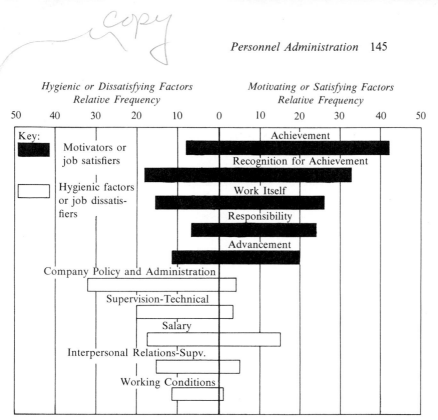

Adapted from Herzberg, F. et. al.: *The Motivation to Work*. New York: John Wiley & Sons, 1959.

Figure 8-3. *Comparison of Motivating and Hygienic Factors*

terms of months or even years. In general, the events that produce satisfaction among all ten factors were of longer duration than those that produce dissatisfaction. The exceptions apparently were recognition for achievement, salary, and perhaps working conditions. Overall, the dissatisfiers produced short-term change in job attitudes and the converse was true of the satisfiers.

Herzberg explained the functional basis of the dissatisfiers or hygienic factors surrounding the job as man's need to avoid pain and discomfort. He related this to the Adamic concept of humanity—the curse placed on man to work and earn his livelihood. In contrast, the motivating factors inherent in work itself and the closely related factors represent a need to achieve and receive recognition for it. This is the Abrahamic concept of humanity in which man feels the need to realize his full potential and grow psychologically.

Based on these two concepts, Herzberg's basic model consists of a two-dimensional need structure: (1) a need system to avoid unpleasantness, and (2) a parallel need system for personal, psychologic growth. While these concepts are not wholly incompatible with Maslow's holistic-dynamic motivational theory, Maslow could hardly accept the dichotomization and compartmentalization of Herzberg's hygienic and motivating factors.

Herzberg's theory has been criticized on the basis that it is technique-bound, that is, the results can be confirmed only if identical methods of research are used. Another criticism is that the responses represent a defensive mechanism of the respondents. These criticisms have some validity, but the criticisms can be explained for the most part.[18] Herzberg's model does provide a practical tool for supervision and motivation primarily because the model is expressed in terms of the job situation.

Herzberg's theory of motivation has been subjected to a considerable number of tests. Allen found the theory applicable to employees of commercial banks.[19] Myers reported that the Herzberg theory held to varying degrees for several occupational groupings—engineers, female assembly line workers, hourly technicians, manufacturing supervisors, and scientists—at the Texas Instrument Company.[20] The company researchers followed up on these findings and as a result, restructured its personnel administration plan to fit the motivation-maintenance theory. Again the Herzberg findings were replicated in public utility firms,[21] a large multi-unit corporation,[22] the Armed Forces,[23] and a large manufacturer.[24]

Vroom has surveyed and analyzed in depth the significant research on motivation.[25] He is critical of Herzberg and related studies on three points. He states the research methods were neither correlational nor experimental in design. He claims the researchers' interpretation of the data was not the only possible one. Finally, he doubts the ability of the subjects to report accurately the conditions causing satisfaction or dissatisfaction, and says that such responses could be the result of a defensive mechanism.

Vroom has evolved his own motivational model based on his own and other research.[26] In Vroom's model a person's choices between alternate courses of action are hypothesized to depend on the relative strength of motivational forces. The relative strength, in turn, was measured by the product of two factors: (1) degree of preference for a particular outcome or result, designated as the *valence;* and (2) the expectancy of the particular outcome or result expressed as a *probability.*

While Vroom's theory stands as one of the leading theories of motivation, its application in practice is severely limited. Herzberg's model provides a better framework for everyday practice. Working conditions, company policy, interpersonal relations, salary, and fringe benefits will prevent employees from becoming dissatisfied, because these are expected in modern society. In contrast, recognition, opportunity to achieve, responsibility, advancement, and work itself will motivate the employees to greater efforts. However, those factors consisting of items of short duration must be repeated more frequently to achieve the objective.

There is no question as to the importance of motivation. Proper motivation effectively eliminates disciplinary problems and makes control of an organization a relatively easy matter.

Staffing Requirements

Since payroll is the single largest expense item and employee wages are variable expenses, pharmacists should be interested in any means of determining the appropriate level of personnel staffing. Queueing theory provides a model by which this can be done.[27]

QUEUEING THEORY MODEL

The queueing theory model may be used to determine the optimum number of personnel for servicing any station at which people may wait to be served on a first-come/first-served basis. Barber shops, telephone switchboards, checkout lanes, and prescription departments are examples of places where the model can be used. The model requires four factors or characteristics.

1. A pattern of probability distribution of the arrivals at the station.

2. A probability distribution associated with the time required to serve the individual.

3. The queue or waiting line (although people do not have to wait in line, only wait their turn) may be organized on a first-come/first-served, or on a random basis. (If a person has to wait too long, he will balk or go to another place for services.)

4. There may be multiple channels for service, but the model requires only one channel of service even though several people can work simultaneously at the station. The number of arrivals must exceed the number served during the period when the theory is applied.

With certain assumptions about these factors, it is possible to apply the theory and determine the behavior of the queue at a prescription department.

First, the arrivals occur in a random pattern within a time unit and the probability of an arrival is independent of the number of arrivals in the previous or the next unit of time. Such a distribution is known as a Poisson distribution or process. It is assumed that the number of prescriptions dispensed per unit of time is also a Poisson distribution. Therefore, the number of arrivals and the number of people served during one hour have no effect on the arrivals or service rate during any other hour; thus, the service rate, which is the reciprocal of the average service time is also independent. Another assumption is that patients will accept service on a first-come/first-served basis. Lastly, the assumption is made that the number of arrivals of prescriptions and the dispensing (service rate) of same are from an infinite universe. This is true in the theoretical sense.

The queueing theory model may be expressed mathematically in the following formula.

$$E_n = \frac{A^2}{S(S-A)}$$

where: E_n = The expected number in the queue

A = the average number patrons arriving per unit of time

S = the average number of prescriptions dispensed per unit of time;

then

$$E_w = \frac{E_n}{A}$$

where: E_w = the expected waiting time in the queue in hours.

APPLICATION OF THE MODEL

Huffman used the queueing model to determine the optimum staffing pattern for a prescription department.[28] The study was conducted during 1969 and 1970 as a part of a doctoral research project and later published by the American College of Apothecaries.[29]

In Huffman's study, the days were segmented by hours, Monday through Saturday, and the average number of prescription arrivals for each hour was computed over a four-week period. The data are replicated in part in Table 8-1.

The average dispensing (service) time was calculated from random sampling of time periods for the existing staffing pattern. It was found that a pharmacist working by himself averaged 6 minutes to dispense a prescription and perform all related paper and clerical work. This time also included other duties such as answering the telephone, if they interfered with the dispensing process. One pharmacist and one clerk reduced the dispensing time to 4.3 minutes; two pharmacists and one clerk, 2.7 minutes, and two pharmacists and two clerks, 2.4 minutes. The respective service rates were 10, 14, 22, and 25 prescriptions per hour, respectively.

Two cost factors enter into the calculation when the model is used. One is the cost of service and the other is the waiting cost. The latter is based on the theory that patients will wait only so long before going to another pharmacy. If a patient waits only five minutes, there is usually little or no consequence. If a patient has to wait for one hour or more, the consequence will be substantial and the patient will probably patronize another pharmacy.

Table 8-1. *Average Number of Prescription Arrivals by Days and Hours*

Time	Mon.	Tues.	Wed.	Thurs.	Fri.	Sat.	4 wk. avg.
8–9 a.m.	4.5	5.0	3.5	3.5	5.0	5.0	4.4
9–10 a.m.	7.0	6.5	12.0	5.5	8.0	16.0	9.2
10–11 a.m.	15.0	18.5	18.0	14.0	16.5	23.0	17.5
11–12	23.0	21.5	22.0	23.5	23.0	22.0	22.5
12–1 p.m.	15.0	16.0	12.5	12.0	12.0	16.5	14.0
1–2 p.m.	11.0	8.5	9.5	5.5	9.0	5.0	8.1
2–3 p.m.	10.0	8.0	13.5	5.0	9.5	4.0	7.7
3–4 p.m.	8.0	11.5	9.0	5.0	11.0	3.0	7.9
4–5 p.m.	5.0	5.0	8.0	5.0	8.0	1.0	5.3
5–6 p.m.	2.0	4.0	2.5	1.0	3.0	1.0	2.3
6–6:30 p.m.	1.0	1.0	1.0	0.5	1.5	0.5	1.0

Adapted from Huffman, D. C.: The Feasibility of Modern Managerial Systems and Innovative Professional Services in a Community Pharmacy. A Case Study. Dissertation. University of Mississippi, University, Miss., 1970.

In the 1969 Huffman study, the following costs were assigned: pharmacists' service @ $5.00 per hour, clerks' service @ $1.50 per hour, and waiting cost @ $10.00 per hour. (The latter figure is a rather subjective one.) However, more realistic figures for the current market would be $7.50 per hour for pharmacist(s), $2.50 per hour for clerks, and $20.00 per hour for the waiting cost. Calculations using the queueing theory model and the more current cost data indicate that one pharmacist working alone can dispense as many as six prescriptions per hour most economically. One pharmacist and one clerk can handle 7 to 11 prescriptions, two pharmacists and one clerk can handle 12 to 18, and two pharmacists and two clerks can dispense 19 or more per hour.

A few calculations will illustrate how the queueing theory model operates in determining staffing patterns. Suppose 13 prescriptions arrive during a given hour quite regularly and the average number of arrivals for that hour is 13. "A" equals 13 with one pharmacist and one clerk and "S," the service rate, is 14; with two pharmacists and one clerk, "S" is 22. Using one pharmacist and one clerk, the total costs are:

$$E_n = \frac{13^2}{14\,(14 - 13)} = \frac{169}{14} = 12.07$$

$$E_w = \frac{12.07}{13} = 0.928 \text{ hour (waiting time)}$$

Service Cost + Waiting Cost = Total Cost

$$\$7.50 + \$2.50 + 0.928 \times \$20.00 = \$29.56$$

Using two pharmacists and one clerk, the total costs are

$$E_n = \frac{13^2}{22\,(22-13)} = \frac{169}{198} = 0.85$$

$$E_w = \frac{0.85}{13} = 0.065 \text{ hour}$$

Service Cost + Waiting Cost = Total Cost

$\$15.00 + \$2.50 + 0.065 \times \$20.00 = \$18.80$

The conclusion is obvious. Two pharmacists should be employed.

Sometimes the difference in total costs is so small that the pharmacist must use judgement in deciding the number and type of personnel. An example of this is the arrival of 12 prescriptions per hour. The pharmacist must decide whether to staff one pharmacist and one clerk or two pharmacists and one clerk. The respective total costs are $18.56 and $18.60—only 4 cents difference! Since this situation usually occurs near the noon hour and the pharmacist will probably favor ample time for patient consultation, he should decide to employ two pharmacists and one clerk.

A study of Table 8-1 indicates that a pharmacist alone can operate the prescription department between hours of 8 to 9 a.m. and 5 to 6:30 p.m. He can also handle the prescription department all of Saturday afternoon. Other considerations also enter into staffing decisions such as work other than direct service to the patrons. Other such work may include stocking shelves, taking inventory on stock record cards (if they are used), rearranging merchandise and displays. These activities are usually done during "slow" periods when few patrons are being served by the prescription department. As a practical matter, a clerk or prescription assistant will normally be present all the time.

The queueing theory model is applicable during the peak period, 9 a.m. to 4 p.m. in this case, when a decision on staffing is critical. Additionally, Kitler and Lamey have reported the potential use of queueing theory to a hospital pharmacy.[30]

Summary

The importance of good personnel cannot be overemphasized. Although purchases represent the largest expenditure, they are an investment that can be recovered if the purchases have been restricted to salable goods. Payroll is the second largest expenditure and the largest single expense item in a typical pharmacy. In contrast to inventory investment, money spent on payroll is gone forever once the checks are written. Only through efficient and effective employees can one hope to reap a return from the money spent on wages and salaries and to achieve business and professional objectives. All phases of employee administration are important, including selection, pleasant working conditions, supervision, compensation, and motivation. A wise proprietor or manager will do well to practice good personnel management.

REFERENCES

1. Slavin, G. F., Jr.: *The Lilly Digest 1972, a Survey of Community Pharmacy Operations for 1971.* Indianapolis: Eli Lilly and Co., p. 7.
2. *38th Annual Nielsen Review of Retail Drug Store Trends.* Chicago: A. C. Nielsen Co., 1971, pp. 7, 8.
3. *NACDS Executive Newsletter.* July 16, 1973.
4. Eiler, L. E., et al.: *Policies and Operational Procedures for Community Pharmacy Managers.* Memphis: American College of Apothecaries, 1972.
5. Peter, L. J.: *The Peter Principle.* New York: William Morrow & Co., 1969.
6. Both books are available in paperback edition published by Bantam Books, Inc.
7. Maslow, A.: *Motivation and Personality.* 2nd ed., New York: Harper and Brothers, 1970.
8. McFarland, D. E.: *Personnel Management: Theory and Practice.* New York: The Macmillan Co., 1968, p. 382.
9. Maslow, A.: *op. cit.,* 1st ed., 1954.
10. Argyris, C.: *Understanding Organizational Behavior.* Homewood, Ill.: The Dorsey Press, 1960.
11. McGregor, D.: *The Human Side of Enterprise.* New York: McGraw-Hill, 1960.
12. Whyte, W. H.: *The Organization Man.* New York: Simon and Schuster, 1956.
13. Porter, L. W.: *Organizational Patterns of Managerial Job Attitudes.* New York: American Foundation for Management Research, 1964.
14. Sayles, L. R.: *Individualism and Big Business.* New York: McGraw-Hill, 1963.
15. Herzberg, F., et al.: *The Motivation to Work.* New York: John Wiley & Sons, Inc., 1959.
16. Vroom, V.: *Work and Motivation.* New York: John Wiley & Sons, Inc., 1964.
17. Herzberg, F.: *Work and the Nature of Man.* Cleveland: The World Publishing Co., 1966.
18. *Ibid.,* pp. 130, 131.
19. Allen, G. R.: Testing Herzberg's Motivation-Maintenance Theory in Commercial Banks. Unpublished doctoral dissertation, Arizona State University, 1967.
20. Myers, M. S.: Who are your motivated workers? *Harvard Business Review, 42*:73–87, 1966.
21. Schwartz, M. M., et al.: Motivational factors among supervisors in the utility industry. *Personnel Psychology, 16*:45–53, 1963.
22. Schwartz, P.: *Attitudes of Middle Management Personnel.* Pittsburgh: American Institute for Research, 1959.
23. Hahn, D.: Dimensions of Job Satisfaction and Career Motivation. *In* Schwartz, *ibid.*
24. Gibson, J. W.: Sources of Job Satisfaction and Job Dissatisfaction as Interpreted from Analyses of Write-in Responses. Doctoral Dissertation, Western Reserve University, 1961.
25. Vroom, V.: *Work and Motivation.* New York: John Wiley & Sons, Inc., 1964.
26. *Ibid.,* pp. 126–129.
27. Spur, W. A., and Bonim, C. P.: *Statistical Analysis for Business Decisions.* Homewood: Richard D. Irwin, Inc., 1967, pp. 403–411.

28. Huffman, D. C., Jr.: *The Feasibility of Modern Managerial Systems and Innovative Professional Services in a Community Pharmacy: A Case Study.* A Doctoral Dissertation, The University of Mississippi, January, 1971.
29. Huffman, D. C., and Smith, H. A.: *Building a Successful Pharmacy Practice: A Case Study.* Memphis: American College of Apothecaries, 1972.
30. Kitler, M., and Lamey, P.: Statistics in hospital pharmacy. *Hospital Pharmacy, 4*:17–21, July, 1969.

REVIEW

1. Discuss the three reasons for emphasizing the importance of personnel administration.

2. Discuss the application of management by objectives to personnel relations, especially supervision, by relating the benefits accruing to both employees and the organization.

3. What are the six *principles* of good personnel administration?

4. Discuss the five major aspects of personnel administration procedures.

5. Define and differentiate between job analysis, job description, and job specification.

6. Describe the four steps in the employee selection process.

7. Explain why the selection process is so critical.

8. Explain the "halo" and "horn" effects and how these influence the selection process.

9. Explain the purpose, importance and basic objectives of orientation of a new employee in a pharmacy.

10. Distinguish between training and educating as it relates to employees in a pharmacy.

11. Distinguish between the two types of training methods.

12. Outline the steps of on-the-job training.

13. Discuss the purpose and use of the conference in employee training and development.

14. Discuss the importance and the role of supervision.

15. Explain the importance of motivation and why motivation is the most difficult aspect of employee relations.

16. Discuss the philosophic basis of Maslow's theory of motivation.

17. Discuss the philosophic basis of Herzberg's theory of motivation and contrast it with Maslow's theory.

18. What were the terms used by Maslow and Herzberg, respectively, to designate their theories of motivation.

19. Contrast the application of the respective models derived from Maslow's and Herzberg's motivational theories.

20. Name the primary methods of evaluating employees, and contrast the two in terms of objectivity, value, and difficulty of implementation.

21. Which of the above means of employee evaluation is better adapted to a system of management by objectives?

22. What are the eight principles of employee evaluation?

23. What are the four methods of employee compensation and the relative merits and disadvantages of each?

24. Describe the types of pharmacies covered by the 1966, 1969, and 1974 Amendments of the Federal Fair Labor Act (minimum wage and hours aspects of the law).

25. Discuss the relationship between MBO and good personnel administration.

26. Discuss the theory and the rationale underlying the queueing theory model.

27. For various average prescription arrivals—5, 7, 11, 14, 18 and 20—calculate the total cost of service and waiting.

9. Purchasing

Good purchasing policies and inventory control are closely interrelated because one cannot be effective without the other. Without the information provided by some type of inventory control system, it is difficult to buy the correct quantities. Conversely, inventory control procedures are of little value unless the information generated is used to determine appropriate quantities to buy. The best policy is to reinforce good purchasing policies and procedures with a good inventory control system, the subject of Chapter 10.

There is an old saying among retailers, including pharmacists, "goods well bought are half sold." Certainly there is much validity in this saying, and pharmacists who neglect the buying function operate under a severe handicap. An extension of this saying is that goods not well purchased cannot be profitably sold. There is another old saying among retailers and pharmacists as well that says "you buy yourself poor and sell yourself rich." Certainly a balance between these two points of view is the best policy.

The specific functions of purchasing are: (1) formulating effective buying policies; (2) determining the demands or desires of the patrons; (3) selecting the best sources of supply; (4) determining and negotiating the terms of purchase; (5) receiving, marking, and stocking merchandise; and (6) transferring the title of the goods, including payment in time to receive maximum discounts.

Formulating Effective Buying Policies

There are *two basic considerations* in formulating buying policies.

1. Buying policies should be *compatible with the general objectives of the pharmacy,* which, in turn, are determined largely by the type of pharmacy and location. For example, a pharmaceutical center stocks fewer merchandise lines, and probably a lesser assortment of merchandise in each line, than a traditional pharmacy. Similarly a traditional pharmacy carries fewer merchandise lines, and a lesser assortment within each line, than a super drugstore. Pharmaceutical companies normally close their books a few days before the end of the month, and the efficient manager places monthly orders just in time for them to arrive at the manufacturer's office on the first day or so of each new discount period.

2. *Needs and desires of the patrons* must be recognized. Obviously, there is an interrelationship between these two basic considerations. The type of pharmacy practice has a substantial influence on the patrons it attracts. The needs and desires of the patrons in a particular market should be the basis for establishing a particular type of pharmacy. The buying policies should reflect basic changes in demographic factors such as age distribution, young families with children, and purchase preference and buying habits caused by both demographic and economic factors.

Determining the Needs and Desires of Patrons

The needs and demands of patrons of a pharmaceutical center or apothecary shop are determined primarily by the prescribers' preferences, which in turn are determined by the prevalence of disease entities, the drugs available to treat these diseases, and the promotional efforts of the producers of these drugs. However, it remains for the proprietor to determine whether certain needs, such as home health care aids and surgical appliances, are to be met. The latter consideration has more relevancy for the traditional pharmacy that stocks rather wide assortments and lines of merchandise, and is even more significant to the super merchandising pharmacy.

Where does the proprietor or manager of a pharmacy find the information on kinds, types, and prices of goods his patrons and potential patrons want? The primary sources are outlined below:[1]

A. Inside sources (in the pharmacy)
  1. Past sale trends by departments and/or lines
  2. Returned goods and adjustment data
  3. Patrons' inquiries—want slip or want book
  4. Suggestions of employees

B. Outside sources
  1. Salesmen's offerings and suggestions
  2. Trade journals and magazines
  3. Survey of patrons' desires and needs
  4. National and local advertisements of manufacturers
  5. Offerings of other pharmacies
  6. Large merchandise marts

Selecting the Sources of Supply

There are basically two kinds of sources of supply, *direct* and *indirect* through either a wholesaler or jobber. A jobber is a wholesaler with limited services and usually limited lines. Before discussing the obvious advantages and disadvantages of each source of supply, we should consider certain similarities and basic marketing functions. These similarities can best be described within the framework of the basic marketing functions, which are outlined below.

A. Exchange function
  1. Buying
  2. Selling
B. Physical supply function
  1. Storage
  2. Transportation
C. Facilitating or Ancillary functions
  1. Standardization and grading
  2. Financing
  3. Risk-bearing
  4. Market information and research, and related services

UNIVERSALITY OF MARKETING FUNCTIONS

Careful consideration of the above functions points to the fact that all of these functions must be performed, if not by the wholesaler, then by either the manufacturer or the pharmacy. This concept is known as the universality of marketing functions. For example, if a manufacturer decides to do all of its marketing, including functions normally performed by the wholesaler, either the manufacturer or the pharmacy must provide additional storage space and pay for the transportation, and the manufacturer must provide a salesman who, in turn, provides the information about the goods offered for sale. Either the manufacturer or the pharmacy must absorb the cost of these functions. Unless there are economies of scale or other economic efficiencies, the only marketing cost that can be avoided by direct selling is the net profit, or risk cost in Peter Drucker's terminology, of the middleman or wholesaler.

In contrast, the wholesaler provides the intrinsic role of a middleman by which inherent economies accrue to society. The middleman role encompasses three related concepts: minimum total transactions, sorting, and market proximity.

MINIMUM TOTAL TRANSACTIONS

This term is used to describe the reduction of the actual number of transactions involving many sellers (manufacturers) and many buyers (pharmacies). This concept can be explained best by an illustration: If each of 1,000 manufacturers were to process one order for each of 50,000 pharmacies each month—a situation that would not be conducive to best inventory management because of out-of-stock situations and possible overstocking—the total number of annual transactions would be six million.[2]

$$50,000 \times 1,000 \times 12 = 600,000,000$$
(pharmacies)   (manufacturers)   (months)   (no. of annual transactions)

If, on the other hand, we assume there were 250 drug wholesalers who ordered weekly from the 1,000 manufacturers and who, in turn, made daily sales to their "share" of pharmacy customers for 255 working days a year, the total number of transactions would be 25,750,000.

$$250 \times 1,000 \times 52 = 13,000,000$$
(wholesalers)   (manufacturers)   (weeks)

$$250 \times 200 \times 255 = +12,750,000$$
(wholesalers)   (pharmacies per wholesaler)   (days)

$$\text{Total annual transactions} = 25,750,000$$

The number of annual transactions can be reduced to almost 4 percent of the original number with the use of the pharmaceutical wholesalers. If we assume that on the average each of the 200 pharmacies will order from two drug wholesalers (255 days/year) and from 15 manufacturers monthly—a more realistic assumption—the total number of annual transactions would be approximately 60,500,000, or approximately 10 percent of the number of annual transactions without the use of wholesalers. This means a reduction in the cost of billing, bookkeeping and freight, and in the number of errors in billing.

SORTING

Sorting is a marketing term composed of two elements or activities, *concentration* and *dispersion*. This is basically what the wholesaler does.

He buys from thousands of suppliers in relatively large quantities. He may buy from several to many gross of a product at much lower distribution cost than could an individual pharmacy. The wholesaler, in turn, may sell only one or a few units of a product to a pharmacy at a given time, but he combines this order with other items, perhaps one to several dozen products, and again economizes in the distribution process. The distribution cost would be tremendous if each pharmacy had to purchase all of its products directly from the manufacturers.

MARKET PROXIMITY

This marketing term simply means being near to the final market. Market proximity is certainly true of drug wholesalers, and has obvious advantages in providing product and market information faster, more frequent deliveries, and an all-around closer working relationship with customers.

All three of these concepts—minimum number of total annual transactions, sorting, and proximity—are interrelated, and together they permit the wholesaler-middleman to perform his unique role.

To better understand the role of the wholesaler-middleman, the marketing concept, *utility,* which largely is the result of market proximity, will be briefly described. There are four types of utility, viz., *time, place, possession,* and *form utility.* The latter is the result of production or manufacturing, which does not concern us here. The first three types are the result of marketing activities. Simply stated, time, place, and possession utility is defined as providing the right good at the right time to the right person at the right place. Dispensing prescriptions is a special, professional case of marketing utility. Of course, the proper dispensing of a prescription includes much more—the correct directions, checking for appropriate dosages and possible drug interactions, and consultation with the patient. Even these activities fall within the marketing function of market information and related services. Thus, the pharmacist assumes a unique professional as well as marketing role.

SERVICES OF DRUG WHOLESALERS

According to Smith,[3] the pharmaceutical wholesaler provides 14 specific services to drug manufacturers. Of more interest to the pharmacist are the services provided to him, many of which are related to those provided to the manufacturers.

Assembly of Goods. The wholesaler has at his disposal trained and experienced buyers who can, and do, purchase and maintain extensive inventories in knowledgeable anticipation of the pharmacist's needs.

Delivery. Not only is regular delivery service available, but a 1962 study showed that more than half of the members of the NWDA maintained separate, more frequent delivery schedules for prescription drugs.[4]

Credit. The value of credit to retailers has already been explored in a previous chapter. This simply means an expansion of working capital for the pharmacist.

Special Services. The pharmaceutical wholesaler has historically provided, free of charge, a number of services to the community pharmacist which are only indirectly related to the product itself. Past and present services of this type include: prescription drug information services, store layout and design, store modernization, location analysis, and traffic-flow analysis.

DIRECT VS. INDIRECT PURCHASING

Table 9-1 compares the advantages and disadvantages of purchasing from the pharmaceutical wholesaler or directly from the manufacturer under normal conditions.

To select the best source of supply one needs to assess all the advantages and disadvantages. If the saving in extra discounts warrants direct purchasing, it is wise to buy in this way. This decision can be made with greater accuracy after studying the economic order quantity phase of inventory control. In general, the typical pharmacy can purchase advan-

Table 9-1. *Sources of Supply*

Item	Purchased From	
	Manufacturer	*Wholesaler*
Inventory size	Larger	Smaller
Turnover rate	Less	Greater
Delivery	Slower; less frequent	Faster; more frequent
Return of goods	More difficult	Less difficult
Availability of goods	Only source for certain lines	Only source for certain lines theoretically
Time involved in ordering	More overall	Less overall
Product information	More complete; possible bias	Less complete; less bias
Available credit	Readily in most cases	Readily if not in default
Cost of handling	More	Less
Cost of product	Lower	Higher

tageously from about 15 to 20 prescription drug manufacturers and about the same number of "out front" manufacturers, including the franchise lines. The remainder of the products should be purchased from one wholesaler primarily, using a second "back-up" wholesaler on a scale to keep him interested in servicing your pharmacy as needed.

COOPERATIVE BUYING GROUPS

Another source of supply, which has become more popular in recent years, is the cooperative buying group. Competition and the profit squeeze have caused pharmacists to forgo some of their independence and form buying groups to survive. Some of these groups have been initiated by drug wholesalers, others by pharmacists. Some restrict their cooperative efforts to buying whereas others include promotion and advertising.

The increasing importance of cooperative buying groups in pharmacy, and even the greater potential they offer the independent practice of pharmacy, warrant more than a passing view of this development. The following discussion of cooperative buying groups is based on a paper by George Grider.[5]

For the past decade the drug trade literature and drug wholesale houses have been discussing the problems and dark future of the independent pharmacist. For several years the National Wholesale Druggists Association (NWDA) and the Federal Wholesale Druggist Association (FWDA) have told the drug wholesaler to develop voluntary chains for the community pharmacist. Not one wholesaler has developed a complete, voluntary chain of group buying and group advertising on a scale comparable to the grocery wholesalers. The independent retail grocery co-op chain and the wholesaler-directed voluntary chain of independent grocery stores realize more than 50 percent of the retail food dollar volume today, whereas 20 years ago they were selling only 30 percent of the retail food volume in this country. They are providing their members with lower prices through group buying and furnishing them an advertising program. Thirty years ago the independent grocery stores were at a crossroad similar to that of community pharmacies today; food chains were rapidly forcing the independent grocery stores out of business, just as the chain drugstores are making it difficult for the community pharmacy to compete in the marketplace today.

Today drug wholesalers are merging, computerizing, offering record-keeping and inventory control service, push-button ordering service, line extension discounts, and across-the-board special discounts to some pharmacies. If the number of community pharmacies continues to decline at the present rate, the drug wholesalers' computer service, push-button ordering service, bookkeeping and inventory control service, and line extension discounts may be of little use.

Some say the pharmacist is too independent and will not join with his fellow pharmacist to form a buying group or voluntary chain. However, there are hundreds of community pharmacies that are members of buying groups and advertising groups, including McKesson and Robbins Economost, a computerized accounting and inventory service as well as a buying and advertising group; Rite-Way Discount System, a Chicago based advertising and marketing firm; Leader Advertising Group in the Cleveland area; and Kentucky Drug Stores, a buying and advertising group in Kentucky.

The purpose of a pharmacy buying group is to promote the economic welfare of independent community pharmacies by utilizing their united efforts for efficient and economical distribution through buying and advertising of products sold in the members' pharmacies. In plain language, it is a large number of pharmacies combining their purchases in order to buy merchandise at the lowest possible price for each member. This is accomplished through a membership organization that may be either a stock corporation or a non-profit corporation.

The next logical question is: how can pharmacists organize a buying group? Following is a brief discussion of how the Kentucky Drug Stores buying group was organized. Originally, five pharmacy owners formed a nonprofit corporation and this corporation contracted with Kentucky Food Stores, a Lexington based grocery buying group of 105 members, to purchase, warehouse, and deliver merchandise to their pharmacies. Next, a manager was selected who had several years of experience as a salesman for a major drug wholesale company and five years of experience in pharmacy layout and design. His job was to help the group to increase its membership and set up the warehouse operation. He was paid a good salary, absolutely necessary if the buying group is going to be successful. The manager for the Drug Store Division was placed in charge of the buying and warehouse operation of the Drug Division and fixture installation for both the drug and grocery divisions. The Kentucky Food Stores' warehouse stocked all types of drugstore merchandise except prescription legend drugs. A contract was negotiated with a full-line drug wholesaler to supply the member pharmacies with prescription legend drugs and other merchandise that was not stocked in the Kentucky Food Stores.

The price of merchandise is the same to each member and is calculated by using actual cost of the merchandise, plus 5 percent operational and warehouse cost, plus 3 percent for transportation. To reduce the net cost of merchandise and operational cost, Kentucky Drug Stores and Kentucky Food Stores buy merchandise and warehouse and deliver it on an integrated basis. Pharmacies with fountains can buy their fountain supplies from the grocery group at a 20 to 30 percent saving. Pharmacy members order once a week and pay for the merchandise the following week. A computer system of purchasing, invoicing, and billing is used for both divisions. An advertising specialist serves both groups on a combined contractual basis for developing advertising, printing of hand-bills, and painting of purchase and window signs.

To finance the pharmacy buying group, each member bought $3,000.00 in Kentucky Drug Stores stock. There are no monthly dues or initiation fees. If a member sells his pharmacy or desires to leave the buying group, Kentucky Drug Stores will buy his stock in the corporation and pay him the original purchase price.

Economics was the basic reason the Kentucky Drug Stores co-op group joined the Kentucky Food Stores. Since Kentucky Food Stores already had an organization, a warehouse, delivery trucks, a computer, and expertise in cooperative group buying, it was patently uneconomical to duplicate these facilities. The Kentucky Food Stores group was happy to have the Kentucky Drug Stores group join them, because this increased their efficiency and productivity simply through economy of scale. The joint venture reduced the initial investment and risk for Kentucky Drug Stores.

Mr. Goodwin Rosen, managing director of National Drug Coopera-tives Associated, an organization of drug cooperatives, franchises, volun-tary chains, and wholesalers from coast to coast, states that the only way for the independent community pharmacy to compete with the chain drugstores is to belong to a buying group or a wholesaler sponsored co-op. Mr. Rosen's organization is composed of 13 cooperative groups in various parts of the country, representing 1,650 independently owned pharmacies.

According to Mr. Rosen, some of the advantages of buying groups are as follows: (1) maximum discounts available through quantity buying; (2) advertising and promotional programs at a much lower cost; (3) special merchandise shows provided for members; (4) the remodeling and in-stallation of pharmacies at savings from 40 to 50 percent; (5) exchange of ideas among members; (6) consulting service providing new methods and techniques of pharmacy operation, in such areas as inventory control, management, financing, individual advertising and promotions, and sales schools for clerks; (7) computer service provided for individual members; and (8) development of a group logo for advertising and pharmacy identification, while the individual member retains his individual phar-macy name.

Buying groups are of great value to the independent pharmacy de-siring a chain store image and, through group buying and advertising, this can become a reality. For those who do not want a chain store image, the buying group will produce a significant increase in profit on mer-chandise purchased from the group warehouse.

SPECIALTY WHOLESALERS

There are other sources of supply that nearly all pharmacists use, depending on the scope of the operation. These are the specialty wholesalers, usually relatively small wholesalers dealing in a limited line of merchandise, but with wide assortments within these lines. Sometimes special services, especially assistance in inventory control, are provided. Examples include veterinary drug wholesalers, tobacco or tobacco and confectionary wholesalers, costume jewelry and gift merchandise wholesalers, suppliers of photography equipment, and leather goods wholesalers. These specialty wholesalers can be of tremendous assistance in the development of special skills departments within a pharmacy.

Determining the Terms of Purchase

The terms of purchase include several important items that are not as generally known as they should be. The significance of the terms is too frequently taken for granted until some misunderstanding develops. The major points in terms of sale include discounts of various kinds, the date payment is due, policy on credit extension, and return of good policy.

Manufacturers' catalogues contain this information, usually in the front portion of the catalogue. Pharmaceutical wholesalers make this information readily available on request. Invoices contain a large portion of this information as a formal part of the sales contract. In this respect, each transaction, whether a $500 drug order or the sale of a ten cent bar of candy, is a sales contract, and every written, spoken, or *implied* bit of information that has any bearing on the consummation of the sale is a part of a binding contract.

DISCOUNTS

Discounts are probably the most frequently discussed aspect of the terms of a sale. Buyers are constantly wanting larger discounts. This is natural and commendable; however, buying the right merchandise that will sell, or the proper quantity of merchandise, can be much more important than a large discount or lower price.

Trade Discounts. There are several kinds of discounts, and each should be understood in terms of its intended purpose. The *trade* (or *functional*) *discount* is given to a firm for performing a level or set of marketing activities. Wholesaling and retailing are examples of marketing levels. The trade discount is not well understood because it is not used directly as frequently as the other types. The trade discount is based on a base line figure known as the *list price,* which is falling into disuse. Some firms use a list price that corresponds to the "suggested" retail or consumer price, while others use what is called a wholesale list price, which confuses the matter. The choice of the type of list price used depends partly on the custom of a particular company and the policy of favoring direct buying by the pharmacist or selling through the wholesaler. A trade discount for a drug wholesaler normally ranges from 15 to 20 percent; for a pharmacy it ranges from 30 to 50 percent. An illustration will explain the two approaches:

Company A sells only through a wholesaler. The catalogue for a drug in a bottle of 100 tablets shows a "retail list" price of $10.00. The pharmacy is given a trade discount of 40 percent and the wholesaler a trade discount of 20 percent. The pharmacist pays the wholesaler $6.00 per hundred [$10.00 − (.40 × $10.00)]. The wholesaler pays the manufacturer $5.80 [$6.00 − (.20 × $6.00)].

In contrast, Company B has a direct selling policy. For a similar drug, costing about the same to manufacture and to market, the company's catalogue shows a "wholesale list" price of $7.00, with a "direct purchase" discount of 15 percent. The pharmacist can buy the drug for $5.95 per hundred [$7.00 − (.15 × $7.00)]. The wholesaler can buy the same drug at a 20 percent "wholesaler's" discount for $5.60 [$7.00 − (.20 × $7.00)]. The wholesaler has to sell the drug to the pharmacist for $6.60 just to break even or make a very small profit. The operational cost of a full-line drug wholesaler ranges from 13 to 15 percent of sales. The economic pressure for the pharmacist to buy direct from Company B is obvious. Trade discounts generally are exclusive of other types of discounts.

Quantity Discounts. Quantity discounts are given when a designated quantity is purchased at one time or when a cumulative dollar volume is purchased over a specified period of time, usually one year. The discount normally ranges from 5 to 20 percent of a base line or quoted "list" price. These discounts are offered to both wholesalers and retailers and are based on economies of larger purchases. Sometimes the discount is given in the form of "free" goods. Often the discounts that include "free" goods and "deals" are misleading. A few examples of the various kinds of quantity discounts will illustrate and explain how they differ and are used in practice.

The most frequent type of quantity discount is a percentage discount from the regular price extended for the purchase of a larger single order. For example, a product that normally sells wholesale at $6.00 a dozen may be offered at $6.00 per dozen less 10 percent in quantities of five dozen. Thus the unit cost is $.45 rather than the usual $.50. Again, the cash discount is not considered here, and often the quantity discount will be inclusive of the usual cash discount. If this were the case in the foregoing example, the actual quantity discount would be less than 10 percent, approximately 8 percent. Sometimes the quantity discount is offered if a designated dollar amount is ordered for an assortment of different products from the same manufacturer. For example, a 5 percent quantity discount on a $50.00 order or a 10 percent discount on a $125.00 order is typical.

Some direct-selling pharmaceutical manufacturers provide a quantity discount during an ensuing year provided a quota was met the previous year. The discount may be 5 to 10 percent in addition to the usual 15 percent "trade" discount for direct accounts. As with all discounts in a series, one does not add the 5 percent to the 15 percent to arrive at an overall 20 percent discount. The basic 15 percent discount is first deducted, then the 5 percent discount is deducted. For example, on a $100 order the pharmacist first deducts $15 ($100 × .15) from the $100 and obtains the difference, $85. Next, the pharmacist subtracts $4.25 ($85 × .05) from $85.00 to obtain the net cost of $80.75, if there is no additional cash discount. The terms of sale indicate whether the 5 percent quantity discount includes the cash discount.

A variation of the above example is sometimes used by companies with a wide variety of drugs—some that are not profitable, such as biologicals, some that are very popular with a high turnover rate, and some that are fairly popular, but with a slower turnover rate. These types of products would be classified as A, B, and C with quantity discounts of 5, 10, and 15 percent, respectively.

The "free" goods or "deal" discount can be misleading, as stated previously. A typical example is a 10 percent quantity discount, including the cash discount, plus four "free" bottles of a four-ounce size of cough syrup with the purchase of one dozen of the four-ounce size and one-half dozen of the eight-ounce size. The eight-ounce size sells for $1.69 each and normally costs $1.13 each. The four-ounce size sells for $.98 and normally costs $.65 each. The regular cost of the dozen four-ounce size is $7.80 and the half dozen eight-ounce costs $6.78 for a total of $14.58. The quantity discount is $1.46, giving a net cost of $13.12. The total sales for the entire deal, provided all units are sold, are $25.82, providing a gross margin of $12.70 or 49.2 percent.

Too frequently the advertisement of the "deal" indicates a discount of $1.46 plus $3.92, the retail value of the four free bottles. The total quantity discount is stated as $5.38, or 36.9 percent, off the regular cost of $14.58 for the dozen of the four-ounce size and the half dozen of the eight-ounce size. This is misleading on two accounts. First, the free goods should be valued at the regular wholesale cost and not at the retail value. Second, the free goods should not be considered a discount until they have been sold. If, for example, two of the four free bottles are never sold, the effective extra discount would be $1.30, and the total *effective* quantity discount would be $2.76, or 18.9 percent, off the regular wholesale price.

Cash Discounts. The cash discount is the smallest discount of all, but it is the most important one. A cash discount is given to a buyer for payment within a time period specified on the invoice or statement. The discount is normally 1 or 2 percent of the regular or *net* amount of the invoice or statement. Note that *net* refers to the amount paid after the designated time period and does not include the cash discount.

The importance of the cash discount can be explained best by an illustration. Suppose a pharmacist finds himself in a financial position in which he is unable to pay his statements for merchandise in time to earn the cash discount. Further assume that the pharmacist purchases $10,000 worth of goods each month. The cash discount rate is 2 percent. Under these conditions, he will lose $2,400 over the entire year. This loss can be prevented by borrowing $10,000 from the bank at 10 percent interest. The $1,000 interest, subtracted from the $2,400 gained in cash discounts, yields $1,400 additional profit. If the pharmacy is being managed appropriately in other respects, it should yield approximately $10,000 normal net profit on an annual sales volume of $225,000. The $1,400 additional profit from cash discounts represents a 14 percent increase in the normal net profit of the pharmacy.

The pharmacist can fare even better than this, provided he has both the financial status and expertise to utilize the financial or money market to its fullest extent. Of course, he would have to have an excellent credit rating and be known as a "prime risk debtor" among financial institutions, a reputation he is not likely to enjoy since he is unable to pay his bills. However, for the sake of students' and practitioners' edification, let us assume these possibilities and determine their net effect. Since the pharmacist normally has until the tenth of the month following the month the goods were purchased to earn the cash discount, he could borrow the $10,000 for 20 days at 10 percent. The interest charges would be only $55.55 for the 20-day period ($10,000 × .10 ÷ 360 days × 20 days = $55.55). If the pharmacist astutely generates sufficient cash from cash sales, collecting accounts receivable, and perhaps reducing inventory levels to pay the $55.55 interest charge and 10 percent of the principal, he possibly could have his note renewed on a 20-day basis. This would result in the liquidation of the debt in ten months at a cost of only $555.55 interest charge.

Let us hasten to warn that the typical pharmacist who has gotten behind in paying his invoices is not likely to receive such favorable treatment in the money market. However, a successful pharmacy, a solvent cooperative buying group, or a chain of drugstores that found itself in a temporary, nonrecurring position of not being able to take the cash discounts could well take advantage of a short-term 20-day loan and yield a handsome return for its effort.

Serial Discounts. The term "serial discounts" is used occasionally in explicit language and frequently in an implicit manner. Students and practitioners should know the manner in which such discounts are computed. Some trades use the term as such and state them as 50, 20, and

5. More often in pharmacy, the series is implied and typically will be 40 percent (trade discount), 10 percent (quantity discount), and 2 percent (cash discount). In *neither* case are the discounts *added* and then multiplied by the amount of the invoice. Rather they are multiplied and subtracted in steps, beginning with the largest discount, which is usually listed first. An illustration will explain how serial discounts are computed.

Step 1. $500.00—Net amount of invoice at retail list
        × .40—Trade discount as decimal
       $200.00—Allowance for trade function

Step 2. $500.00
     −200.00
     $300.00
      × .10—Quantity discount
     $ 30.00—Allowance for quantity purchased

Step 3. $300.00
     − 30.00
     $270.00
      × .02—Cash discount
     $ 5.40—Allowance for paying invoice by specified time

Step 4. $270.00
     − 5.40
     $264.60—The amount the pharmacist pays

DATINGS AND CREDIT TERMS

There are a number of terms and notations that pertain to the delivery of goods, date of payment and cash discounts. Collectively, these are usually referred to as "datings." Following are the more common terms with definitions. The last definition is the most common set of cash and dating terms encountered in pharmacy.

AOG or ROG	Arrival of goods or receipt of goods
COD	Collect on delivery
EOM	End of the month
FOB; FOB (city)	Free on board; free on board at designated city
N	Pay the net or full amount
N/30	Pay net 30 days from date of invoice
N/10 EOM	Pay net within 10 days after the end of the month

2/10, N/30	Deduct 2 percent within 10 days after invoice date; otherwise pay net within 30 days after the invoice date
2/10 ROG, N/30	Deduct 2 percent within 10 days after receipt of goods; otherwise pay net within 30 days after receipt of goods
2/10 EOM c̄ 60 extra	Deduct 2 percent within 70 days after the end of the month in which the goods were purchased
2/10 EOM, N/30	Deduct 2 percent cash discount if paid within 10 days after the end of the month; otherwise pay net within 30 days after the end of the month

RETURN GOODS POLICY

Another important sales term is the return goods policy. The pharmaceutical industry is very generous in this respect. Most company catalogues contain a statement on the return of goods in the front of the catalogue as a part of the general statement on policies, credit terms, and the like. There are limitations placed on the return of goods, the most common being broken packages (i.e., a part of the contents has been used); mishandling of stored goods, and a time limitation for credit, usually five years, but this varies with the company. Each pharmacy should have a new product section in the prescription department, and this should be checked weekly. If a new product has not been used in three or four months, it should be returned for credit. To maintain an orderly and efficient goods return system, each pharmacy should build a series of small bins in the stock room with each labeled for the respective manufacturer and wholesaler from whom the goods were purchased. All return goods—wrong merchandise, wrong size, damaged, or nonsalable—should be placed in the appropriate bin, and a list maintained of these items.

Receiving, Marking, and Stocking Goods

This aspect of purchasing may seem to be ordinary and not too important, but this is not the case at all. Each invoice should be checked for the appropriateness, both quality and quantity of the merchandise, the terms of the sale, and the accuracy of the extension of the cost (number of units multiplied by the unit cost). Then goods should be marked appropriately. The latter should include the cost per unit (in code), the source, the date, and quantity received. Then the merchandise is placed on the shelf or display with new, fresher products placed behind the older products.

There are hundreds of *cost codes.* Only two will be indicated, one a letter code, the other a simple system of straight lines in two planes or directions. The first, the best known of all cost codes, is an aberration of the spelling of pharmacist.

$$P \ H \ A \ R \ M \ O \ C \ I \ S \ T$$
$$1 \ 2 \ 3 \ 4 \ 5 \ 6 \ 7 \ 8 \ 9 \ 0$$

(It should be noted that this code is not, and probably never was, the official code of the NARD.)

The second code uses a vertical line for zero, a horizontal line attached but extending to the right to represent one (∟), and extending to the left to represent two (⌐), and so on as follows:

$$1 \quad 2 \quad 3 \quad 4 \quad 5 \quad 6 \quad 7 \quad 8 \quad 9 \quad 0$$

Letters are usually used to designate the source, for example, A, B, and C represent three wholesalers that the pharmacist frequently utilizes, and D is used when merchandise is purchased direct. Most pharmacists also indicate the date the merchandise was received, either by number (1/4/74), letter (A-Jan.) or different colors of stickers to indicate the year of purchase. Some use five or six colors and change the color of the sticker every quarter. The quantity frequently is indicated by an arabic numeral preceded by a dash (-). All of these codes may be put together as a composite such as (PAM)D 1/4/74-12, meaning that twelve units of a product were purchased directly from the manufacturer at a cost of $1.35 per unit and were received the fourth of January, 1974.

A final word of advice on marking the cost of merchandise. It is the best policy, in most instances, to mark the exact cost per unit to the nearest whole cent after allowing for all discounts, including free goods. The exception would be when the accounting system included an account for discounts and rebates, which is not a very common practice. Also, the cost of freight and postage should be evenly distributed over the order unless, again, a separate account is maintained for freight and postage. In this regard, most merchandise is shipped to the pharmacy with the freight prepaid.

Title to Goods

As a general rule, the intention of the parties determines when the title passes. Difficulty arises in that the parties may not express any intention on this point. When the parties fail to do so, the law, with the aid of certain assumptions, must decide this question for them. There are about a dozen such assumptions under the law, but discussion will be limited to only those instances most applicable to pharmacy.

If the goods are to be shipped to the pharmacy with freight prepaid, the title passes to the pharmacist when the goods arrive in *good condition.* If there is any damage or shortage, a notation to that effect must be made on either the bill of lading or freight bill (even if it is a prepaid freight bill) before signing for the receipt of the merchandise in order to protect the interest of the purchaser.

If the goods are sold without reference to delivery or prepaid freight and they are in a deliverable state, title passes immediately. If, on the other hand, the terms of sale include a statement that the merchandise will be delivered FOB at the railroad depot in Chicago, title passes when the goods arrive in Chicago in good condition.

When goods are delivered on *consignment,* they remain the property of the supplier, and the pharmacist is required to pay for only the amount he sells. Unfortunately, this includes merchandise that may be stolen, because the pharmacist is the legal custodian of the goods.

REFERENCES

1. Duncan, D. J., and Phillips, C. F.: *Retailing Principles and Methods.* 6th Ed., Homewood, Ill.: Richard D. Irwin, Inc., 1963, p. 266.
2. Smith, M. C.: *Principles of Pharmaceutical Marketing.* 2nd Ed. Philadelphia: Lea & Febiger, 1975, p. 202.
3. *Ibid.,* pp. 204–206.
4. *Pharmaceutical Distribution Plus,* New York: National Wholesale Druggists Association, 1962, p. 9.
5. Grider, G. W.: Advantages of a Buying Group. A paper presented in a seminar at the University of Kentucky College of Pharmacy, Sept. 24, 1971.

REVIEW

1. Discuss the two points of view or philosophies of purchasing.

2. Name and discuss in detail the six purchasing functions.

3. Discuss the two basic considerations in formulating purchasing policies.

4. Outline the sources of information for determining the kinds and types of goods patrons want.

5. Outline the various marketing functions and relate each to purchasing activities in a pharmacy.

6. Discuss the advantages and disadvantages of purchasing from a wholesaler and directly from a manufacturer.

7. Explain the concept of the universality of marketing functions.

8. Explain and give an illustration of the concept of minimum total transactions.

9. Define and explain the significance of the following terms: sorting, market proximity, and time, place, possession, and form utility.

10. Name and describe four services the full-service drug wholesaler provides to a pharmacy.

11. Discuss cooperative buying groups, including the two basic types (or manner they are initiated), the advantages of a cooperative buying group, and especially the economics of joining an existing cooperative group in another trade.

12. Describe and give examples of specialty wholesalers.

13. Define and be able to work problems relative to the following kinds of discounts: trade, quantity, cash, "deals" with free goods, and serial discounts.

14. Define or explain the following dating and credit terms: AOG; ROG; COD; EOM; FOB; N; N/30; N/10 EOM; 2/10, n/30; 2/10 ROG, N/30; 2/10 EOM c̄ 60 extra; and 2/10 EOM, N/30.

15. Explain the value of a new product section and special return goods bins in a pharmacy.

16. Discuss and be able to describe the procedure of receiving, checking, marking, and stocking an order of merchandise.

17. Explain the conditions that determine when the title of goods transfers to the buyer.

18. Explain the term consignment.

10. *Inventory Control*

Among the many problems facing pharmacy today, the challenge of maintaining the appropriate inventory investment and providing superior pharmaceutical services at a competitive price is perhaps the most critical. Inefficient use of capital in general, and inventory specifically, is the cause of many of the problems in pharmacy. Utilizing capital more effectively, especially better control of the inventory investment through more efficient control techniques, can provide the necessary funds to offer *new* and traditional pharmaceutical services at a competitive price.

In one reported study,[1] a majority of the 5,000 pharmacists surveyed indicated they did not consider inventory to be a major problem. Surely these pharmacists were not fully aware of the significance of inventory control or the magnitude of the investment in inventory. According to *The Lilly Digest*[2] inventory investment exceeds the investment in any other single asset by nearly fourfold. The average investment for the 1,823 pharmacies reporting for 1972 in *The Lilly Digest* was $41,435.[3] Proper inventory control can reduce the inventory investment from 10 to 25 percent, depending on the degree of overstocking. In one research project,[4] the inventory was reduced by 22 percent over a nine-month period.

A simple example will illustrate the significance of an inventory control system by reducing the inventory investment from $40,000 to

$30,000, a 25 percent reduction. If we assume a sales volume of $250,000 and a net profit of $10,000, both of which are typical, the significance of inventory reduction on both the return on investment, and the length of time to liquidate a debt that may have been incurred in purchasing the inventory, can be readily demonstrated. Assuming all other factors remained constant, the reduction in inventory would have increased the return on the inventory investment from 25 percent to 33 percent. Also, disregarding the interest charge, the debt incurred by financing the inventory on credit could have been liquidated with the net profit in three years instead of four. Another aspect of the savings resulting from inventory control is the interest that could have been earned if the inventory had been financed with cash (or equity funds) by the pharmacist-proprietor. In the example above, the $10,000 inventory reduction would earn $750 per year at 7.5 percent simple interest. The $10,000 would have more than doubled if the 7.5 percent interest charge were compounded for ten years.

Methods of Inventory Control

There are at least six methods of inventory control, ranging from the elementary and ineffective to sophisticated and effective methods.

INTUITIVE METHOD

The first method is designated as the intuitive method, aided by the well-known *wantbook*. This is the most common method in practice today and surely the least effective. Items are recorded in the wantbook when the number of units in stock reaches one to three, and the amount ordered is the best estimate of the pharmacist-manager or proprietor.

SYSTEMATIC WANTBOOK METHOD

The second method is a set of systematic wantbooks. In this case, there is a wantbook for each direct account and each major wholesaler. Items are recorded in the appropriate wantbook based on the need as indicated by an order card located with each product, or a strip of cardboard on the edge of the shelf. The information on the card or strip simply indicates the minimum/maximum quantities—the number at which the item is ordered and the quantity to order to bring the inventory to the maximum level. The selling price and sometimes the cost, in code, are also included. The items are ordered at the appropriate time, at which point the quantities and date of the order are recorded in the wantbook. When the order is received, notation is made of shortages and related information. Reviewing the data in the wantbooks aids greatly in the establishment and refinement of the minimum and maximum quantities.

PERPETUAL INVENTORY METHOD

Perpetual inventory is the most accurate and effective method of inventory control. Before this method can be economically feasible, the use of computers and a practical and economical computer terminal, possibly as an extension of the cash register, must be available. Some of the large department store chains are using this system now, and the entire supermarket industry is about to launch an industry-wide program adopting this technology. The fact that there have already been several pharmacies experimenting with variations of a completely computerized record system is evidence of the merit of the method.

OPEN-TO-BUY BUDGET SYSTEM

One of the simplest and easiest inventory control systems to implement is the open-to-buy (O-T-B) budget method. The rationale underlying this method is simply to adjust each month's purchases based on the increases or decreases in the sales of the previous month in comparison to the corresponding monthly sales a year ago, and to make adjustments of any overbuying or underbuying during the previous month. Based on this premise, a purchase budget is established for each month.

When a purchase is made, it is subtracted from the balance of the purchase budget maintained in a separate purchase journal or register. In this manner, the pharmacist-manager can determine whether he is buying too much or too little by referring to his budget balance in his purchase journal during the month. This part is easy to do, but establishing the purchase budget for each month requires more skill. To assist students and practitioners in developing a monthly purchase budget for the prescription department, Table 10-1 was constructed to explain each step in the process.

As illustrated in the table, the pharmacist-manager implemented his O-T-B budget system in January. Note that no adjustment was made for January's purchase budget because the sales for the month were not known until January 31, and the purchase adjustments necessarily are based on the events of the prior year and month. To illustrate the system, we will follow each step taken to establish the adjusted purchase budget for February:

First, the sales for January this year were $500 more than for January of last year. This figure was multiplied by .50, the decimal form of the 50 percent cost of goods sold, to transform the increased sales figure to a purchase figure of $250. Second, we note $500 less was purchased during

Table 10-1. Open-to-Buy Budget Method for Inventory Control

Month	Sales Past Year	Sales This Year	Unadj. Purchase Budget[a]	Adjustment: Sales[b] + Purchases[c] = Adj.	Adj. Purch. Budget	Actual Purchases	Monthly Balance in Budg.[d]
January	$10,000	$10,500	$5,000	NA[e] + NA = NA	$5,000	$4,500	$+500
February	10,500	10,500	5,250	(+500 × .5) + 500 = 750	6,000	5,500	+500
March	11,000	10,500	5,500	(0 × .5) + 500 = 500	6,000	5,750	+250
April	10,500	11,000	5,250	(−500 × .5) + 250 = 0	5,250	5,250	0
May	9,500	10,000	4,750	(500 × .5) + 0 = 250	5,000	5,250	−250
June	10,000	10,500	5,000	(500 × .5) − 250 = 0	5,000	4,750	+250
July	9,000	10,000	4,500	(500 × .5) + 250 = 500	5,000	5,000	0
August	8,500	9,000	4,250	(1000 × .5) + 0 = 500	4,750	5,000	−250
September	8,500	9,500	4,250	(500 × .5) − 250 = 0	4,250	4,500	−250
October	9,500	10,000	4,750	(1000 × .5) − 250 = 250	5,000	5,000	0
November	10,500	11,000	5,250	(500 × .5) + 0 = 250	5,500	5,000	+500
December	11,000	12,000	5,500	(500 × .5) + 500 = 750	6,250	6,250	0
TOTAL	$118,500	$124,500	$59,250	-------	$63,000	$61,750	$ 1,250

[a] Based on a 50 percent cost of goods sold for the same month one year before.
[b] The difference in sales between the previous month and the same month a year ago.
[c] The difference between the adjusted purchase budget and the actual purchase of the previous month.
[d] A positive monthly balance in the purchase budget indicates an inventory depletion of the same magnitude, and vice versa.
[e] No adjustment is made the first month the method is implemented.

January than had been budgeted. This means that there was a balance in the adjusted purchase budget, and an additional amount of $500 should be included in February's adjusted budget to bring the inventory up to the proper level. Third, the $250 ($500 multiplied by .50) should be added to the $500 budget balance to arrive at the $750 adjustment, as shown in the adjustment column. Finally, we note that February sales for last year amounted to $10,500, which when multiplied by .50 provided an unadjusted purchase budget of $5,250, to which the $750 adjustment was added to obtain the final adjusted purchase budget for February of $6,000.

The O-T-B budget system may be applied in several ways. It may be used for one or more departments or the entire pharmacy, or for the slower moving drugs in the prescription department when the inventory of the faster moving prescription drugs is controlled by a more sophisticated system, for example, the stock record card system.

To implement the O-T-B budget method, a pharmacist should set up a format similar to the one illustrated in Table 10-1 and obtain the following information: (1) sales for each month for the unit being controlled, and (2) the percent cost, or at least a fairly accurate estimate, of goods sold.

For the latter estimate, a sample of 360 prescriptions can be drawn by taking the first 30 of each month over the year for the prescription department. It would be preferable to take the first 30 prescriptions dispensed on Monday in January, the first 30 prescriptions on Tuesday in February, and continuing this rotation through June, but skipping Sunday, and repeating the days of the week beginning with July. The total cost of ingredients (drugs) for the 360 prescriptions is divided by the total sales for the same prescriptions to estimate the percent cost of goods sold. In addition, the sales and purchases for the current year have to be recorded each month and the adjustments calculated as outlined above. This procedure requires little additional time or information for most pharmacies.

The real value of the O-T-B budget system is that it is much easier to make twelve small adjustments, one each month, than to try to make one large adjustment at the end of the year when the physical inventory is taken. To illustrate further, let us assume a pharmacy had an inventory of $41,000 and a turnover rate of 3.4 per year with a cost of goods sold of $140,000. The pharmacist-manager decided that his inventory was too high and should be reduced to at least $35,000 during the following year to provide a turnover rate of 4. The $6,000 reduction in inventory represented 14.6 percent of his current inventory. Each month after the pharmacist calculated his adjusted monthly purchase budget as outlined above, he deliberately reduced this adjusted budget by an additional 14.6 percent. On the average the reduction was $500 each month.

STOCK RECORD CARD SYSTEM

Even though one can control the inventory investment for major departments by means of the open-to-buy budget, he cannot use this system to determine the optimum number of individual units of a product to be ordered. To determine the optimum number of individual units for each product in each major department, a more formal control, such as the stock record card system, must be utilized. A stock record card system, as illustrated in Figure 10-1, has proved to be very effective. Ideally, the stock record card should have at least 12 columns to record data for each month. The heading of the stock record card normally shows the manufacturer's name and address, the discount, and other sale terms such as the date the company closes its books.

After the general information has been recorded for a company, the name, size, cost per unit, and the minimum and maximum quantity of the product to be stocked are recorded as indicated by the column headings. Figure 10-1 demonstrates that the pharmacist in our example stocks tetracycline syrup in pints, tetracycline 250 mg. capsules in 1000s, and meprobamate 400 mg. tablets in 500s.

This stock record card system was begun in January and the first inventory taken was on January 25. On January 25, the pharmacist had one pint of tetracycline syrup, and the pharmacist recorded the value 1.0 in the upper part of the block under the date, January 25. On this date he also had 2 units of tetracycline 250 mg. capsules and 2 units of meprobamate 400 mg. tablets, plus various other products. Based on the minimum and maximum quantities the pharmacist had previously estab-

Name: Manufacturer A

Address: 1428 W. 22nd St., New York, N.Y. (Use Self-Addressed Order Form when available)

Discount Terms: 2% 10 days E.O.M., Net 30. Books are closed on 28th each month.

Item	Cost	Size	Inventory minimum/maximum	Inventory and Purchases by Date								
				1/25	2/25	3/25	4/25	5/25	6/25	7/25	8/25	9/25
Tetracycline Syrup	3.42	Pt.	1 / 2	1 /	<1 / 1	.5 / 2	.5 / 2	1 / 2	1+ / 1	1.5 / 1	0.5 / 0	1 / 2
Tetracycline 250 mg. Cap.	6.17	1000	1 / 3	2 / 1	1 / 2	1 / 2	2 / 1	1 / 2	2 / 1	2.5 / 0	1.1 / 2	1.5 / 2
Meprobamate 400 mg. Tab.	18.50	500	1 / 3	2 / 1	1.5 / 2	1 / 2	.5 / 2	1 / 2	2 / 1	1.5 / 1	1 / 2	1 / 2

Figure 10-1. *Typical Stock Record Card*

lished from experience, he decided to purchase one pint of tetracycline syrup and the number of units of other products as indicated. This information was recorded in the lower part of the block. Upon completing the order the manager can ascertain whether he has purchased the minimum amount necessary to receive the maximum discounts available. This can be easily determined by multiplying the units ordered times the cost per unit, totaling the costs, and comparing the total with the manufacturer's minimum order requirement. On February 25 and each month thereafter, the pharmacist again recorded the quantity of items in inventory and repeated the process.

Some product lines do not warrant the additional time required to maintain the inventory on stock record cards because of their small investment and slow turnover rate. The pharmacist must decide which products warrant stock record cards and which should be controlled with the open-to-buy budget. As a starting point for setting up the stock record card system, it is suggested that the system include all prescription products purchased directly from the top 10 to 20 major pharmaceutical manufacturers and all other prescription drugs with a high turnover rate purchased from wholesalers, especially if the product appears in the top 200 products listed in the National Prescription Audit.[5] Stock record card inventory control of the top 200 prescription drugs will include the investment of about two-thirds of the prescription sales volume. Another consideration is that most of these drugs are routinely inventoried and ordered monthly by a majority of community pharmacists. The stock record card system should be restricted to prescription drugs in the beginning because the average investment in major lines of prescription drugs is usually greater than the average investment per line of non-legend drugs or other merchandise.

By maintaining stock record cards on prescription drugs with high turnover rates, the pharmacist is in a position to place a larger order at the end of the month and thus have the suppliers finance the inventory investment for as long as 40 to 45 days. The system also ensures the earning of cash discounts on the products controlled by the system and provides more cash for other investments. The extra cash can be invested in other products with a high gross margin and/or high turnover rate or can be invested in securities or other property. Also, the additional money may be used to improve patient services, for example, a patient medication record system.

THE ECONOMIC ORDER QUANTITY

The basic problem of inventory management is having the right amount of stock on hand, neither too much nor too little. Fundamentally, inventory control is deciding how much to buy and when. The economic order quantity (EOQ) deals with both *how much* to purchase and the appropriate reorder point, or *when* to buy. Also, the EOQ is the amount to buy that will keep total costs at a minimum.

There are two sets of costs involved in purchasing, *procurement* costs and *carrying* costs. Procurement costs vary with the number of orders and may be reduced for any given item by placing fewer and larger orders. However, the result is an increase in inventory and consequently in the other set of costs, the carrying costs. Procurement costs vary directly with the number of orders and inversely with the amount of investment. On the other hand, the carrying costs may be reduced for any given item if smaller orders are placed. However, the result will be an increase in the number of orders and consequently an increase in the first set of costs, the procurement costs. Carrying costs vary directly with inventory investment and inversely with the number of orders.

The various individual expenses of the two sets of costs are:

PROCUREMENT COSTS | CARRYING COSTS
Checking inventory | Interest, imputed and/or real
Purchasing | Obsolescence
Receiving the merchandise | Loss through theft
Marking the merchandise | Deterioration or damage
Paying for the merchandise | Storage (insurance and property tax)

The EOQ model provides a level of inventory at which the combined costs of procuring and carrying inventory are at a minimum. For example, Table 10-2 shows how total costs are affected by the size of the order with a procurement cost of $4.00 per order and a carrying cost of 10 percent of the average inventory investment, on a product with annual cost of goods sold of $720.

First, if an order for $720 is placed only once each year, the total cost of procurement is $4. Since the average value of the stock will be $360, or one-half of the value of the order, the carrying costs will be 10 percent of $360, or $36. The sum of the two costs will be $40.

Table 10-2. *How the Value of Orders Determines Total Costs*

Value of Order	No. Orders Per Year	Procurement Costs	Average Active Inventory	Carrying Costs	Total Cost
$720	1	$ 4	$360	$36	$40
360	2	8	180	18	26
240	3	12	120	12	24
180	4	16	90	9	25
144	5	20	72	7	27
120	6	24	60	6	30

If two orders are made each year, the value of each order will be $360. This will double the procurement costs and reduce the carrying costs to one-half. Total costs will be $26 instead of $40. However, by placing 3 orders of $240 each, the total cost will be the least of all. Beyond this point the increase in procurement costs will always be greater than the decrease in carrying costs, as can be seen in the table. The total cost is at a minimum when the procurement costs and carrying costs are equal. For practical considerations, the two sets of costs may be only approximately equal.

For any one item, a reduction in *one* set of costs causes an increase in the other set. This is also true for a group of items under ordinary purchasing practices. The application of EOQ to any group of stock items will cause the sum of the two sets of costs to be lower than under any other system of purchasing. This will happen in one of the following ways: (1) by balancing or equating the two sets of costs; or (2) by reducing one set of costs without increasing the other. (This latter possibility is not a likely event under normal purchasing practices.)

Any other order quantities may: (1) produce a certain stock turn, but at unnecessarily high costs; (2) reduce procurement costs by increasing carrying costs; or (3) reduce carrying costs by increasing procurement costs.

Under many replenishment systems, items are ordered at regular intervals. Such systems result in maintaining on the average a constant level of supply for all items in the group. Under other systems, the number of orders may vary according to demand. For items with a high dollar demand, orders may be placed more frequently than for low dollar demand items, in which case, fewer and larger orders, relative to demand, are placed. In addition, under some of these systems, consideration is properly given to special characteristics such as limited shelf life, space requirements, and seasonal demand. But after all these characteristics are considered, the questions still remain, how many orders per year is the right number for any given item? How much should be ordered at a time? How much stock should be maintained?

The economic order quantity (EOQ) equation is difficult to derive but not difficult to use. The model is expressed by the following equation:

$$Q = \sqrt{\frac{(2)\,(C_p)\,(D)}{C_h}}$$

where Q = the economic order quantity;
  C_p = procurement cost;
  D = the demand for the product expressed either in dollars or physical units; and
  C_h = the holding or carrying cost of the investment.

Table 10-3. *Table of Square Roots*

Number	Square Root	Number	Square Root	Number	Square Root	Number	Square Root
1.0	1.0	10	3.2	100	10	1,000	32
1.2	1.1	12	3.5	120	11	1,200	35
1.4	1.2	14	3.7	140	12	1,400	37
1.5	1.2	15	3.9	150	12	1,500	39
1.6	1.3	16	4.0	160	13	1,600	40
1.8	1.3	18	4.2	180	13	1,800	42
2.0	1.4	20	4.5	200	14	2,000	45
2.5	1.6	25	5.0	250	16	2,500	50
3.0	1.7	30	5.5	300	17	3,000	55
3.5	1.9	35	5.9	350	19	3,500	59
4.0	2.0	40	6.3	400	20	4,000	63
4.5	2.1	45	6.7	450	21	4,500	67
5.0	2.2	50	7.1	500	22	5,000	71
6.0	2.4	60	7.7	600	24	6,000	77
7.0	2.6	70	8.4	700	26	7,000	84
8.0	2.8	80	8.9	800	28	8,000	89
9.0	3.0	90	9.5	900	30	9,000	95

To find the square root of a number larger than 9,000, simply drop the last two numbers. Find the square root of this resulting number and add a zero to it.

Suppose the value of the yearly demand of an item is $29,750. Rounding to 30,000 and dropping the last two numbers, you get 300. You will find in the table that the square root of 300 is 17. Adding a zero, you get 170. This is approximately the square root of 30,000.

To find the square root of a number less than 9,000 not in the table, take the square root of the nearest number or one in between. For example, use 25 for the square root of 640, which is between 600 and 700. The approximate square roots you will get will be accurate enough for determining EOQ.

Table 10-3 is a modified table of square roots, and contains instructions for its use in determining the EOQ.

One important consideration in using the EOQ equation is that both D and C_h must be expressed in comparable terms with respect to time and quantity. For example, if D is expressed as the amount in dollars that will be purchased in one year, the C_h must be expressed as the annual percent in decimal form which represents the holding (carrying) cost. Currently, this cost will range from 10 to 12 percent in most pharmacies. However, if D is expressed as the number of physical units that will be purchased in a period, for example one month, C_h must be expressed as the holding cost for the average cost per unit purchased each month. The following examples explain how to calculate the EOQ using monthly and annual data.

Assume that a pharmacy purchased $3,000 worth of goods from one company in a year, with an average of 50 physical units of the various products each month. It was determined with the aid of a stop watch that, on an average, 20 minutes were required to inventory and place an order from this company. If this were done by a pharmacist with a salary of $9.00 per hour, the procurement cost (C_p) would be $3.00 ($9.00 × 20/60 minutes). It was determined that the average cost per physical unit of the product mix ordered during the year was $5.00. The carrying cost per unit per month (C_h) can be calculated as follows: $5.00 × 0.10 ÷ 12 = $0.0416. Substituting in the equation, we solve for Q as follows:

$$Q = \sqrt{\frac{(2)\,(C_p)\,(D)}{C_h}}$$

$$Q = \sqrt{\frac{2 \times \$3.00 \times 50}{\$0.0416}}$$

$$Q = \sqrt{\frac{300.00}{0.0416}}$$

$$Q = \sqrt{7,211.54}$$

Q = 84.92 or 85 units in round figures because the dollars in the numerator and denominator cancel each other.

When the number of units is converted to dollars, the EOQ is $424.50, or approximately $425 in round figures. The idealized average investment is one-half the EOQ value or $212 to the nearest whole dollar. The optimum turnover rate is 14.2 ($3,000 ÷ 212).

The economic order quantity may be calculated by use of annual data—the total amount purchased per year, the same procurement cost per order, and the 10 percent carrying cost for the year. The calculations are as follows:

$$Q = \sqrt{\frac{2\,(C_p)\,(D)}{C_h}}$$

$$Q = \sqrt{\frac{2 \times \$3.00 \times \$3,000}{.10}}$$

$$Q = \sqrt{\frac{\$18,000}{.10}}$$

$$Q = \sqrt{\$180,000}$$

$$Q = \$424.26$$

The difference between the $424.50 and the $424.26 results from rounding. The average inventory investment to the nearest whole dollar and the optimum turnover rate remain the same.

Now let us calculate the EOQ, using the yearly demand in dollars for the same company but under a different set of conditions. Instead of having the pharmacist take the inventory and place the order, the pharmacist-manager hired a stock clerk for $3.00 per hour to do the job. (He found the clerk could do this chore just as efficiently after two months of training.) Procurement cost (C_p) was $1.00 ($3.00 × 20/60 minutes). The holding cost remained the same. The yearly demand (D) remained $3,000. Substituting into the equation:

$$Q = \sqrt{\frac{2\,(C_p)\,(D)}{C_h}}$$

$$Q = \sqrt{\frac{2 \times \$1.00 \times \$3,000}{.10}}$$

$$Q = \sqrt{\frac{\$6,000}{.10}}$$

$$Q = \sqrt{\$60,000}$$

$$Q = \$244.94 \text{ or } \$245 \text{ in round figures.}$$

Under these conditions, the idealized average inventory investment is $122.50 (1/2 × $245.00). The optimum turnover rate is now 24.5. This latter set of conditions is more realistic and represents a "money-saving" approach to the problem. It is readily apparent that the inventory investment has been reduced by 42 percent, and if other cost factors remain the same, the percentage return on the investment in inventory would increase significantly.

The economic order quantity model will determine the optimum quantity to order, in terms of either dollars or physical units, and the optimum turnover rate. This can be applied to a line of merchandise or to an individual product. Since the actual number of units of each product that a pharmacist can expect to dispense during a given month can be rather closely estimated by inspection of the stock record card, it is more feasible to apply the model to the monthly order of the entire manufacturer's line. This, of course, requires that the EOQ model use the stock record cards or a computerized counterpart.

Once the EOQ for the line has been calculated, quantity adjustments among the various products may be necessary to obtain the most economic product mix for each order. In any case, the company's minimum direct order quantity must be considered, especially if the minimum direct order quantity exceeds the EOQ by a considerable amount. This could be a good indication that this company's line of products may be purchased more economically through the wholesaler. Of course, the discount for direct buying should enter into the decision.

A simple example illustrates a way to approach such a decision. Assume a pharmacy has a low sales volume of $200 per year for a small manufacturer's line. Also, assume a 50 percent cost of goods sold (CGS) and gross margin (GM) and a net profit of 10 percent of sales. The manufacturer requires a $100 order for direct purchases with a 10 percent quantity discount. Under these conditions, the CGS is $100, the average investment in inventory is $50.00 (1/2 × $100 CGS) and the net profit (NP) is $20.00. The return on the investment in inventory is 60 percent ($20.00 NP + $10.00 in discount divided by the $50.00 average investment).

However, the EOQ is calculated to be $33.33 purchased every four months. The average investment is now $16.67 (1/2 × $33.33 CGS), but the net profit is only $20.00 since the pharmacist-manager must forgo the discount. His return on investment is now 120 percent ($20.00 ÷ $16.67); he has doubled his percentage return on the inventory investment. It should be noted, however, that his actual net profit declined by $10.00, and the real issue is whether the pharmacist could have invested the difference in the average inventories ($33.33) in some other venture and earned more than the $10.00. This could have been achieved by investing the $33.33 in a product with a 40 percent gross margin, with four turnovers per year and a net profit potential of 5 percent of sales. This investment would yield $11.11 in net profit.

Selection of the Optimum Method(s)

No one method of inventory control is the most appropriate for every pharmacy. The least any pharmacist-manager should do is to maintain a systematic set of wantbooks to assist him in ordering more nearly the appropriate quantities of merchandise. This will only approximate the desired results, but it is an improvement over the usual use of wantbooks.

The larger pharmacies, those with annual sales over $100,000, can use the more sophisticated methods profitably. Any pharmacy can use the open-to-buy budget method for the pharmacy department, or any of its other major departments. This method, however, only provides control of the dollar amount of the inventory. Together with a system of wantbooks, with appropriate entries in them, the O-T-B method will be fairly effective for small pharmacies with sales volumes of $100,000 or less.

The stock record card system should be used for those products or lines of goods on which the economic order quantity model indicates the feasibility of the system. Under most conditions, the carrying cost ranges between 8 and 12 percent. When interest rates are normal and fairly stable, carrying costs are also stable at approximately 10 percent. The feasibility of the S-R-C system depends more directly on procurement costs than any other factor.

The following example illustrates the way to determine the feasibility of using the S-R-C system and the EOQ model. A pharmacy purchases $500 worth of drugs annually from Company A. The minimum order is $100, providing a 15 percent discount. Judicious purchasing from a local drug wholesaler provides a 10 percent quantity discount on line extension of $10 per product, a 5 percent difference. If a trained clerk checks the inventory and does the ordering, procurement cost is $1.00 per order. If a pharmacist does the job, the cost is $5.00. Carrying cost is 10 percent.

When the clerk is used, the EOQ is $100. The total cost for the year is $10.00. The procurement cost is 5 × $1.00 and the carrying cost is 10 percent of $50, the average inventory investment. The difference in quantity discount for the year is $25, a net gain of $15.

When the pharmacist does the ordering, the EOQ is $225 in round figures.

$$Q = \sqrt{\frac{2 \times \$5 \times \$500}{0.10}}$$

$$Q = \$223.61, \text{ or } \$225 \text{ rounded.}$$

In practice, the pharmacist orders $250 twice a year. The procurement cost is $10 and the carrying cost is $12.50, 10 percent of the average inventory of $125. The total annual cost is $22.50, just $2.50 less than the difference in quantity discount. This difference is hardly worth forgoing the convenience of buying locally from the drug wholesaler.

The crux of the problem is the procurement cost. If a pharmacist installs an efficient S-R-C system with a well-trained stock clerk, or a combination of a stock clerk and a prescription aide, annual purchases of as little as $300 can be profitable. Only with stock record cards and the EOQ model is the pharmacist able to determine with a high degree of accuracy the most advantageous quantity and frequency per order.

The stock record card system, maintained either manually or with a computer, together with the EOQ model, can be used to control the inventory for individual products when used in large volume. This situation may be found in large pharmacies, in institutional pharmacies using a formulary, and in warehouses of chain drugstores or drug wholesalers. Unit control is feasible under these conditions and an example will illustrate this.

A hospital pharmacy uses 1,200 units annually at a cost of $2.00 per unit for a total dollar volume of $2,400. The procurement cost is $1.00 and the carrying cost is 12 percent annually. The EOQ is $200 or 120 units.

$$Q = \sqrt{\frac{2 \times \$1.00 \times \$2,400}{0.12}}$$

$Q = \$200$; 100 units or 12 orders per year.

The same result is obtained by substitution of the demand in units per month for annual dollar demand and $0.02 for 12 percent as the carrying cost per month per unit cost.

Effect of Inventory Control

A professional pharmacy was located in a medical building in a city of approximately 40,000 population.[4] Fifteen physicians and an oral surgeon practiced in the building. About 65 percent of the $245,000 sales volume was derived from prescriptions and physicians' supplies. The pharmacy was heavily overstocked with prescription drugs. The inventory for the prescription department was $34,866 before a program of purchasing and inventory control was implemented. The turnover rate for the previous year was 1.6 for the prescription department.

During the initial preparatory stage of the project, 51 percent of the inventory was returned to the suppliers or written off as nonsalable and nonreturnable merchandise. The balance of the inventory of $16,970 was considered to be usable and constituted a well-balanced prescription drug inventory for this pharmacy.

At this stage of the project, two inventory control methods were implemented, the stock record card system and the open-to-buy budget system. Product lines of eleven manufacturers were selected for stock record card control based on the observed utilization rate during the preparatory stage and the policy of direct selling to pharmacies. It had been observed that at least the minimum order quantity was purchased monthly from each of the companies during the preparatory stage. The EOQ was used to determine the optimum order quantity.

The inventory controlled by the stock record card system was reduced by an additional 17 percent during the six months' test period. The turnover rate increased to 6.1, on an annual basis for the first three months, and 8.0 on an annual basis for the second three months. The inventory controlled by the open-to-buy budget method was reduced by 4 percent. The turnover rate for this group of drugs increased to 2.4 on an annual basis. Overall, the turnover rate for the prescription department increased from 1.6 to 3.22, a two-fold increase.

It was determined that, on an average, only 24 seconds were required to inventory and place an order for a single product among all the products of the eleven manufacturers controlled by the stock record card system. An additional 36 seconds were required to check, mark, and stock a product on receipt of the order—for a total of 60 seconds. The out-of-stock rate was almost exactly the same for each method and averaged 1.2 prescriptions per day.

REFERENCES

1. Cullman, W. A.: What Pharmacists Think. *NARDJ, 88*:24–34, 1966.
2. Slavin, G. F.: *The Lilly Digest, 1972.* Indianapolis: Eli Lilly and Company, 1973, Table 31.
3. *Ibid.,* p. 7.
4. Huffman, D. C., Jr.: *The Feasibility of Modern Managerial Systems and Innovative Professional Services in a Community Pharmacy: A Case Study.* Dissertation, University of Mississippi, January, 1971.
5. *National Prescription Audit General Information Report,* Dedham, Mass.: R. A. Gosselin Division of Lea Associates, Inc. This information is published in several pharmaceutical journals each year.

REVIEW

1. According to the *1973 Lilly Digest,* what was the average investment in inventory in 1972 (nearest $1,000), and how did this investment compare with other items of assets?

2. Describe the six methods of inventory control.

3. Given the necessary data, complete a table of open-to-buy budget inventory control including the adjustments, adjusted purchase budget, and the monthly balance in the adjusted purchase budget.

4. Discuss the procedures and be able to devise and complete a system of stock record card inventory control.

5. Explain the concept of the economic order quantity (EOQ) including the terms of the formula and the specific information it provides the pharmacist.

6. Given the appropriate data, calculate the EOQ in either units per order or dollar value per order, the reorder point, and the optimum turnover rate for a given line of products or for a company. Table 10-3 has been included to assist in determining square roots.

7. Given the necessary data, including quantity discount rates, determine when a minimum direct order, example $100, is feasible using the EOQ model.

8. Discuss the various situations (size of pharmacy, sales volume, etc.) under which each method of inventory is most feasible.

9. Discuss how the turnover rate is indicative of a good inventory control method.

10. Discuss the relationship between the return on investment in inventory and the efficiency of an inventory control method.

11. *Pricing and Professional Fees*

General Pricing Considerations

BASIC FACTORS

When a pharmacist makes a determination of the pricing philosophy, policy, and method(s) for his pharmacy, he must consider at least five basic factors that affect his decisions.

Philosophy. The philosophy of the pharmacist is a primary consideration. This philosophy is a product of the pharmacist's socioeconomic background, the market in which he practices, and his education. In the final analysis, however, the philosophy is determined by the pharmacist's volition.

Competition. This factor is certainly a major consideration. Since it has already been discussed in some detail, the point of emphasis here is that the pharmacist can deal effectively with various forms of price and non-price competition through a well-designed strategy of market segmentation. The application of the principles of economics and marketing is the principal tool in this case.

Merchandise Cost. The cost of merchandise is a necessary factor that must be considered in determining methods of pricing and the pricing of individual merchandise or services. The cost of the merchandise forms the fundamental base line for determining prices. Cooperative buying groups and other buying methods are important in determining prices and profits. Again, the application of economic and marketing principles is necessary to purchase merchandise in a manner to be competitive.

Expenses. The control of expenses is another essential element in price determination. Control of expenses, especially variable expenses, provides one of the bases for more competitive pricing. In the long run, prices must cover all expenses, and more, to yield a profit. The application of accounting and economics can assist the pharmacist in reducing unnecessary expenses, and thereby to price competitively.

Legal and Social Constraints. These combined forces make up the fifth basic factor in price determination. There are franchise agreements that prohibit the pharmacist from charging less than the stipulated or suggested price. Certain lines of cosmetics are sold exclusively through franchise agreements. Fair trade laws are largely inoperative now, but may still be in effect for certain lines in certain jurisdictions. These operate more in the nature of a franchise, through individual contractual agreement, than through the general operation of statutory law, with the exception of the sale of alcoholic beverages. In addition, certain goods sell for a certain price because of long-standing custom. Although inflation has largely displaced these "customary prices," there is still some residual constraint to sell some candy bars, for example, for five cents—the manufacturers just make the candy bars smaller. This latter socioeconomic constraint and the fair trade laws are included here more for a historic purpose and to apprise the reader of the necessity to consider this overall factor, especially franchise agreements, in price determination.

There are many factors, policies, and strategies which must be considered in the making of pricing decisions. These considerations vary with the market, the type of pharmacy practice, and the pharmacist himself.

COMPETITIVE STRATEGY

As discussed in Chapter 1, competition has been a problem in American pharmacy from the beginning. The report of a recent study by the Dichter Institute for Motivational Research, Inc.,[1] commissioned by the American Pharmaceutical Association, may provide the pharmacist with some useful insight into the design of a competitive posture for his pharmacy. The research revealed that in purchasing prescriptions, the public is not so much *pulled* toward discounters by their price advertising as it is being *pushed* away from the regular community pharmacy by a sense of alienation. The community pharmacists are not communicating and consulting with their patrons and showing a genuine concern for their welfare, which the public so desperately desires. The public perceives prescription and comprehensive pharmaceutical services as a vital part of their health care and have very deep-seated feelings about the services provided and concern shown in providing these services.

Types of Competition. The two major types of competition are *price* and *non-price.* Non-price competition takes several forms of promotion in which price is not a primary factor. These include advertising, displays, broad lines and assortments of merchandise, extra services (both professional and nonprofessional), and, probably the most important form of all, a vast number of competing units vying for the consumers' dollars for the same or similar products and services. This latter form of competition may be divided into non-drug firms and the various types of pharmacies and drugstores. The large discount emporium with a prescription department and a drug counter can be classified in either category, but traditionally it is not considered to be a "regular" pharmacy or drugstore and, therefore, is placed in the non-drug class. This type of firm is found in the larger cities where competition, both price and non-price, is the severest.

Market Segmentation. Non-price competition, in many ways, is associated with the concept of market segmentation. Market segmentation is the strategy of identifying a segment of the market who are desirous to purchase a particular, and frequently unique, line of goods and/or services. The pharmacist attempts to measure the extent of the demand for the special line of goods and/or services and offers the line and/or services if the demand seems to warrant it.

Market segmentation can range from stocking a single product, such as a very expensive imported perfume, to the design, decor, stock and services of an entire pharmacy, such as the pharmaceutical center. In the first instance, the pharmacist is appealing to a small number of wealthy female patrons. In the latter instance, the pharmacist is appealing to a much larger number of people of both sexes who prefer a highly personalized, professional service. Other market segments include a complete home health care, convalescent, and orthopedic department; hypoallergenic cosmetics; complete veterinary drug and pet department; a complete baby department supervised by a licensed nurse; a professionally operated medication record system; and a clinical laboratory—just to mention the more common lines and services that appeal to particular segments of the market. The stocking or implementation and promotion of these special lines and/or services are viable examples of non-price competition.

Quasi-Price Competition. In addition to direct price competition, there exists a technique known as quasi-price competition. The trading stamp is a classic example of quasi-price competition. Another example of this technique is the inclusion of a product "free" with the purchase of another product. This is more frequently done at the manufacturer's level and passed on to the customer. Another example is providing coupons in a newspaper ad or circular that permit a person who tenders the coupon to purchase an item at a reduced price *provided* he or she purchases goods costing a designated amount, for example, $5.00. There are many variations of this, but they are not used in pharmacy to the extent that they are used in supermarkets. While quasi-price reduction is not a true, direct price reduction on a product, it is similar in some respects to price competition.

Direct Price Reduction. Direct price reduction on a particular product is the most obvious mode of price competition. Direct price reduction may take several forms also. The broadest form is the *across-the-board* reduction of prices below normal or average market price on all the merchandise. At least two chain drugstore firms have adopted this approach.

A second form of direct price reduction is the *loss leader.* In this case, the management selects a group of products and reduces the prices below the market norm by a significant amount. This practice was once restricted to "out front" merchandise, but now it is used extensively by "discounters" and some other pharmacies on *popular* or *maintenance* prescription drugs.

Another approach is to use *weekend "specials,"* offering a significant discount on selected products from Thursday evening through Saturday or Sunday. The group of products is selected each week from a larger, master list of popular shoppers' items. This also gives the impression that the drugstore or pharmacy offers substantial discounts over a wide range of products, while in fact, the range of products discounted is less than the image created—at least that is the objective of the promotional method. This method of competition has been designated "shadow boxing."

A fourth method of price competition is to have *sales* or *"special events"* coinciding with holidays (e.g., Washington's birthday), anniversaries, seasons, and the so-called close-out sales. Usually there are discounts on the prices of selected merchandise, but sometimes the "sales" are at the regular price. Some firms even buy special sale merchandise, usually not a regular line of goods, and sell them at the usual or regular margin, but marked to indicate a discount price. This is practiced more frequently in the dry goods trade. Needless to say, this practice is unethical, if not fraudulent. Any false close-out sale also comes under this indictment.

Last, there is the famous annual or semi-annual *one cent sale.* This type of sale was introduced by Rexall many years ago, and it later was used by Walgreen drugstores. The original concept was that the purchaser could buy a second unit of a product for one cent provided the first unit was purchased at the regular price. The Federal Trade Commission stopped the use of the phrase "one cent sale" and a somewhat different title is used today. However, older consumers still associate the sale with the "old-time one cent sale."

The foregoing discussion covers competitive practices ranging from selective non-price, service-oriented programs to "hard-hitting" across-the-board discounting, as well as the once traditional "one cent sales." The pharmacist must select the competitive posture he should adopt. The choice, of course, will depend on the individual, the type of pharmacy, and the market.

PRICING POLICIES

The pharmacist's pricing policies correspond to the competitive strategy of his pharmacy. He may choose from among the following approaches to pricing merchandise or use a combination of these approaches for various departments or product lines: (1) traditional or regular pricing, (2) competitive pricing, (3) price leadership, (4) pricing based on an estimation of what the market will bear, (5) odd pricing, and (6) professional discount.

Traditional Pricing. Traditional or regular pricing simply means that, for a particular product or merchandise line, the pharmacist used a markup that has become the general custom or practice over the years. The markup varies with the nature of the product and its turnover rate. The markup percentages are always based on the selling price equaling 100 percent. These range from approximately 10 percent on tobacco products up to 50 percent on products with high service requirements and relatively slow turnover rates. These various percentages are estimated on the basis of the turnover rate, the service costs, the carrying costs, and the procurement costs. These intuitive estimates, derived through many years of experience, parallel the marketing theories of Professor Aspinwall.[2] Pharmacists who practice this approach are not considered either to be very competitive or to have extremely high prices. Many pharmacists who have good locations and provide superior professional pharmaceutical services and use market segmentation strategy have been very successful. In contrast, pharmacists with an inferior location or who provided inferior professional pharmaceutical service have faced bankruptcy as a result of this pricing policy in a highly competitive market.

Competitive Pricing. Competitive pricing approximates fairly well what has come to be known as the game plan by sophisticated managers. Game theory, a mathematical and statistical model, is designed to guide managers in decision-making. However, experts in game theory admit the impossibility of encompassing all of the varieties of economic behavior in their model. The theory presumes that people pursue their own interests, whatever they may be, and each individual has a preference pattern among the available options and follows the pattern rather consistently.[3] Statistically, this theory is sound, but in practice it is subjective individuals who make the decisions, and their choices are subjective, isolated acts that often cannot be treated as aggregates. Thus, the game plan is a rather tenuous method of long-range planning. However, the game plan works well in the area of competitive pricing. The following cases illustrate the application of the game plan on a scale that is practical.

One drug company tabulates the advertisements of its competition, most of which are the weekend specials variety. A chart is constructed to show what products, by classes or categories, are advertised with the quoted price by firm and week. These charts are updated continuously, and the general, composite pattern of advertising behavior of the competition is easily discernible. The management of this company simply selects the product mix and the price of each product to convey a competitive image and not a deep-cut discount image. The company provides many services not offered by the larger competitors. This game plan is successful because it is directed toward a specific objective; it is based on data that provide a fairly high degree of predictability of the behavior of the competition; and finally, it is flexible enough to permit desired changes in the plan. This game plan is in sharp contrast to a long-term game plan based on data providing less predictability and designed to achieve broad and general objectives.

Two other mini-cases illustrate the concept on a much smaller scale. In a small town of approximately 6,000 with four pharmacies, one of the pharmacists was rather aggressive from a professional viewpoint (or progressive from a business viewpoint) and ran "weekend specials" advertisements in the weekly newspaper. One of his colleagues, or competitors if you prefer, consistently cut out the advertisement and taped it on the front door of his pharmacy with the notice that he would match all of the prices advertised for the items that he also stocked.

The other case is a little more subtle in the game plan used. A pharmacist who operated a traditional pharmacy with a professional orientation and atmosphere and a large prescription volume suddenly found himself in a highly competitive market. He designed an attractive poster that indicated that he offered competitive prices consistent with the services he provided on those products he stocked. The notice indicated the average cost for charge service, delivery service, patient medication record system, and personal professional consultation. It also indicated that for those who did not want these services, a cash and carry price would be quoted. Since most of his patrons wanted these services, he had few inquiries about the cash and carry price. The pharmacist was able to satisfy those few patrons in his trade area who were especially price oriented without loss of patronage or profit.

Price Leadership. This is the most aggressive approach to pricing policies or price competition. As the term implies, the management of the pharmacy or firm attempts to have the lowest prices in the market. This is characteristic of the discounters and some well-known department stores such as R. H. Macy and Company of New York. Some chain drugstore companies practice this policy.

Most of these firms have several characteristics in common: (1) they buy in large volume and search out the lowest possible price; (2) they cut their expenses as much as possible, both by carefully controlling necessary expenses and by not offering many services such as credit, delivery, and personalized attention or selling; (3) many use the least expensive fixtures and furnishings; (4) many carry only the fast turnover products or sizes and styles. Most of these firms practice price leadership on all merchandise, while some use price leadership on a large portion of their stock, but not necessarily on a majority of the items. Few pharmacists, including those employed by traditional chain drugstores, are advocates of this type of pricing policy.

People other than pharmacists condemn this "cut throat" type of practice. Mr. J. C. Penney, founder of the company that bears his name, had this to say about the practice: "The item we sell at 79 cents is a 79 cent item. We neither expect nor want customers of ours to think either that we are such poor business people as to believe we can sell them a dollar item for 79 cents, or we think them of such poor intelligence that they would actually think we could do so."[4]

What the Market Will Bear. Pricing based on what the market will bear is the worst of all approaches to pricing. First, it is the most inconsistent pricing policy of all. Second, it shows a lack of social responsibility and sensitivity *unless* the practitioner makes allowances for the indigent, which would require great astuteness and a sense of fair play. Third, the policy is undemocratic in that the practitioner takes advantage of both the ignorant and the rich—if he can get away with it—without adequate information to determine a just price.

Unfortunately, some pharmacists have been practicing on the fringe of this policy with respect to prescription charges because they did not have a logical method of prescription pricing, but priced them in a haphazard manner. Although the prescription pricing surveys that have appeared in several newspapers and *Consumer Reports* were poorly designed with faulty analysis and conclusions, the wide divergence in prices for the same prescription in different pharmacies is cause for some apprehension in the minds of thinking pharmacists as well as the less-informed public. When these discrepancies in prices appeared for the same prescription dispensed from the same pharmacy, there was indeed cause for alarm![5] This latter inconsistency, together with severe competition on popular and maintenance drugs from discounting pharmacies in a nearby city, caused one independent pharmacist to adopt the professional fee for prescriptions.[6] For these reasons, the policy of "what the market will bear" should be discouraged.

Odd Pricing. This is an old gimmick that has been used for so long that it has lost most of its potency in accomplishing its intended purpose. Odd pricing is simply using an odd figure, for example 49 cents, instead of the round figure of 50 cents, in the belief that the public would think the price difference was more than one cent. The basis of this theory is that 49 cents is associated with the decimal class of 40s in contrast to the decimal class of 50s, a 10 cent difference. In other words, 49 cents carries the connotation of being less in price than the one cent difference it really is. Also, it is supposed that the public thinks the merchant is pricing the item as low as possible by reducing the price a penny to its lowest possible level.

Odd pricing probably was first used by price leaders and later by those who priced competitively. Odd pricing became so common that it became a characteristic of traditional or regular pricing. Although odd prices are still prevalent for many products sold in pharmacies, at least one chain drugstore company has discontinued its use for clerical reasons. The company found that fewer errors and greater efficiency were achieved at the cash registers when rounded prices were used.

Professional Discounts. Most pharmacies generally adhere to a one-price policy except for special or professional discounts. Professional discounts have been a problem for pharmacists for many years. Most pharmacists, if not all, will agree that professional discounts are good if used on a reciprocal basis. The crux of the problem is that prescribers in general, and physicians in particular, expect discounts on drugs and other pharmaceutical products, but they do not reciprocate for their services in many instances. Furthermore, professional discounts do not stop with the prescribers but are extended to nurses, receptionists, and others, either by request or voluntarily. The question is where the professional discount should stop. Many pharmacists gladly extend these discounts when requested in the hopes of enhancing their professional relations with the prescribers and those associated with them. The ultimate goal, however, is the increase in the number of prescriptions from these sources. Other pharmacists actively seek the opportunity to offer professional discounts to prescribers and their associates.

It is the abuse of the professional discount that demeans pharmacy, and some logical and fair guidelines or policy should be established in every pharmacy. In addition, pharmacists in each market should establish a uniform policy or guideline and abide by it. Since the discount is based on professional courtesy, I do not see such an agreement as a violation of the Anti-trust Laws; however, such activity should be reviewed by an attorney in each case.

Sometimes, special discounts are offered to ministers, policemen, and others. In my opinion, there is no rational basis for these discounts.

Pricing Methods

Having discussed the various competitive markets and competitive strategies to deal with the market situations, let us turn our attention to pricing methods. The competitive strategy and pricing policy of a pharmacist provide the theoretic and philosophic framework for price determination. However, the actual mathematical or non-mathematical methods of pricing constitute the final step of price determination.

Non-Mathematical Methods. These methods of pricing are used under various circumstances described in the discussion of competitive strategy and pricing policies. They include the suggested selling price for products sold under a franchise agreement, fair trade laws where they are operative, and certain circumstances of competitive pricing in which the competitor's price is simply emulated. The haphazard pricing used in an attempt to get the price the market will bear is determined without the benefit of rational arithmetical calculation.

Mathematical Methods. The use of mathematics is a rational approach to price determination. The mathematical calculations should be based on a thorough understanding of management's objectives and policies, operational costs, and financial analysis of the financial statements. The *mechanics* of mathematical methods of pricing is based on the equation representing the relationships found in the profit and loss statement. The equation is expressed as follows:

$$SP - CGS - Exp = NP$$

where: SP = the selling price
CGS = the cost of goods sold
Exp = the expenses
NP = the net profit

The basic equation may be broken down into two other equations:

$$SP - CGS = GM$$
$$GM - Exp = NP$$

where: GM = the gross margin.

In pharmacy, contrary to many other occupations, the selling price always equals 100 percent, unless otherwise specified, just as net sales volume equals 100 percent in the profit and loss statement. The combined equations above may be illustrated by percentages and dollars as follows:

$$SP - CGS = GM \quad \text{and} \quad GM - Exp = NP$$
$$100\% - 65\% = 35\% \quad \text{and} \quad 35\% - 31\% = 4\%$$
$$\$5.00 - \$3.25 = \$1.75 \quad \text{and} \quad \$1.75 - \$1.55 = \$0.20$$

The relationships as illustrated above are such that the desired selling price may be calculated if any one of the other terms of the equation and its corresponding percent are known. The dollar value is divided by the percent, expressed as a decimal, for example, $3.25 ÷ .65 = $5.00. The selling price in the above example may be calculated algebraically as follows:

Let X equal the selling price: then,

$$(X)(.65) = \$3.25$$
$$.65X = \$3.25$$
$$X = \$5.00$$

Pharmacists have devised short cuts or easy methods for arriving at the selling price, given the unit cost, to provide a desired percent gross margin. An overview of the more commonly used short cuts should be valuable to the reader. To yield a 50 percent gross margin, double the cost; for a 40 percent gross margin, take two-thirds of the cost and add this figure to the cost, or divide the cost by 6 and multiply the quotient by 10; for a $33^1/_3$ percent gross margin, take one-half of the cost and add this value to the cost; for a 25 percent gross margin, take one-third of the cost and add this figure to the cost; and for a 20 percent gross margin, take one-fourth of the cost and add this value to the cost. In each instance, the resulting selling price will yield the specified or desired percent gross margin.

PRICING OBJECTIVES

The mathematical method of pricing will permit the pharmacist to mark up a product or product line to accomplish specific objectives and to adjust the percent gross margin to compensate for turnover rates and other variables.

Return the Usual Net Profit. One pricing objective is to cover average expenses and usual net profit. The *Lilly Digest* percentage total expenses was 32.5 for 1972, and the estimated percentage for nonprescription sales was approximately 28 to 29 percent. The NACDS *Lilly Digest* average percentage for total expenses was 23.7 for 1972, and the estimated percentage expenses for nonprescription sales was approximately 20 to 21 percent. The percentages net profit were 3.6 and 4.4 and for gross margin, 36.1 and 28.1, for independent and chain pharmacies, respectively. Thus, the independent pharmacist sets his percentage gross margin for the bulk of nonprescription products at 33 percent, whereas the management of the chain drug firms targets the percentage markup of the bulk of nonprescription products at 26 percent.

Promotional Image. Another pricing objective is to cover variable expenses and sometimes the desired net profit. If the objective is to cover variable expenses only, then the general purpose is to project a promotional or low price image with little or no extra cost. If the objective is to include a net profit, then the purpose is to maintain profits while projecting a promotional or low price image. For the purpose of this discussion, the following expense items are classified as *variable expenses,* even though they may be fixed to an extent for a given pharmacy: advertising, bad debts, employees' wages, and miscellaneous expenses. Employee wages and miscellaneous expenses are semi-variable, but they are classified as variable expenses for the purpose of delineating all expenses into two categories. Variable expenses for independent pharmacies were estimated at 17 percent from *Lilly Digest* data for 1972. For nonprescription sales, the variable expenses were estimated at $16\frac{2}{3}$ percent. If a pharmacist wishes to cover variable expenses only, he can take one-fifth of the unit cost and add this figure to the unit cost. If he wishes to make about 3.5 percent net profit on sales, he can add one-fourth of the unit cost to the unit cost. This method of pricing is used mostly for promotional, nonstaple merchandise.

It should be understood that pricing merchandise to cover variable expenses is *not* pricing at the marginal cost. The two are somewhat similar concepts, but the economics as well as the method of arriving at the marginal cost are quite different.

This type of pricing is *not* the true "loss leader" type of pricing whereby a product is priced at or near cost and sometimes below cost. The *objective* of the *loss leader* method of pricing is to create a definite low price image. Both special and staple goods are used for loss leaders.

Turnover Rate Variations. The percent gross margin should vary with the turnover rate of a product. Turnover rate is determined by dividing the cost of goods sold by the average inventory investment. Table 11-1, composed of hypothetical data, illustrates how gross margin and turnover are inversely related while achieving the same annual net profit.

The same principle can be illustrated by actual data derived from the *Lilly Digest.* The pharmacies were divided into two groups for comparison—those with low turnover rates and those with high turnover rates. The gross margin, total expenses, proprietor's total income, and inventory were related to the respective turnover rates as shown in Table 11-2.

Even though the data in Table 11-2 are a few years old, an analysis clearly indicates the relationship between increased turnover rate and proprietor's total income. This is achieved with a smaller percent gross margin and a smaller investment in inventory. The percentage of total income as a return on the investment in inventory is increased 3.3-fold as the turnover rate is increased 3.3-fold. If the proprietor's salary is subtracted from total income, the percentage return on investment is even more dramatic—yielding a 4- to 5-fold increase.

With a good inventory control system, the turnover rate can be

Table 11-1. *Relationship Between Gross Margin and Turnover Rate*

Turnover Rate Per Unit	1.5		3		6	
Selling price	$1.00	100%	$1.00	100%	$1.00	100%
Cost	.50	50%	.60	60%	.65	65%
Gross margin	$ .50	50%	$ .40	40%	$ .35	35%
Expenses	.30	30%	.30	30%	.30	30%
Net profit	$ .20	20%	$ .10	10%	$ .05	5%
Annual NP	$ .30	—	$ .30	—	$ .30	—

determined for certain products and product lines. The pharmacist is in a good position to price wisely, be competitive when necessary, and still maintain realistic profits.

Prescription Pricing

The pharmacist should not be misled into believing that prescription prices are of little or no concern to the public. In fact, there is a relationship between trusting the pharmacist as a professional person to provide the necessary advice and the correct drug (including avoiding drug interactions and allergies), and trusting him to charge a reasonable price. If the trust is not fulfilled with respect to price, the pharmacist will lose the professional trust, and *vice versa.*[7] Since only a few popular maintenance prescription drugs, some 15 to 20, are discounted in most instances, this is one of the best arguments for using a reasonable professional or dispensing fee, a method that will yield a charge that is both competitive and defensible.

HISTORY OF PRICING

Attempts to establish fair and adequate dispensing or professional fees go back into the antiquity of pharmacy. These efforts have been both private and public. As discussed in Chapter 1, one of the earliest public

Table 11-2. *Relationship Between Turnover Rate and Other Operating Data*

Turnover Rate	6.7	2.0
Gross margin	33.9%	38.7%
Total expenses*	21.1%	26.2%
Proprietor's total income	13.8%–$21,875	12.5%–$19,814
Inventory	— $15,376	— $46,128

*Total expenses excluding the proprietor's salary.
Adapted from: Olsen, P. C., Hecker, F. C., Chagaris, C. H., and Ford, W. L., *How to Decide How Much to Buy.* New York: National Wholesale Druggists Association.

attempts to regulate prescription prices was the edict of Frederick II.[8] Griffenhagen traced the early private attempts to promote "Fair Trade" in prescription pricing.[9] He described the *Catalogue of the Materia Medica and of Pharmaceutical Preparation with Uniform Prices of the Massachusetts College of Pharmacy* published in 1828. It included 40 pages and 700 items. It was the first such American catalogue with printed prices. A unique feature was a compounding pricing schedule, which included the following examples: Pills: 2 to 4, 12 cents; 6 to 8, 19 cents; 10 to 18, 25 cents; and 1 cent each over 30. There was a schedule for powders, liquids, ointments, and plasters. Clearly, this schedule was a type of compounding or professional fee. Griffenhagen noted earlier catalogues, but he emphasized the uniform pricing and pricing schedule aspects of the Massachusetts catalogue.[10]

No doubt interest in prescription pricing has occupied the thinking and deliberations of pharmacists over the years since 1828. McEvilla reviewed briefly some of the early history of the changing attitudes toward prescription pricing between World War II and the 1950s.[11] Myers provided a more extensive review of the changing attitudes and approaches toward the professional fee in an article entitled, "Professional Fee: Renaissance or Innovation?"[12] Nitardy made one of the earlier contributions to rational prescription pricing when he developed the "Prescription Pricing Schedule" for the National Association of Retail Druggists (NARD) in 1908.[13] The schedule was based on the cost of ingredient(s), doubling this, and adding a compounding charge as a reward for professional skills and knowledge. Almost every pricing schedule developed since the Nitardy schedule contained a dispensing or professional fee, which included either a nominal or a substantial amount, for the professional function.

Myers briefly described two other prescription pricing schedules devised by Cutts and the Minnesota Pharmaceutical Association in 1893 and 1903, respectively.[12] The proliferation of prescription pricing methods was beginning to take place. Chase also noted that chaos and diversity of prescription prices existed from the use of the many different schedules and rules.[14] In 1915, he found that some pharmacists were "getting whatever they think the customer will stand for . . ."

Until World War I, the cost of ingredients generally was not the major factor in pricing prescriptions. The labor cost and professional skills involved were the major considerations. Therefore, most of the various pricing schedules and rules contained a significant professional fee component. This began to change with the high cost of drugs and chemicals during World War I. These higher costs resulted from the fact that most drugs and chemicals were imported and Germany was the world's largest producer. The price of acetophenetidin increased as much as 2,000 to 3,000 percent.[12] As a result, a flat-rate system of pricing was no longer feasible.

In 1915 the APhA appointed a committee to investigate the matter and suggest a proper manner of pricing prescriptions. The Committee, under the chairmanship of Harry B. Mason, made its report, and the House of Delegates adopted Evans' rule as the preferred method of prescription pricing. Evans' rule was rather simple and did not confuse the issue greatly. It simply stated that a pharmacist should double the cost of the ingredient(s) in the prescription and add $1.00 per hour for the time consumed in compounding the prescription. Ironically, one of two papers presented by title only at the same session was written by Nitardy, who had devised the NARD Schedule, and who advocated that a fee for the professional services of the pharmacist be incorporated into the formula or schedule.[12]

From this historic moment until the present day, at least *five* major developments have increased the emphasis on the cost of the drug and the percent markup, with de-emphasis on the professional component of prescription services. First, the industrial revolution in the pharmaceutical industry brought about a reduction in the number of compounded prescriptions, with a corresponding reduction in the utilization of the manipulative skills of the pharmacist. Second, the revolution brought about a proliferation of potent, prefabricated pharmaceuticals with a high ingredient cost to the pharmacist. Third, with the gradual expansion of the merchandising function of the pharmacist, there was a gradual carry-over tendency to apply the markup concept more directly in the prescription department. Fourth, the enactment of the fair trade laws in the 1930s and their application to prescription legend drugs had a most profound and direct influence on the philosophy of prescription pricing. The minimum fair trade price was based on a percentage markup. Last, the various prescription pricing schedules, devised during the 1950s as a timesaving convenience, emphasized the markup aspect, but retained a substantial or nominal professional fee as a part of the final prescription price.

ANALYSIS OF PRICING SCHEDULES

Many prescription pricing schedules were devised during the years between World War II and the 1960s. Although these schedules claimed a rationale, they generally were short on sound logic. Kendall and Lee attempted to correct this deficiency by analyzing various schedules and developing an improved formula.[15] They found that most schedules used one of the two following formulas:

1. *Computation type—*

$$M + C + CF = SP$$

where: M = the material cost plus a markup;
C = the container cost with or without a markup;

CF = the compounding fee, determined by multiplying the compounding time by $1 to $3, depending on the pharmacist's hourly salary;

SP = the selling price.

2. *Computation plus a flat rate—*

$$C + S + M = SP$$

where: C = the compounding fee;
    S = a flat service charge;
    M = the material cost plus a markup;
    SP = the selling price.

The markup varied from $33^1/_3$ to 50 percent of the cost, depending on the value of a unit. The improved formula of Kendall and Lee varied little from previous formulas except that an average service fee, SF, was established, based on the average time for experienced pharmacists to compound a given number of units of a dosage form. For prefabricated prescriptions, one-half of the service fee was used. The revised formula was:

$$M + C + SF = SP$$

where: M = the cost of materials plus a markup of $33^1/_3$ to 50 percent;
    C = the cost of the container, which was doubled;
    SF = a flat rate based on the number of units dispensed;
    SP = the selling price.

There are basically four methods of computing prescription charges.

> Percent gross margin (GM)
> Sliding scale gross margin
> Professional fee
> A combination of these

Analysis of several prescription pricing schedules revealed the following variations and combinations of the four basic methods. One schedule used a fixed percent GM and a fixed dispensing fee to determine the total prescription price. Another schedule applied a decreasing percent GM with increments of cost of the quantity dispensed without a dispensing fee. A third schedule used a decreasing percent GM with increments of the cost of the quantity dispensed plus a variable fee which increased with the increments of quantity dispensed. Four schedules utilized a decreasing percent GM based on the quantity dispensed, without respect to cost of the drug, plus a percentage dispensing fee added to the GM. Three other schedules utilized some form of professional fee concept. None of the other possible combinations of the basic pricing methods was observed.

All of the schedules examined made provision for a professional fee for compounded prescriptions. One schedule provided a fixed professional fee of $2.00 added to the cost of ingredients. The same device provided six variable percent gross margin schedules for a wide range of choices. The variable percentage markups decreased at a decreasing rate with increasing number of units dispensed. It supposedly followed a "curve" rather than a step-wise progression.* One other schedule also utilized a "curve" in establishing the gross margin to which a fee could be added, but all the other schedules were based on a decrease in percent gross margin, ranging from a minimum of two to ten steps. Some had a fee built into the selling price as shown in the schedule, while others suggested a fixed or variable fee to be added to the "commodity" value of the prescription drug as shown in the schedule.

There are several objections to most of the existing pricing schedules:

1. The price of small quantities of inexpensive prescriptions frequently is not sufficient to cover the amount of fixed costs of dispensing. This "deficit" is made up on larger quantities and expensive prescriptions which causes a hardship on the patrons affected.

2. The use of some of the schedules requires interpolation, especially for the more expensive drugs.

3. Some schedules vary the percent gross margin in a manner that causes inequities in prescription charges among patrons. For example, 50 tablets that cost $2.00 per 100 sell for $2.35, while 10 tablets costing $10.00 per 100 sell for $2.85. This is a 50 cent difference in price for a $1.00 ingredient cost in each instance, but fewer doses are provided in the more expensive prescription.

Professional Fees

REVIVAL OF PROFESSIONAL FEES

A serious attempt to determine the cost of dispensing prescriptions was made by Jefferies.[16] He established norms for dispensing prefabricated prescriptions using time and motion studies. An average overhead or expense per prescription was computed, which was applicable to most pharmacies. The study further indicated three levels of labor cost (5, 6, and 7 cents per minute, respectively) depending on the marketing area. He devised three sliding charts corresponding to the three different labor costs per minute which, when set at the combined cost of the ingredient and container, would indicate the breakeven cost over eleven different

---

*The publisher of the schedule stated the selling price was calculated "on a curve." The ingredient cost varied by a fraction of a cent in the low cost range, but the ingredient cost varied by discrete intervals (in excess of one cent) in the higher cost range and by one cent intervals in the mid-range.

time intervals required to dispense the prescription. To the breakeven cost, the pharmacist could add a flat or percentage fee, representing the net profit for each prescription dispensed. This chart was made available to pharmacists by Becton, Dickinson and Company.

Evanson's economic analysis of prescription departments provided basic operational data that gave further insight into the economics of prescription pricing.[17] In 1952, Apple published another method of calculating prescription charges.[18] His method included both a significant professional fee and a commodity value. In 1957, a student of Professor Fuller first advocated a simple, all inclusive single professional fee for all prescriptions filled in a particular pharmacy.[19,20] Since then, much has been written for, and against, the professional fee concept.[21] It generally is believed by those who have made a serious study of the fee concept that a professional fee *is* possible. It can be simple to use and is easy to adjust to meet competitive conditions or to maintain a desired profit structure.

PHILOSOPHY

Before one can really appreciate and understand or use the professional fee concept, one must examine the three basic tenets of its philosophy. They are:

1. A prescription drug is not an ordinary article of trade that the public may buy or sell at their pleasure. Prescription drugs are developed and produced to alleviate human suffering. They are potent compounds and are subject to misuse and abuse in unskilled hands. Therefore, laymen may possess these drugs only through competent professional people, including the pharmacist, after diagnosis of the illness, prescribing and proper dispensing of the indicated drug.

2. Neither the dispensing cost nor the benefit derived from such prescription is a function of the cost of the ingredient(s) in a prescription.

3. Neither the professional and legal responsibility nor the time incurred in dispensing a prescription is a function of the cost of the ingredient(s) in a prescription.

Having accepted these three tenets, one can proceed to examine the pros and cons of the fee concept.

PROS AND CONS OF PROFESSIONAL FEES

Advantages. First, there are several economic advantages to the professional fee:

1. The fee concept tends to stabilize prescription prices, protecting the pharmacist from a profit squeeze due to prescriptions of less expensive brands or generic drugs, and protecting the public from high prescription charges resulting from a markup on expensive new drugs.

2. The pharmacist is able to recover all expense and a fair return on *each* prescription dispensed on a fee basis.

3. The professional fee permits a competitive charge for expensive, maintenance prescriptions.

4. The fee, being fixed, saves time and prevents miscalculations and errors.

5. The fee may be used to improve professional relations. Physicians have been enthusiastic in accepting the fee concept.

6. Since most patients accept the fee concept wholeheartedly, it will, when properly used, promote good public relations and image.

7. The fee could have legal advantages in negotiations with third-party payers, since it more nearly defines the professional services of the pharmacist than does the markup method.

Potential Problems. Some of the potential problems, and their resolutions, which a pharmacist may encounter with the fee are:

1. How does one price refills of prescriptions already on file? The answer to this question lies in not raising the price on any refill, but rather, adjusting downwardly the price of expensive refills.

2. What does one do about requests for refills of multiple or fractional amounts? The fee remains the same unless a certain defined upper limit is exceeded. This will discourage refills for one-half or one-fourth amounts, which are seldom economic. Such requests have been eliminated largely by third-party payment programs. Exceptions are made in the case in which only a few doses are needed until the next appointment with the physician. The fee is retained for all larger quantities up to the size of the regular stock bottle. An adjustment of the fee is added for the second or fraction of each additional stock bottle quantity dispensed. This rule is designed solely to protect the pharmacist economically from someone deliberately prescribing or requesting unusually large quantities.

3. What about new prescriptions for very large quantities? The answer is the same as discussed above.

4. How does one compute the fee for a compounded prescription? Simply add to the regular price the appropriate rate for the pharmacist's time spent in compounding. This occurs in less than one percent of the prescriptions.

5. How does the fixed fee cover the cost plus a return on the investment in inventory? The answer is that only about 10 to 12 percent of the overhead expense can be related directly to inventory investment. Most expenses are fixed on an annual basis. Average return on the inventory investment can be calculated for each prescription, and this is the only way of ensuring the proper return on inventory investments.

6. Isn't the fee unrealistic for prescription ingredients costing $5.00 or more? The answer is that only a small percentage of the prescriptions cost $5.00. The supposed deficit on expensive prescriptions is adequately

compensated by the increased revenue from the less expensive prescriptions.

Regardless of the method used to determine the prescription charge,
consideration must be given to three basic factors: (1) the cost of the
ingredient and the container; (2) the cost incurred in dispensing the
prescription; (3) the profit necessary to sustain the practice and to permit
its growth.

The first of these is always computed in the same manner, regardless
of the pricing method used. The second and third factors are combined
and an average value per prescription is computed to arrive at the
professional fee. The markup method is based on the theory that the sum
of factors two and three is a function or percentage of factor one. Since
this is not true, the markup is not a logical method. The major difficulty
lies in how much the professional fee should be, but this difficulty also
exists with the markup method. Several methods of determining the
professional fee have been proposed.

Fuller's Formula.[22] Fuller offered the following formula:

$$\frac{(AE - PS)\,(R_xS \div TS)}{TR_x} + LC + NP = PF$$

where: AE = All expenses
   PS = Proprietor's salary
   R_xS = Prescription sales
   TS = Total sales
   TR_x = Total number of prescriptions dispensed
   LC = Direct labor cost ($0.50 in the original formula)
   NP = Desired net profit
   PF = Professional Fee

Applying this formula to 1972 *Lilly Digest* data, the average professional fee for all the pharmacies is $1.56 plus desired net profit. The value
is $1.54 plus desired net profit for prescription-oriented pharmacies with
85 percent prescription sales to total sales.

Abrams' Formula.[23] Abrams has suggested the following formula:

$$\frac{(AE - PS)\,(R_x \div TS) + PS}{TR_x} + NP = PF$$

If this formula is applied to the same two groups of *Lilly Digest*
pharmacies, the professional fees are $1.84 plus desired net profit and
$1.70 plus desired net profit, respectively.

Jacoff's Method. Jacoff and Evanson computed an average burden rate of $1.39 per prescription for 1960 *Lilly Digest* pharmacies.[24] The burden rate was 43.5 percent of the average prescription charge. If this percentage is applied to the average prescription charge reported in the 1972 *Lilly Digest,* the burden rate would be $1.91. To this figure the desired net profit must be added. It should be noted that $1.91 may not be the burden rate per prescription for 1972 *Lilly Digest* pharmacies, if the burden rate is recalculated by means of the technique of Jacoff and Evanson.

Jacoff and Evanson applied the cost accounting technique to 1958 data derived from a prescription-oriented pharmacy.[25] Their burden rate was $1.00. Again, extrapolating the percentage of the burden rate to the average prescription charge for pharmacies with 83.4 percent prescription sales in 1958, the estimated 1972 burden rate would be $1.43.

Knox's Method.[26] A trial and error method of computing a professional fee was suggested by Knox. This method requires the use of a representative sample of prescriptions—both new and renewals—dispensed during the previous year. From the sample, an average prescription charge is computed. A professional fee is selected and added to the ingredient cost of each prescription. The average of the prescription charges using the fee is computed and compared with the average of the original prices. The fee is adjusted so that the same average charge, gross margin, and net profit potential are realized. A simpler approach would be to compute the average gross margin for a representative sample of original prices and round to the nearest five cents or quarter. This gives a professional fee that ensures approximately the same net profit.

An average cost of dispensing a prescription of $1.69 was reported in 1968.[27] This study, sponsored by the NARD, was based on 1,638 usable questionnaires, which were purported to represent the U.S. pharmacies.

Smith's Method.[28] Smith applied cost accounting principles to 1964 *Lilly Digest* data and computed a burden rate per prescription ranging from $.85 to $1.75 when the data were classified by sales volume and number of prescriptions dispensed per day. Addition of a net profit of $.50 per prescription to the burden rates resulted in professional fees ranging from $1.35 to $2.25. The cost allocation method used in this study involved the following steps.

STEP 1. ALLOCATION OF LABOR COST. This step consists of two parts: (A) the employed pharmacist's(s') salary is allocated to the prescription department (number of hours employed pharmacist works times the average hourly salary for the area); and (B) the amount of proprietor's salary is calculated to equal the number of hours the pharmacy is opened less the number of hours the employed pharmacist works times the average hourly salary for pharmacists in the area. The sum of A and B is the direct labor cost of rendering professional services.

STEP 2. OCCUPANCY COST. The product of multiplying the sum of the cost of rent, heat, light, and power times the ratio of the square feet of the prescription department to the total square feet is allocated to the prescription department. This is the occupancy cost.

STEP 3. GENERAL AND ADMINISTRATIVE COST. All expenses, other than salaries, wages, rent, heat, light, and power—but including the remainder of the proprietor's salary—are multiplied by the percentage of prescription sales to total sales and allocated to the prescription department. This is the administrative and general cost, and includes the cost of carrying the inventory. It does not include imputed interest for carrying the inventory, but it does include a proportional amount of the actual interest charge.

STEP 4. SUMMATION OF TOTAL COST AND AVERAGE BURDEN RATE. The sum of Steps 1, 2, and 3 is divided by the number of prescriptions dispensed to ascertain the average burden rate per prescription.

STEP 5. DETERMINATION OF PROFESSIONAL FEE. The average burden rate plus the desired net profit equals the professional fee. Figure 11-1 illustrates how the average dispensing cost is calculated.

Modified Cost Allocation Methods. The Kansas Department of Social Welfare modified and refined the cost allocation method published by Smith, and the modified method is applied to each pharmacy that wishes to participate in the Kansas Title XIX Program.[29] The modifications in the Kansas Form require that: (1) any direct expense that can be identified as a direct prescription department expense is allocated directly to that department, for example, prescription bags; and (2) insurance premiums and property taxes are allocated to the prescription department on the basis of prescription inventory divided by total inventory and prescription fixtures and equipment divided by total fixtures and equipment, respectively. A further refinement of the Kansas Form was published in *The Kentucky Pharmacist.*[30]

When judgments were required, the concept of standard cost was used. A standard cost is the best judgment of what the cost should be, everything considered, and not what the cost actually is. An example of this is the hourly salary for the pharmacist for which $7.50 was selected in application to the 1972 *Lilly Digest* data. Of course, standard cost should be close to the average costs for the industry and area.

When Smith's method was applied to two groups of pharmacies reported in the 1972 *Lilly Digest,* the 160 prescription-oriented pharmacies with an average of 85.1 percent prescription sales to total sales and the total sample of 1,823 pharmacies, the respective burden rates were $1.48 and $1.64. The difference between the two rates may be attributed to the efficiency of prescription-oriented pharmacies with high levels of prescription volume concentrated in a relatively small area.

The cost allocation method was subjected to a validity test by a comparison of the $1.48 burden rate for prescription-oriented pharmacies, with the burden rate derived from the same data adjusted to 100 percent prescription sales. If a pharmacy derived all its income from prescriptions,

1972 Lilly Digest Data	U.S. Average (*1,823 Pharmacies*)		*Example of Calculations*
Sales			1. *Professional Labor Cost:*
Prescription	$112,777	46.6%	
Other	129,133	53.4%	a. Pharmacist's Professional
Total	$241,910	100.0%	Labor Cost: ($7.50/hr. rate) 40 hrs. × $7.50 ×
			52 wks. = $15,600.
Cost of goods sold	154,566	63.9%	b. Proprietor's Professional
			Labor Cost: ($7.50/hr.
Gross margin	$ 87,344	36.1%	rate) 69 hrs. − 40 hrs. =
			29 hrs. proprietor serves
Expenses			as pharmacist. 29 hrs.
Proprietor's or manager's salary	$ 20,304	8.4%	× $7.50 × 52 wks. =
Employees' wages	29,104	12.0%	$11,310. Total of a. and
Rent	6,077	2.5%	b. is $26,910, total pro-
Heat, light, and power	1,878	0.8%	fessional labor cost.
General and administrative expenses	21,266	8.8%	
Total expenses	$ 78,629	32.5%	
			2. *Occupancy Cost:*
Net profit (before taxes)	$ 8,715	3.6%	$6,077 + $1,878 × .14 =
			$1,114.
Add proprietor's withdrawals	20,304	8.4%	
Total income of self-employed proprietor (before taxes on income and profits)	$ 29,019	12.0%	3. *General and Administrative Cost:*
Value of inventory at cost and as a percent of sales			a. $78,629 − ($20,304 + $29,104 + $6,077 +
Prescription	$ 13,969	12.4%	$1,878) = $21,266.
Other	27,466	21.3%	b. $20,304 − $11,310 =
Total	$ 41,435	17.1%	$8,994, remainder of proprietor's salary.
Annual rate of turnover of inventory		3.8 times	c. $21,266 + $8,994 = $30,260, total general
Size of area and sales per square foot*	sq. ft.		adm. cost.
Prescription	334	$335.96	d. $30,260 × .466 ℞/total
Other	2,055	62.56	sales = $14,101.
Total	2,389	100.84	
Sales per dollar invested in inventory			
Prescription		$8.07	4. *Average ℞ Dispensing Cost:*
Other		4.70	a. Sum of 1, 2, and 3:
			$26,910 + $1,114 +
Net profit per dollar invested in inventory		$0.210	+ $14,101 = $42,125.
			b. $42,125 ÷ 25,743 ℞'s =
Number of prescriptions dispensed			$1.636, $1.64 rounded.
New	11,823	45.9%	
Renewed	13,920	54.1%	
Total	25,743	100.0%	5. *Add Desired Net Profit/℞:*
Prescription charge		$4.38	$1.64 + $.50 (e.g.) = $2.14 or $2.15 rounded.
Number of hours per week			
Pharmacy was open		69 hours	
Worked by proprietor		52 hours	
Worked by employed pharmacist(s)		40 hours	

*Based on averages of pharmacies that reported all data

Figure 11-1. *Application of Cost Allocation*

the problem of cost allocation would not exist. Since prescription sales in the 160 prescription-oriented pharmacies averaged 85.1 percent prescription sales to total sales, there should be a relatively low order of error in adjusting the data to 100 percent prescription sales. The remaining 14.9 percent of sales were converted to prescription sales without any adjustment in the total expense structure. The $21,261 nonprescription sales are the equivalent of 4,532 additional prescriptions using the average prescription charge of $4.47—making an adjusted total of 31,826 prescriptions. The adjusted burden rate was calculated to be $1.60.

The five-step method of cost allocation described above may be criticized on the grounds that none of the wages of the employees, other than the pharmacist, was allocated to the prescription department. Counterbalancing this possible weakness is the fact that none of the pharmacist's salary was allocated to other departments. This counterbalancing principle was followed because it was felt the pharmacist's activity in other departments did, in fact, balance the contribution of other personnel to the prescription department.

Perhaps the main weakness of the cost allocation method used here is the absence of a direct allocation of all the specific costs incurred in the prescription department. For example, delivery cost was not allocated directly to the prescription department. However, the unadjusted burden rate for the 160 prescription-oriented pharmacies in the study accounted for 92.5 percent of all the costs and the services rendered.

PRACTICAL IMPLICATIONS AND EXPERIENCES

The methods of determining the cost of dispensing a prescription presented in this chapter are meant to serve as a practical guide for those pharmacists desiring a rational approach to determining a professional fee for their practice. The amount to be added to the dispensing cost of burden rate is an individual matter for each pharmacist.

With all cost allocation methods, and in the application of any method, judgment must be used in computing burden rates and professional fees. Any professional fee that may be adopted by a practitioner should be designed for his practice and may have to be modified to accommodate certain unusual circumstances. These include requests for fractional or multiple quantities of the original prescription, prescriptions for drugs commonly sold without a prescription, renewals of old prescriptions, and competitive conditions. These situations can be handled satisfactorily by a pharmacist who is convinced of the economic and professional soundness of the professional fee.

Additional prescription dispensing cost studies are needed to determine the best method(s) and a more precise estimate of the cost of dispensing a prescription. A pilot project of developing and testing a uniform cost accounting system for pharmacies was performed in Michigan during 1973. The next step will be to extend this project to a national sample representing all types of pharmacies. This is necessary to validate the system and determine its application to various types of pharmacies and limitations, if any.

REFERENCES

1. *Communicating the Value of Comprehensive Pharmaceutical Services to the Consumer.* Washington: Amer. Pharm. Assoc., 1973, p. 14.
2. Aspinwall, L. V.: *Four Marketing Theories.* Boulder, Colo.: Bureau of Business Research, University of Colorado, 1959.
3. Odiorne, G. S.: *Management Decisions by Objectives.* Englewood Cliffs: Prentice-Hall, 1969, p. 170.
4. *Supermarket Merchandising,* Nov., 1960, p. 83.
5. The same prescription means two or more prescriptions for the same quantity, the same drug and the same strength.
6. Anon. by request, personal communications.
7. *Communicating the Value of Comprehensive Pharmaceutical Services to the Consumer.* Washington: Amer. Pharm. Assoc., 1973, p. 28.
8. Sonnedecker, G.: *Kremers and Urdang's History of Pharmacy.* 3rd ed., Philadelphia: J. B. Lippincott Co., 1963, p. 39.
9. Griffenhagen, G.: Fair Trade in 1828. *J. Amer. Pharm. Assoc., Pract. Pharm. Ed., 20*:156, 1959.
10. *Ibid.*
11. McEvilla, J. D.: Pharmacy and the professional fee in theory and practice. *J. Amer. Pharm. Assoc., NS 2,* 520, 1962.
12. Myers, M. J.: Professional fee: renaissance or innovation? *J. Amer. Pharm. Assoc., NS 8,* 628–631, 1968.
13. Nitardy, F. W.: Prescription pricing schedule. *NARD Notes, 6*:17, 1968.
14. Chase, W. M.: Prescription prices in Detroit. *J. Amer. Pharm. Assoc., 4*:1357, 1915.
15. Kendall, H. L., and Lee, C. O.: Rapid method for determination of prescription fees. *J. Amer. Pharm. Assoc. Pract. Pharm. Ed., 5*:130–35, 1944.
16. Jeffries, S. B.: *The Universal Prescription Costing and Pricing Calculator.* Rutherford, N.J., Becton, Dickinson & Co., 1953.
17. Evanson, R. V.: *An Economical Study of Prescription Departments in Indiana Pharmacies.* Dissertation, Purdue University, 1953.
18. Apple, W. S.: Prescription Pricing. *Wisconsin Commerce Reports, 3,* No. 3 (Aug., 1952).
19. Fuller, H. J.: *Bulletin of the Ont. Coll. of Pharm., 6*:43, 1957.
20. Fuller, H. J.: *Canad. Pharm. J., 90*:418, 1957.
21. For a comprehensive review of the professional fee see *J. Amer. Pharm. Assoc. NS 2,* No. 9 (1962); *J. Amer. Pharm. Assoc., NS 8,* No. 12 (1968); *Am. J. Hosp. Pharm., 23,* No. 9 (1966); and *Hosp. Pharm., 2,* No. 1, pp. 11–20 (1967).
22. Fuller, H. J.: *Bull. of the Ont. Coll. of Pharm., 13*:80, 1964.
23. Abrams, R. E.: *Focus on Pharmacy, 1962.* Detroit: Wayne State University College of Pharmacy, March, 1962.
24. Jacoff, M. D., and Evanson, R. V.: An expense-cost analysis for professional fee planning. *J. Amer. Pharm. Assoc., NS 2,* 525–28, 1962.
25. Jacoff, M. D., and Evanson, R. V.: An Application of Cost Accounting to Prescription Pricing. Paper presented to the Section on Pharmaceutical Economics, APhA Annual Meeting, Washington, D.C., (Aug. 1960).

26. Knox, H.: Procedure for setting professional fee. *J. Amer. Pharm. Assoc., NS 2,* 530, 1962.
27. Anon.: NARD prescription cost study. *NARDJ, 90*:17, 1968.
28. Smith, H. A.: Determining the Professional Fee. *J. Amer. Pharm. Assoc., NS 8,* 646–49, 1968.
29. Miller, Jacob: Personal Communication.
30. Smith, H. A., and Billups, N. F.: Survey form to determine the cost of dispensing a prescription. *The Kentucky Pharmacist, 36*:20, 1973.

REVIEW

1. Discuss and differentiate between price and non-price competition and give examples of each in the practice of pharmacy.

2. Explain market segmentation strategy and give several examples in the practice of pharmacy.

3. Define and give several examples of quasi-price competition in a pharmacy.

4. Discuss and give examples of five types or levels of price competition.

5. Explain the push-pull effect on the public of prescription price advertising.

6. Explain each of the five basic factors that enter into pricing decisions. Include the underlying principles and concepts of each.

7. Discuss each of the six pricing policies and describe how they differ.

8. Explain and give examples of the application of the game plan to competitive pricing.

9. What is wrong with pricing according to what the market will bear?

10. Why has odd pricing lost the potency it had originally?

11. Given the appropriate data, calculate the selling price, cost of goods sold, gross margin, expenses, and net profit, in terms of both dollars and percentages.

12. Given appropriate data, calculate the selling price required to achieve the following pricing objectives: (a) average expenses and net profit, (b) variable expenses and usual net profit, and (c) variable expenses.

13. Explain the usual relationship between turnover rate and percent gross margin and given appropriate data, calculate the effect of turnover rate on total annual net profit.

14. Discuss the history of prescription pricing and the professional fee. Include: (a) the action of the APhA House of Delegates in 1917, (b) Nitardy's NARD "Prescription Pricing Schedule," (c) Evans' "Simple Rule of Determining Prescription Prices," and (d) the Kendall and Lee formulas of prescription pricing.

15. Describe five reasons the percentage markup became the usual method of prescription pricing after World War I.

16. Outline the variations and modifications of the percentage markup, with or without a fee, used in the many prescription pricing schedules.

17. Discuss the three tenets of the professional fee philosophy.

18. Given the Fuller and Abrams formula for prescription pricing and the appropriate data, determine the prescription price by each method and explain the essential difference between the two formulas.

19. Calculate the breakeven cost of dispensing a prescription using the cost accounting method as published by Smith in the JAPhA.

20. Describe the basic differences between Smith's cost accounting method and the Kansas Medicaid formula.

12. *Pharmacy Patronage*

Pharmacy patronage is a complex subject. Many types of motives are involved in any specific purchase or patronage decision. There is no simple explanation of motivation; it is a complex of many economic, social, and psychologic forces, both rational and emotional. This is true of both purchasing and patronage motivations.

Among the many studies on motivation, relatively few have dealt with pharmacy purchases and patronage. A study by the Dichter Institute for Motivational Research, Incorporated, provided some interesting and nontraditional insights into the deepseated, underlying motives of consumers with respect to their image and patronage of pharmacies.[1] The research utilized depth interviews, psychologic tests, and projective techniques. The depth interviews, Phase I of the research, were conducted in two waves of 27 interviews each. Wave I was performed to test some hypotheses and to construct new ones through a comprehensive analysis of the findings. Wave II was performed to validate the hypotheses and to quantify them to a degree. The psychologic tests and projective techniques were performed with 447 respondents in 33 geographically diverse locations to provide further data and insight into the public's image of pharmacy. Another study by Benson and Benson provided additional, but more traditional, information and insight into pharmacy patronage.[2]

Pharmacy's Public Image

A *key concept* emerged from the Dichter study—namely, the pharmacist has lost contact with his patients. It was found that the patients expect, and deeply desire, personal contact and attention, and genuine professional services from the pharmacist. It is a feeling of isolation and alienation that prompts patients to be *pushed* away from the independent pharmacist rather than *pulled* by lower prices to the mass merchandisers. The American consumer has an uneasy feeling which permeates the entire shopping situation.

The researchers probed the respondents to determine how this feeling developed. The respondents felt that they had been abandoned by the new breed of pharmacists. This parallels the changes that have taken place in medicine, and apparently these changes are symptomatic of the cool, aloof, and scientific manner of dealing with patients today. It appears that while developing sound scientific curricula for our health practitioners, we have neglected the socioeconomic and behavioral aspects of the health professions. The famous medical historian and sociologist, Henry Sigerist, was keenly aware of this deficiency.[3] Sigerist labeled medicine a social profession; surely pharmacy is none the less a social profession. An awareness and a commitment to pharmacy as a socioeconomic institution is incumbent on both educators and practitioners if change is to be made in the orientation and behavior of pharmacists, who in turn will be able to alter the perception their patients have of them.

LOSS OF PUBLIC CONTACT

The Dichter researchers associated the alienation that patients feel toward their pharmacists with a basic instinct, the instinct for survival as represented by their health needs. Where alienation has occurred, the perception of loss is felt deeply, whether consciously or not.

The results of the motivational research revealed that the pharmacy is in a unique and complex shopping category.[1] It provides products and services that affect the well-being, even the very life, of its patrons, while offering a wide range of non-health products for the convenience of patrons. This peculiar mixture of professional service and commercialism produces a degree of confusion in the minds of the public. It is difficult to perceive the pharmacist as a professional on the same plane as the physician or attorney. The latter serve their patients or clients in an office type of environment, whereas the pharmacist performs his professional service in a commercial context. However, the "ideal pharmacist," as perceived by the respondents, closely resembles the "doc" of the past decades, especially when the pharmacist was friendly, approachable, and concerned about his patrons.

The depth probes revealed that the public wants more than the old-fashioned, friendly "doc"; they want a proficient pharmacist who will protect their health with medication profiles and one who strives to prevent allergic reactions and drug conflicts of all types. The key to the latter, more sophisticated role is to fill the first role—that of the friendly pharmacist who has personal contact with the patient and calls him by name. Although the physical environment and the diverse merchandise in the pharmacy can have a negative effect on the attitude of the public toward the pharmacist, it is the *attitude* and *behavior* of the pharmacist himself that exert the greatest influence with the public. When the friendly druggists of the thirties were considered the family doctor substitute, or simply "doc," the typical pharmacy realized only about 10 to 20 percent of its income from prescriptions and sold a wide assortment of non-health products, and the soda fountain, the antithesis of professionalism, was an integral part of most pharmacies.

An understanding of behavioral and sociologic phenomena, such as the sick role, is a necessary prerequisite to the development of expertise in the broader new roles of the pharmacist. A better and deeper understanding of the profession as a unique social institution is also a prerequisite to assuming these new roles. A pharmacist with internal role conflicts of his own can hardly instill confidence and trust in the patients he serves. He must understand the profession-business complex in which he works and his role within it, if he is to contribute to the public confidence in the profession. "Surely no one would deny that the role of the pharmacist is crucial to the success of the pharmacy enterprise because it is he, more than any other employee, who can effectively build patron loyalty."[4] He should not be providing professional services one moment and pushing household goods the next, especially for the same person.

"It is also clear from the research that, for the most part, the pharmacist has not properly communicated with the public. As a result, the public is almost completely in the dark with regard to what the pharmacist really does. One of the public's most *prevalent perceptions* is that the pharmacist hides behind a specialized counter in a corner of the establishment, makes a little bit of noise, and comes up with a small bottle and a large bill."[4] This image must be reversed if pharmacy is to regain its credibility.

There are some interesting comparisons between the findings of the Dichter motivational research and the earlier study by Benson and Benson.[2] There are points of agreement and disagreement, which can be attributed largely to the changes in the public's attitudes and pharmacy itself during the eleven intervening years. Part of this is due to the differences in methodology used in the two studies. The Benson and

Benson study used both structured and nonstructured depth interviews with a sample of consumers located from coast to coast. The number of respondents was not reported, but it is thought to include 200 or more.

RANKING OF PHARMACISTS

Both the Dichter motivational study and the Benson and Benson study attempted to rank pharmacists among other professions and occupations. Unfortunately, the two studies did not make congruent comparisons possible. The Dichter study used fifteen occupations, whereas the Benson and Benson study used eight occupations plus a "no opinion" category. The Dichter study included dentists and optometrists; the Benson and Benson study used clergymen. The latter researchers specified "high school teacher," but the former used the term "school teacher." The Dichter group divided the respondents into two groups. They used the word "druggist" with 218 respondents (Group A) and "pharmacist" with 229 respondents (Group B). In contrast, Benson and Benson used both words together as "druggist/pharmacist." Table 12-1 indicates the relative rank of the top seven professions in the Dichter and the Benson and Benson studies. Bear in mind the many incongruencies in the techniques employed.

It is interesting that the combined term "druggist/pharmacist" ranked fifth among the top five occupations in the Benson and Benson study, while the term "druggist" ranked sixth among the top six occupations in group A and the term "pharmacist" ranked fourth among the same six occupations in group B of the Dichter study. People apparently perceive a difference between a "pharmacist" and a "druggist," and this perceived difference was verified in the Benson and Benson study. The

Table 12-1. *Relative Ranking of Professions in Two Studies*

Profession	Benson and Benson Study	Dichter Study Group A	Dichter Study Group B
Physician	1	1	1
Dentist	–	2	2
Attorney	2	3	3
Pharmacist	–	–	4
Optometrist	–	4	5
School teacher	3	5	6
Clergyman	4	–	–
Druggist/pharmacist	5	6	–

Adapted from *Communicating the Value of Comprehensive Pharmaceutical Services to the Consumer.* Washington: American Pharmaceutical Association, 1973; and from *How to Win Friends and Influence Customers.* New York: Sterling Drug Co.

respondents were asked if, in their opinion, there was a difference between a druggist and a pharmacist. Forty-eight percent responded "yes," 42 percent said "no," and 10 percent had no opinion.[5] When the respondents were asked what the difference was, the answers focused on the pharmacist's roles of compounding and dispensing prescriptions and his education and licensure requirements; in contrast, the druggists had roles of ownership and dealing in many matters that were not health related.

Although Knapp et al. found that the provision of information by pharmacists to patrons failed to make a strong attitudinal impact on the patrons,[6] Yellin and Norwood found the opposite.[7] The latter researchers concluded that "an improvement in public attitude may be realized more through increased pharmacist-patient contact than any other means, especially when this leads to increased communication regarding health matters."

ROLE CONFLICT

In an earlier chapter, sociologic data were cited which indicated the divergent roles and role conflicts in pharmacy resulting from its institutional, professional, and business complexity. The Dichter group sought to determine the public's attitude toward a pharmacist as a professional versus a business person.[8] They used a modified version of the semantic differential technique, which positioned two opposing statements with a six-point scale between them. The two statements were as follows: "Pharmacists are more businessmen than they are medical men," and "Pharmacists are more medical men than businessmen." The results are shown in Table 12-2.

The reasons given for the nonprofessional perception of pharmacists, shown via the probe technique, can be categorized as follows: (1) pharmacists were not professional in the sense that physicians, dentists, and attorneys are professional; (2) the place of practice is more a business than an office, usually having proximity to grocery and similar stores; (3) pharmacies sell many non-health products; (4) the attitude and behavior of pharmacists show a lack of concern, which seemed to be paramount to the respondents; and (5) the public doesn't expect the

Table 12-2. *Pharmacists as Businessmen or Medical Men*

Businessmen	1	2	3	4	5	6	Medical Men
% of Respondents	15	22	17	23	13	10	

Adapted from *Communicating the Value of Comprehensive Pharmaceutical Services to the Consumer.* Washington: American Pharmaceutical Association.

pharmacist to be *ultra* professional, but rather more concerned and helpful. Some of the respondents called this "professional interest," "common courtesy," and "devotion to duty."

Paul interviewed 200 consumers in Pittsburgh concerning their patronage preferences.[9] He found that approximately 47 percent thought that there was a difference between a pharmacy and a drugstore. As the income of the respondents increased, the percentage of those who thought there was a difference between a pharmacy and a drugstore also increased.

PERCEIVED ATTRIBUTES OF PHARMACISTS

For the pharmacist, professionalism is an elusive concept. It is a mixture of the friendly "doc" of past years and the knowledgeable, concerned modern pharmacist of today who gives advise about drugs, and watches for contraindicated drugs and drug interactions. The friendly, reliable, and accessible attributes of pharmacists were much in evidence in the Benson and Benson study,[10] as shown in Table 12-3.

The concept of a personal pharmacist who is concerned and knowledgeable appears to be the answer to pharmacy's public image.

Table 12-3. *Words Used to Describe Druggists/Pharmacists*

Question to Consumers: Please go through all the cards and pick the ones that might be used to describe the average (druggist) (pharmacist).

Characteristic	%
Reliable	82.0
Friendly	82.0
Intelligent	78.0
Helpful	76.0
Hard working	63.0
Sincere	57.5
Public spirited	40.0
Clever	29.0
Generous	22.5
Charitable	19.5
Greedy	7.5
Crafty	5.5

(Multiple answers are included in the above table.)

Source: *How to Win Friends and Influence Customers.* New York: Sterling Drug Co. (in cooperation with the NARD), 1962.

Consumer Patronage

PATRONAGE MOTIVES

In the traditional context, patronage motives are primarily rational motives, although not entirely. Most textbooks on marketing or general retailing provide the following list of patronage motives: (1) *convenience*—rational, and traditionally the single most important motive in pharmacy patronage; (2) *reputation of the seller*—both rational and emotional motives; (3) *services rendered*—rational motive; (4) *breadth of assortment and quality of goods*—rational motive; (5) *price*—rational motive; and (6) *appearance and general appeal*—both emotional and rational motives.

Pharmacy is not an ordinary retail business, but is a professional institution as well. One might expect different factors to be influential in pharmacy patronage compared to grocery or department stores. The Benson and Benson research group sought to determine the reasons for consumers patronizing a particular pharmacy. The results of this research are tabulated in Table 12-4.

In comparing the results of the Benson and Benson study with the traditional and general patronage motives, there is remarkable agreement. Convenience stands out as the single most important reason for patronizing a particular pharmacy. If the various types of conveniences mentioned are additive, convenience as a patronage motive totaled 42.5 percent, not counting "convenient, unspecified," which had a 19 percent response. Most of the other reasons listed can be categorized under one of the other traditional motives. "Know, friendly with owner, druggist, clerks" drew a 29 percent response as a main reason for shopping most at a particular pharmacy. This reason had the *second highest* response rate, and when combined with the other reasons associated with reputation, the combined percentage was 50. Services had a combined response of 25 percent.

The Benson and Benson study dealt with pharmacy patronage in general. A much different set of motives (reasons) would be expected to influence people in deciding where to purchase their prescriptions. This question was investigated in the Dichter study. The respondents were given a list of seven factors and requested to put the number corresponding to each factor in one of seven unequal segments of a circle or pie. The unequal segments were designed to give a relative weight to each factor. After all the computations were performed, the seven factors were ranked as shown in Table 12-5.

Perhaps more useful information could have been derived from the test shown in Table 12-5 if professional services had been divided into distinct and meaningful segments. Professional service is such a broad category. Also, the convenience factor should have been included as well. Convenience has been found to be a significant factor in nearly every research project on pharmacy patronage to date.

Table 12-4. *Reasons for Shopping at Pharmacy Patronized Most*

Question to Consumers: What are your main reasons for shopping most at this drugstore?

Motive	Response Item	%
Appearance and general appeal	Clean store, uncluttered	1.5
Breadth of assortment and quality of goods	Good, wide stock; have what is needed	12.5
	Has a soda fountain	.5
	Carries groceries	.5
Convenience	Close to home, neighborhood pharmacy	34.5
	Convenient, unspecified	19.0
	Close to doctor's office	5.0
	Close to other stores, shopping district	2.5
	Close to work	.5
Price	Reasonable prices, economical, sales	15.0
Reputation of the seller	Know, friendly with owner, druggist, clerks	29.0
	Reliable, reputable, recommended to me	20.5
	Druggist is public spirited	.5
Services rendered	Good service, prompt, helpful, courteous	15.5
	Have delivery service	6.5
	Convenient hours	1.5
	Credit available	1.5
Other	No drugstore patronized most	4.5
	No reason	1.0

Multiple answers are included in the above table.

Adapted from *How to Win Friends and Influence Customers.* New York: Sterling Drug Co. (in cooperation with the NARD), 1962, p. 9.

Table 12-5. *Factors Determining Choice of Pharmacy*

Rank	Factor	Weighted Score	%
1	Professional service	2,302	18.5
2	Lower prices	2,192	17.6
3	Personal attention	1,970	15.8
4	A pharmacist who knows your MD	1,653	13.3
5	A ready source of drug information	1,632	13.1
6	A large variety of merchandise	1,437	11.6
7	Advertised drug prices	1,259	10.1
	TOTAL WEIGHTED SCORE	12,445	100.0

Adapted from *Communicating the Value of Comprehensive Pharmaceutical Services to the Consumer.* Washington: Amer. Pharm. Assoc., 19, p. 37, Table 13.

By way of comparison with the "high" score given professional service, a very broad category, lower prices, were only about one percentage point lower, and advertised drug prices, the lowest score of all, were only 8.4 percent lower than the professional service score. The personal attention score was 2.7 percent lower than professional services, whereas the ready source of information score was 5.4 percent below the professional service score.

In another semantic differential test, the Dichter study indicated that consumers are more concerned that prescription prices be posted than that they be advertised. Also, more people believed that they were being overcharged than believed that prescription prices were high.

Herman and Wills investigated community pharmacy patronage in a metropolitan city.[11] They found that people preferred an apothecary type of pharmacy to a traditional pharmacy, and a service-oriented pharmacy to a price-oriented pharmacy. However, these preferences were not indicated as being statistically significant. Older people appeared to prefer apothecaries over traditional pharmacies as indicated by the chi-square test. Eighty-two percent of the respondents gave closeness to their residence as the reason for their preference of the location of a pharmacy. Closeness to physician's office was rated second, as indicated by a 12 percent response.

Paul sought to determine the type of pharmacy that consumers preferred and actually patronized in purchasing their prescriptions.[9] The data from this research are summarized in Table 12-6.

The difference between the preferences and actual purchases has a message that is consistent with the general theme of most of the data in the other two studies. Pharmacists should emphasize their strong suit, namely, the provision of genuine professional service (for example, monitoring drug utilization and preventing therapeutic conflicts) in a warm, friendly manner, in pleasant surroundings, and at reasonable, defensible prices. This does not mean that every pharmacy has to divest

Table 12-6. *Types of Pharmacies Consumers Preferred and Actually Patronized for Prescriptions*

	Percentage of Consumers	
Type of Pharmacy	*Actually Patronized*	*Preferred*
Neighborhood, community	75.0	61.0
Prescription type	8.5	19.0
Chain type	13.5	8.5
Other types or no opinion	3.0	11.5

Adapted from: Paul, S. H.: Pharmacies: how do you know what the customer wants? *Marketing Insights*, pp. 12–14, Feb. 6, 1967.

itself of all non-health related products. On the contrary, it is attitude and behavior, and the actual delivery of true professional services that are important.

Before a pharmacist can devise a strategy for obtaining or increasing his patronage, he must have some idea of factors and services that influence the patrons most. Then he can proceed to make his patrons aware of these services.

DESIRED PHARMACEUTICAL SERVICES

The Benson and Benson study investigated a wide range of available features and services that influence the consumers' patronage of a pharmacy. The results are shown in Table 12-7.

The more recent study by the Dichter Motivational Research Associates investigated respondents' awareness of, and desire for, a narrower range of pharmaceutical services. The people were asked which services they were most familiar with and which services they would most like to have. Each person was given a list of services to be evaluated. The results are reported in Table 12-8.

It is difficult to make direct comparisons between the data in Tables 12-7 and 12-8. The question asked in the Benson and Benson study was open-ended, providing the opportunity for a wide variety of responses, 18 in all. In addition, the question was asked in a manner to elicit responses at two levels of importance, very important and most important. The responses across the two levels are not additive. It would appear that in the Benson and Benson study, the responses at the most important level were mutually exclusive, except for a 10 percent discrepancy over the total percentage of responses. Otherwise, both studies permitted multiple responses. In addition to the above differences, the manner in which the questions were asked of the respondents and the total context of the two studies were quite different. Given these differences in methodology, only rough comparisons can be made.

The combined services of longer hours, deliveries, Sunday and emergency service in the Dichter study closely corresponded to the separate listing of being open late at night, delivery, being open seven days, and 24-hour prescription service in the Benson and Benson study. Fifty-eight percent of the Dichter respondents indicated that these were services they would most like to have, while a range of 33 to 47 percent of the Benson and Benson respondents indicated that these services were very important. Although these latter percentages are not additive, their combined effect probably would have matched the 58 percent in the Dichter study. Moreover, the respective percentages of people who indicated that these services were most important totaled 40 percent, which with some reservations are additive. It is interesting that only 48 percent of the Dichter

Table 12-7. *Importance of Services and Features Influencing Pharmacy Patronage*

Questions to Consumers: What features and services often available at drugstores would you consider very important in influencing your selection of a drugstore in which to trade?

Which one of these things is most important to you?

Features and Services	Consumers' Rating	
	Most Important (%)	*Very Important* (%)
Pricing	21	62
24-hour prescription service	21	47
Friendliness of druggist	12	61
Clean and neat inside	9	72
Delivery service	9	41
Quick service	8	55
Professional advice on health aids	8	38
Being open 7 days a week	6	41
Being open late at night	4	33
A wide variety of brands	3	32
A wide variety of types of merchandise	2	29
Availability of credit	2	18
Friendliness of clerks	1	46
Clean and neat outside	1	41
Ample parking space	1	25
Self-service	1	7
Professional advice on beauty aids	1	4
Trading stamps	–	4

Multiple answers are included in the above table.

Adapted from *How to Win Friends and Influence Customers,* New York: Sterline Drug Co. (in cooperation with the NARD), 1962, p. 10.

respondents were aware of the availability of these services, while in fact they are available in most pharmacies, especially the neighborhood type of pharmacy.

The conclusion that can be drawn from the foregoing data is that these services are traditional, but they are still considered important to the public. The Benson and Benson study indicated 24-hour prescription (or emergency) service was the most important of the group, which if actually provided and promoted, would mitigate the necessity of very late or long hours and being open all day on Sundays.

The Dichter study combined credit with accounting services for tax purposes and elicited 54 percent response as a service the public would most like to have. This response is 36 percent greater than the 18 percent of the people in the Benson and Benson study who thought credit alone was very important. Given the importance of tax deductions these days, it would not be surprising to find that a tax record service would elicit a 36 percent additional favorable response.

The only other two categories that are at all comparable are the "dispensing of information not directly related to prescriptions" and "professional advice on health aids." The former service was one that 48 percent of the Dichter respondents stated they would most like to have,

Table 12-8. *Consumer Awareness of and Desire for Pharmaceutical Services*

Items Evaluated	A %	B %	Net Change %
Maintains a complete inventory of drug products which physicians may prescribe for treatment. a. Properly stores same	62	47	−15
Maintains a medication record for each prescription-filling customer.	57	57	None
Makes certain the prescription drug is "right" for the patient, questioning a. Drug conflict b. Patient allergies	30	70	+40
Guarantees drug's high quality and "freshness."	57	57	None
Packages, dates, and labels patient's prescription with directions.	87	39	−48
Supplies patient with special information, i.e., to be taken on an empty stomach, X-times daily, and similar instructions.	51	62	+11
Dispenses information not directly related to prescriptions.	24	48	+24
Provides credit and accounting services for tax purposes.	51	54	+ 3
Offers longer hours, deliveries, Sunday and emergency service.	48	58	+10

Note: Column A represents "services most familiar with" and Column B is "most like to have."

Source: *Communicating the Value of Comprehensive Pharmaceutical Services to the Consumer.* Washington: American Pharmaceutical Association, 1973.

and 38 percent of the Benson and Benson respondents thought the latter service was very important. Eight percent of the respondents in the Benson and Benson study thought this service was most important. Unfortunately, only 24 percent of the Dichter respondents were aware of the availability of information about health and nonprescription drugs from pharmacists. Even worse, this lack of awareness may reflect the true state of the activities of pharmacists.

The Paul study indicated those services preferred by 50 percent or more of the people interviewed were, in the order of decreasing importance, as follows: acceptance of telephone orders, public telephones, delivery service, parking facilities, record-keeping for tax deductions, and the profitless sale of postage stamps.[9] The services desired by less than 50 percent of the respondents, in descending order, were: "free orders," gift wrapping, giving premium stamps, and charge accounts.

The supplying of information about prescriptions and other health information was explored further by the Dichter motivational research group with the use of the modified semantic differential technique. Two sets of opposing statements dealing with the actual and potential use of pharmacists as a source of information were used. The results are shown in Figure 12-1.

The Dichter study emphasized professional services and focused on special services and features. It was surprising that 57 percent of the people interviewed thought pharmacists maintained a medication record system, and the same percentage of people wanted this service. This is a strong message to pharmacists, a signal to fulfill this need and desire, or else suffer the consequence of greater degradation of their public image.

Actual Medical or Drug Questions							
"I frequently consult a pharmacist on medical or drug questions."	1	2	3	4	5	6	"I never consult a pharmacist on medical or drug questions."
Percent of Respondents	12	17	17	12	18	23	
Potential Sources of Medical Information							
"Pharmacists are not physicians and, therefore, are not good sources of medical information."	1	2	3	4	5	6	"Because of their profession, pharmacists often are good sources of medical information."
Percent of Respondents	11	13	12	23	26	16	

Figure 12-1. *Pharmacists as Actual and Potential Sources of Health Information.*

As great or probably greater opportunity in the professional service area involves the prevention of drug conflicts (drug-drug interaction) and patient allergies. The 40 percent difference between expectation and the awareness of this service is probably understated. It is doubtful that 30 percent of the people are now receiving this type of service. It should be noted that an individualized medication record profile system is requisite for preventing drug-drug interactions, patient allergies, and other adverse effects.

Purchasing Motives

CLASSIFICATION OF MOTIVES

Product purchasing motives may be classified along three dimensions or in three different ways. The first is time- and/or age-oriented. Therefore, the first classification of purchasing motives is *latent* or *dormant,* and *conscious* motives. Many motives are latent (lie dormant) in the mind until some effect, for example a display, arouses the desire to make the decision to purchase the item. The things that cause a latent motive to become a conscious one vary with circumstances and especially with age. As other types of motivations are discussed, it should be apparent that these have greater impact on each of us at various ages and circumstances.

The second way to classify purchasing motives is related to the primacy of the motive. Thus, a purchase may be classified as either *primary* or *selective.* These two types of motives have their counterpart in the context of the *generic* versus *branded* product controversy. A good example of this classification is the purchase of a headache remedy. The first or primary motive is to purchase a remedy to relieve the headache. Because of the influence of an advertisement or advice, the purchaser may become selective and demand a particular brand of aspirin. The technique of product differentiation, both real and contrived via adver tising, is the basis for actuating a selective purchase motive.

The third classification, and perhaps the most pertinent of all, is based on the rationality of the purchaser's behavior. Thus, purchasing motives are classified as *rational* or *emotional.* Most of us think we behave rationally almost all of the time, including the way we spend our money. Not so! Research has shown that the majority of purchases are really actuated by appeal to our emotional motivations. A careful study of advertisements, using the technique of content analysis, would reveal the degree to which emotional appeal is used in the majority of the ads. The complexity of the entire purchasing process must be recognized, and it must be noted that a combination of motivational appeals, both rational and emotional, is used in most advertisements.

RATIONAL MOTIVATIONS

Rational motivations may be further classified and described in the following manner:

1. *Dependability* or *confidence* is one of the strongest rational motives.

2. *Economy,* which refers to the "best buy" or "greatest value," not necessarily the lowest price. People often confuse economy with the lowest price.

3. *Low price* (or simply *price*) is an appeal to the rational process. Although people are sometimes misled, it is still a rational appeal, and only the lack of information is the basis of a "bad buy."

4. *Money gained* is related to the economy motive above, but it differs in that the appeal is to future gains or benefits to be derived from the purchase. An example would be a well-fitted suit for a salesman.

5. *Convenience* is rational in nature and it relates to the ease of use, repair, and related characteristics. This is one of the strongest motives for patronage of a pharmacy, as previously discussed.

EMOTIONAL MOTIVATIONS

Emotional motivations are numerous and complex. They are designed to appeal to both our innate and our acquired appetites and desires. Not all appetites and desires are bad, and values are not to be inferred from this classification. However, our value system will play a large role in the effectiveness of emotional appeals; in fact, it may completely negate the effect of certain advertisements or displays on some people. Emotional motives may be classified as follows:

1. *Pride* traditionally has been one of the most common and strongest emotional motives among Americans. It may focus on the individual, his family, an organization, or any entity with which a person identifies.

2. *Emulation* is the basis of fashion changes. The expression, "keeping up with the Joneses," is a good illustration of this motive, which may well replace pride as the number one motive in this country.

3. *Innovation* probably is the second fastest growing motivational appeal in the advertising industry. The concept of avant-garde, borrowed from the French, plays an important role in modern American life. Many advertisements appeal to this type of life style, which, of course, is symptomatic of the affluence of our society.

4. *Comfort* and *recreation* are two somewhat related motives. One may argue that they contain an element of rationality, and they probably do. They are not identical, but both theoretically are directed toward a sense of well-being. However, neither, and especially recreation, may produce the desired results. Many purchases are based on these two appeals.

5. *Conformity* or *sameness* is still a common motive among Americans. This motive is related to emulation, but it goes one step beyond. It is

based on the desire to be "lost in the crowd" as opposed to emulating the new or the latest style.

6. *Sex* is the most used motivational appeal today. The term is not even listed in the older marketing textbooks. The use of this basic and often base appeal is a matter of concern among a portion of our society, while other parts of our society see sex and its use in motivating as a "healthy liberation" of humanity. The manner in which sex appeal is used in advertisements is to draw attention to a product, and to this end it no doubt is successful. Whether such appeals have long-term or even actuating force is a subject that awaits interesting and profound psychologic research.

7. *Love* is the last of our emotional motives in this classification. Love is a complex emotion and is represented by two opposite extremes—*self-love* or *ego,* and *altruism.* Self-love cuts across and underlies all of the above ego-oriented motives. Altruism is somewhat old-fashioned, but it is a force that happily still exists in our society. For example, if not from habit, then altruism is the motive underlying the sale of many boxes of Valentine candy.

With a basic understanding of product purchasing motives, the pharmacist is better qualified to construct an advertisement or display. He certainly will be able to consult with the advertising manager of his local newspaper. This latter statement is particularly important, since most pharmacists do not have either the time or sufficient knowledge to develop their entire advertising program.

INTERRELATIONSHIP OF MOTIVES

The public's image of pharmacy, pharmacy patronage, and product purchasing motives are all interrelated. The understanding of each, in

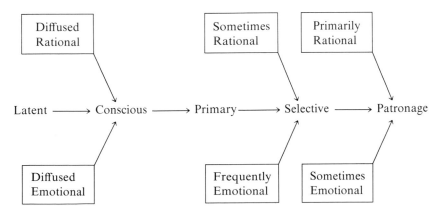

Figure 12-2. *The Interrelationship Among the Various Purchasing Motives.*

turn, has an effect on the efficient application of the other and implications for the development of promotional strategies. The interrelationships are depicted in Figure 12-2.

The subject matter of this chapter is the most complex of all the facets of pharmacy management and practice. More definitive research is needed. Past research has produced a great amount of data and some much needed insight into the subject; however, much more research is needed. There are many facets of public image and consumers' motives about which we know little.

REFERENCES

1. *Communicating the Value of Comprehensive Pharmaceutical Services to the Consumer.* Washington: Amer. Pharm. Assoc., 1973.
2. *How to Win Friends and Influence Customers.* New York: Sterling Drug Co. (in cooperation with the NARD), 1962.
3. Sigerist, H. E.: The medical student and the social problems confronting medicine today. *Bulletin of the Institute of Medicine,* 4:411–22, 1936; also Sigerist, H. E.: *A History of Medicine.* Vol. I, New York: Oxford Press, 1955, pp. 3–37.
4. *Communicating the Value of Comprehensive Pharmaceutical Services to the Consumer. op. cit.,* p. 14.
5. *How to Win Friends and Influence Customers. op. cit.,* p. 3.
6. Jang, R., Knapp, D. A., and Knapp, D. E.: Reactions of the public to the pharmacist as drug advisor. *Amer. Pharm. Assoc.,* Unpublished Paper, 1970.
7. Yellin, A. K., and Norwood, G. J.: The public's attitude toward pharmacy. *J. Amer. Pharm. Assoc., NS 14,* 61–65, 1974.
8. *Communicating the Value of Comprehensive Pharmaceutical Services to the Consumer. op. cit.,* p. 23.
9. Paul, S. H.: Pharmacies: how do you know what the customer wants? *Marketing Insights,* pp. 12–14, Feb. 6, 1967.
10. *How to Win Friends and Influence Customers. op. cit.,* p. 5.
11. Herman, C. M., and Wills, R. A., Jr.: Community pharmacy patronage. *J. Amer. Pharm. Assoc., NS 14,* 66–70, 91, 1974.

REVIEW

1. Discuss the purposes of Wave I and Wave II of Phase I of the Dichter motivational research and explain the technique(s) used in Phase I and Phase II of the research.

2. What was the *key concept* that emerged from the Dichter motivational research?

3. Explain how this developed over the years and the basic instinct underlying the feelings of consumers.

4. Explain the interdependence of the performance of the modern professional service the consumer desires and the role of the friendly pharmacist of past decades.

5. What are the public's most *prevalent perceptions* of the modern pharmacist?

6. Given the various professional categories used in the Dichter and the Benson and Benson studies. Rank pharmacists and/or druggists in reference to other occupations.

7. What are the five major categories or reasons why pharmacists are not considered by consumers to be professional, as shown in the Dichter study.

8. What were the terms used to describe the average druggist/pharmacist by over 50 percent of the respondents in the Benson and Benson study?

9. What were the top seven services or features that the respondents in the Benson and Benson study considered to be *most important* in selecting a pharmacy?

10. In the Dichter study, the respondents were asked which of nine services they were most familiar with and which they would most like to have. Of which services did the respondents have greater expectations than awareness?

11. What are the six traditional patronage motives?

12. Identify the 17 reasons for patronizing a pharmacy given in Table 12-4 with the 6 traditional patronage motives.

13. What reason was most frequently mentioned for patronizing a pharmacy in the Benson and Benson study (Table 12-4)?

14. Rank the 7 factors for purchasing a prescription in a particular pharmacy as listed in Table 12-5.

15. Is posting or advertising prescription prices more important to the public?

16. Is it the high prices of prescriptions or the feeling of being overcharged for prescriptions that concerns consumers the most?

17. What was the basis for the preference of a pharmacy location in the Herman and Wills study?

18. What factors did Yellin and Norwood find to be the most significant in improving patrons' attitudes toward pharmacy?

19. Distinguish between (a) latent (dormant) and conscious; (b) primary and selective; and (c) rational and emotional purchasing motives and show by a schematic diagram the relationships among these motives.

20. Given a list of emotional and rational purchasing motives, identify them as either rational or emotional.

13. *Promotion*

The age of consumerism is here and likely to stay.[1] Advocates of consumerism, as exemplified by Ralph Nader, have obtained a high degree of sophistication and acceptance. The new consumerism has taken many forms including picketing, boycott, publicity of various causes, and lobbying for legislation. Two well-known expressions are indicative of the public's concern for health or the lack of it, namely, "health as a fundamental right" and "the right to know." It should be apparent that the public will have input into the decisions affecting matters related to health. This principle should be in the minds of pharmacists, both individually and collectively, as a philosophic guide when they are developing promotional programs of all types.

With this increase in consumerism and the public's awareness of health needs and costs, it is more important now than ever before that pharmacists begin to communicate with their patrons and develop positive promotional programs.[2] Pharmacists need to implement innovative services, and make these, as well as traditional services, visible to the public through all the various media of promotion. If pharmacists choose not to advertise prices, they should be prepared to defend them.

Objectives

The specific objectives for a particular pharmacy depend to a large degree on the type of pharmacy or practice and location. However, there are general promotional objectives for any pharmacy in any location: (1) to develop a public image and public acceptance of the pharmacy; (2) to attract new patrons to the pharmacy; (3) to maintain patronage of present patrons and thus maintain a competitive position; (4) to gain acceptance of a new service or line of goods; and (5) to induce both new and old patrons to purchase more merchandise and services.

Classification of Promotions

All of the various types and modes of promotion are either *institutional* or *merchandising* in nature. The former tend to be *professional* and the latter *commercial,* but not necessarily.

INSTITUTIONAL APPROACH

Institutional promotions focus on the firm or organization and its services and characteristics. An institutional advertisement is used to tell the public of a new service such as a patient medication record system, or it may make the public aware of a unique characteristic such as "Serving the community for over 100 years." Direct patient contact by the pharmacist is the most effective means of institutional promotion, although the promotional program may well use other methods simultaneously.

MERCHANDISING APPROACH

In contrast, merchandising promotions focus on merchandise offered for sale, depicting special features such as dependability or convenience of use, or a special price. Merchandising advertisements may emphasize weekend specials, special events, such as anniversary or holiday sales, a new line of goods, or a combination of products. The term *sales promotion* is used synonymously with merchandising promotion because of its familiarity and similarity in most contexts.

MODES OF PROMOTION

There are several modes of promotion, each with its purpose, advantages, and disadvantages.

Public Relations or Publicity. Public relations and publicity are used synonymously in most instances. One technical difference is the case in which a public relations program is launched with the expenditure of funds, whereas publicity, by definition, is free. This criterion also distinguishes publicity from advertisements.

A public relations or publicity program is community oriented. It may be a local program such as sponsorship of a local civic event or program, which may be either athletic, academic, or cultural in nature. Other types of programs support national drives or campaigns, usually health-related. National Poison Prevention Week, National Diabetic Week, and National Pharmacy Week are just a few of the many examples a pharmacy can use as a basis for a good public relations program.

Personal Selling. Personal selling may range from ordinary sales activities of clerks to professional consultation with patrons by the pharmacist. The public is hungry for this type of personal attention, as documented in Chapter 12. The success of professional consultation depends on: (1) genuine concern or empathy, (2) friendliness and accessibility of the pharmacist, and (3) a patient medication record system, especially when the consultation involves prescriptions or other drugs that may interfere with their effectiveness.

Sales Promotion. The term "sales promotion" is used to provide a convenient label or umbrella for a large number of specific promotional activities. Sales promotion may be defined as the coordinated use of advertising, displays, direct mail, and miscellaneous promotional activities such as contests, coupons, and trading stamps. These activities usually are directed toward the sale of merchandise and should be coordinated with personal selling efforts.

Developing a Promotional Program

PROMOTIONAL PLAN

The first decision in developing a promotional program is to determine the type of promotional program that is most compatible with the type of pharmacy, its location, and its objectives. Basically, the pharmacist/ manager must decide whether to use the institutional or merchandising approach, or a combination of the two. The promotional program must be compatible with the philosophy of the pharmacist, the pricing policy, and the strategy of the pharmacy. To do otherwise may dilute the promotional efforts, confuse the public image, and nullify the results of previous promotional programs. However, traditional pharmacies have used a combination of the two approaches, placing the greater emphasis on the type of promotion that best characterizes the practice, although the success of the dual approach is at least questionable.

Promotional Strategy. Based on the above considerations, the pharmacist/manager should divide the pharmacy into three major segments to provide the basis of the promotional strategy.

The first segment, the professional areas, includes the prescription department, prescription accessories, orthopedic and surgical supplies and appliances, home health care aids, and "ethical" nonprescription drugs.

The second segment, the general merchandise departments, includes proprietary drugs, cosmetics, toiletries, and traditional drug sundries. Special skill departments also may be included in this segment or in the professional segment, depending on the nature of the department and the promotions used.

The third segment, the promotional and traffic-building departments, includes special promotional merchandise, the tobacco department, magazines, candy, and the fountain.

The pharmacist selects one of the major segments as the primary basis of his promotional strategy, depending on the type of pharmacy. Some pharmacists/managers utilize all three segments when developing a promotional strategy, especially in a large traditional or super drugstore. The promotional strategy incorporates the pricing policy and competitive strategy, discussed in Chapter 11. The amount of market segmentation and quasi-price reduction, and the amount and type of direct price reduction also must be included in the promotional strategy.

Promotional Budget. Developing the promotional budget is one of the most important but difficult steps in the promotional plan. The problem is to budget enough money to get the market penetration desired without overspending, which is wasteful. There is not a magic formula to use in developing a budget. Using an average percent of sales, as reported in publications such as *The Lilly Digest,* is not the answer, although it is better than a "guesstimate." *The Lilly Digest* for 1972 reported a range of 1.2 to 1.4 percent of sales, while the *NACDS-Lilly Digest* reported a range of 1.4 to 1.7 percent of sales.

The first step is to estimate the full market potential for your location and type of pharmacy. If the full market potential has not been reached, an upward adjustment in the budget is indicated. If, on the other hand, the full market potential has been obtained, a "set" promotional budget should be used to maintain the competitive position.

Next, the budget should be segmented into seasons and months based on a calendar of events. Extra money should be budgeted for certain months because of special events such as "back to school days" for a merchandising promotional plan, or National Pharmacy Week for an institutional-professional promotional plan. Then the budget should be divided according to the major segments of the pharmacy or departments that will be featured each month. Finally, the budget should be divided between money spent on displays and the various advertising media. Once the budget has been established, adherence to it is recommended.

Calendar of Events. The calendar of events is the master guideline for the week-to-week promotions. The National Wholesale Druggists Association (NWDA) publishes a Planning Calendar which can be used or easily adapted for most pharmacies. The Planning Calendar indicates all the special weeks and months, such as National Pharmacy Week, National Cancer Month, and many more. It also indicates national and religious holidays and the birthdays of important people. In addition, the calendar lists four departments or lines of products that are suitable for promotion each month. With the addition of local events and the anniversary of the pharmacy, the NWDA Planning Calendar provides the basis for developing an excellent promotional calendar of events.

The NWDA Planning Calendar, or some other calendar of events, should be selected to provide the detailed guidelines of the promotional strategy. This in turn will depend on the type of pharmacy and promotion, institutional or merchandising. Professional and health-related events and campaigns naturally should provide the basis of a promotional program for a pharmaceutical center or apothecary shop. A traditional pharmacy could use both health-related and other special events, with the emphasis dictated by the percentage of sales derived from the prescription and other health-related departments. A large merchandise pharmacy would make more use of Valentine's Day, Mother's Day, Father's Day, "Back to School" events, weekend specials, and related types of promotion.

Executing the Program

STEPS IN IMPLEMENTATION

After developing the promotional program, including the strategy, budget, and calendar of events, specific steps have to be taken to put the program into effect. The promotional budget should indicate the amount that has been budgeted for displays, the various advertising media, direct mail, and miscellaneous promotional methods. If not, this is the *first step* in executing the promotional program.

The *second step* is to select the proper mix of products and/or services to be promoted. If promotional or seasonal merchandise is selected, the best source of supply must be sought. The amount to be purchased should be based on experience. This points to the importance of *step three*, complete records of promotions, including the amount purchased, the cost of the promotion, and the success in terms of the sale of promotional and staple merchandise.

The *fourth step*, and the most critical, is to inform all sales personnel of the details of the promotion. Without the knowledge and energetic support of the sales personnel, any promotion will fail to achieve the desired results. Failure to keep all personnel informed happens in too many instances.

Finally, a schedule, including the date of each step, should be developed and followed. Execution of the promotional program may be summarized as follows: (1) selecting and stocking the appropriate merchandise or service; (2) selecting the various modes of promotion; (3) informing the sales personnel; (4) making and following a schedule; and (5) keeping records of the results.

ADVERTISING

Advertising is any paid publication of information, which reaches beyond the confines of the pharmacy, and appeals persuasively to the public to patronize a pharmacy and/or purchase its merchandise or service. Any of the various media may be used. The pharmacist may select from newspapers, direct mail, handbills or circulars, billboards on highways or moving vehicles, radio, and television. The pharmacist must select the medium or media which will serve his purpose best. This depends largely on the type of promotion and pharmacy practice, but it also depends on the scope of the circulation and the hearing or viewing area as compared with the pharmacy's trading area. Whereas a regular or cooperative chain may use a large advertisement in a large city newspaper or on television profitably, the small independent pharmacy cannot.

Smaller pharmacies may profitably use radio spot announcements, sponsor a short, community-oriented radio program such as birth announcements or hospital news, and place small institutional ads in the larger papers. Rural pharmacies can profitably use the weekly county newspaper.

Direct mail is one of the best media for professional, institutional ads directed to both lay patrons and prescribers. Direct mail costs more than prepared handbills or circulars, but it can be better controlled to reach the specific target people.

The use of announcement cards, which may be reproduced in the newspaper or used as a spot announcement on television, is an ideal method for introducing a new service such as a patient record system, diabetes screening program, or the monitoring of hypertension for selected patients with approval of the patient's physician.

Types of Advertisements. Merchandising advertisements are one of three types: *omnibus*—made up of many unrelated items; *related items* or product line advertisement; and *single product* advertisement. As previously stated, an advertisement may be institutional, which informs the public of one or more services or unique characteristics of a firm.

Larger merchandising independents and the regular or cooperative chain drugstore most often use the omnibus ad. Frequently, these contain an institutional component, usually relating to services of the prescription department. Often a product line or a single product ad is a cooperative advertisement, purchased in part by the manufacturer.

Psychology of Advertising. The psychology of advertising can best be illustrated by the use of the acronym AIDA, the title of a well-known opera.

A—Attract attention, usually with headline and sometimes an illustration.

I—Induce interest, usually with an illustration, price, or overall layout design.

D—Develop desire to buy, appealing to the various purchasing motives.

A—Actuate to buy, usually with special message, e.g., "Available only through _____."

Preparation of the Advertisement. The first step is to decide on the type of advertisement and the general message or theme that is to be conveyed. The theme may be institutional in nature, a special event, an anniversary sale, a weekend special, or a value or price reduction message. This may involve one or more services, a product, a product line, or group of unrelated products. Once this decision is made and the necessary product(s) assembled, the headline is written. This step is critical.

Next, the copy is written and it may be elaborate, constituting the major portion of the ad, or it may be as simple as notice of a reduced price.

The logo, which is the one permanent or constant component of every ad, is the trademark that identifies the pharmacy or firm. It is usually placed at the top or bottom of the ad and must be well coordinated with the headline. Illustrations, if they are to be used, must be drawn or selected from available sources.

Finally, the layout of the various components of the advertisement must be arranged: the headline, the logo, the size and shape of the ad, the arrangement of the illustration. Product, price, and message must be arranged to meet the four criteria of advertising psychology. Not only should the ad catch the reader's attention, it should hold it long enough to cause the reader to peruse through the entire ad. Obviously, this requires talent when one considers the great amount of competition for the reader's attention. Most pharmacists should consult with an expert in advertising when developing any other than a simple ad.

DISPLAYS

Displays are known as point-of-sale advertising. There are various types of displays, each serving different secondary purposes with the one common purpose of increasing impulse sales.

Types of Display. The more common types of display are: (1) window displays, (2) "shadow-box" displays, (3) showcase displays, (4) counter displays, (5) "hot-spot" or high-traffic displays, and (6) mass displays.

Window displays are used for professional displays and seasonal merchandise. It is recommended that window displays be kept sufficiently low to provide full view of the interior of the pharmacy. The "shadow-box" displays are small window displays, usually 3 feet by 4 feet, located on the side of the store. They are frequently used to display a line of cosmetics or some other special line or service.

Showcase displays are the oldest type of display and are used for cosmetics, costume jewelry, cameras, and other expensive items.

Counter displays have been used for years and may be used for seasonal products, a new product or product line, and fast moving staple goods. These are often the three- or four-tier displays adjacent to the cash register, often referred to as a "selling console."

"Hot-spot" displays are usually floor displays placed in high-traffic areas. They are often specially built by manufacturers to display their seasonal or new products. This type of display is used for special promotional merchandise—nonstaple merchandise purchased in large quantities at a special reduced price.

Mass displays are used on gondolas, on the top of the wall shelving, and sometimes on the "selling console." A large amount of merchandise is normally used with multiple facings of each item and each size of an item. The theory is that the massiveness of the display will attract attention of patrons and create the image that it is a popular and highly desired product. This image is often enhanced by a price reduction or special price.

Psychology of Displays. The psychology of displays is the same as that for advertising and is also illustrated by the acronym, AIDA. There are additional psychologic factors of which the pharmacist should be aware in constructing displays. The display should be one dominant theme. Good use should be made of color and lighting effects, and the display should reflect order but not nessarily symmetry.

Constructing the Display. The *first step,* as trite and simple as it may be, is to remove the old display and thoroughly clean the display area.

The *second step* is to select the theme, which usually includes the merchandise to be displayed or the service to be illustrated or demonstrated.

The *third step* is the assembly of the physical materials for the display, which may include: background material (especially in window displays), fixtures (regular or special such as boxes), accessory items (cloth, paper, show cards, price tickets, professional equipment, or animated devices), and the merchandise.

The *fourth step* is to sketch the display on paper when appropriate.

Sometimes the display can be visualized without the benefit of a sketch.

The *fifth step* is to arrange the display as sketched or planned. Often this may require that parts of the display be rearranged several times to obtain the desired effect.

Selecting the Merchandise. There are several factors influencing the choice of merchandise, the most obvious being the nature and type of display. There are other factors to be considered such as the value, bulk, perishability, and attractiveness of the merchandise. Other factors such as the season, the calendar of events, and "tieing in" the display with national promotion should also be included in the consideration.

DIRECT MAIL

Direct mail normally is used for personalized and professional messages. It is one of the most effective methods of reaching a particular group of people, and is the recommended method of reaching prescribers in the area. Professional newsletters or bulletins are included in this category for convenience. Direct mail is an excellent means of introducing a new line of goods or services. Some examples include a new line of cosmetics, a new and complete line of orthopedic and surgical appliances and supplies, a medication record system, or a screening or diagnostic laboratory service. It is perhaps the best single promotional method for a pharmaceutical center or a prescription shop. A good up-to-date mailing list is an essential part of all direct mail promotions.

MISCELLANEOUS PROMOTIONS

There are dozens of promotional methods that fall into the miscellaneous category. This broad category includes samples, gifts for babies, posters and banners, push merchandise (PMs), drawings for prizes, coupons, trading stamps, brochures or package inserts, and contests just to name the more common forms. Some are useful; others are not recommended.

Most of these promotional methods have their place in the various types of pharmacies; however, trading stamps are neither profitable nor economic in the long run except for the trading stamps producer and the manufacturers of the premium products. Trading stamps are an expensive means of promotion, and they lose their competitive advantage as soon as the competitors adopt other stamps. The producers of the stamps and the premiums reap a windfall from the unredeemed stamps alone. The goods offered as premiums usually can be purchased at a lower price in regular stores.

In my opinion, PMs are not a good method of promotion because of the tendency to divide loyalties and promote an overly aggressive attitude among the sales personnel.

It is suggested that banners and window signs be used judiciously so that they do not lose their effectiveness when the full impact is needed. Less frequent use prevents a continuous cluttered appearance which obscures the total effect of well-organized displays and a good layout design of the pharmacy.

The miscellaneous professional promotional programs are excellent. These include patient medication record system, a record of the expenditures for drugs for income tax deduction, health information brochures on various diseases, record of immunizations, special printed instructions for medications with complicated instructions, standardized measuring spoons, and a list of prescription accessories that may be needed with certain prescriptions. This list is only the more common means of professional promotion.

Coupons in newspaper ads can be valuable in measuring market penetration and the effectiveness of a promotion.

PERSONAL SELLING

Personal selling is the personal assistance given a patron to achieve his desired satisfactions and to meet his real needs. Of course, this ranges from the simple act of taking his money to the complicated process of helping the patron select the proper product and providing the appropriate advice.

Fundamentals of Personal Selling. The fundamental principles of professional personal selling or consultation are: (1) know your patrons and patients; (2) know drugs and other products; (3) understand and use patronage and purchasing motives; (4) develop empathy; and (5) provide prompt, courteous, and helpful service.

A person's name is to him the sweetest sound on the earth. Forgetting the names of the people who patronize our pharmacies is one of the most common failings among a large majority of pharmacists. There are a few rules, *if used,* that will greatly assist in overcoming this problem. The first rule is to have a personal interest in the patron as an individual. The second rule is to be sure to understand his name, even if it requires his repeating it several times. Repetition of the name is itself the third rule. The fourth rule is to write or type the name. Seeing the name in print is a powerful reinforcement in the remembering of names. Last, associate the name with something about the person, his appearance, his occupation, or something such as an event that is *unique,* not something that is common.

Pharmacists should know the products they sell and should know drugs thoroughly. The important thing is to think of the indications, side effects, dosage, and other information in terms of the individual. For example, is a drug contraindicated because a particular patient, Mrs. Clark, has diabetes; this should be remembered or available for recall from the patient medication record. The pharmacist should strive always to be judicious, as well as objective and truthful, in consulting with patients and patrons.

Patronage and purchasing motives have been discussed in the previous chapter. The important point is to personalize this knowledge and understanding when dealing with clients. It should be realized that it is the results—the ease of pain, comfort, attractiveness—not the product, that the patron is really buying.

Developing empathy is not easy for most of us. We are too self-centered. Empathy comes from really putting oneself in the place of the other person. Some will argue that one loses objectivity when this happens. It is my contention that sufficient objectivity *can* be retained while one is developing empathy for another.

With genuine interest in the objectives of the pharmacy—achieved via MBO (management by objectives)—and empathy, pharmacists and clerks alike are ready to provide prompt, courteous, and helpful service. The process is almost automatic and supervision is reduced to a minimum.

Meeting Objections. There are at least three methods of answering objections. First is the "yes, but" method which consists of agreeing with a customer as far as possible without argument. The clerk then proceeds to present the goods from another perspective and to obtain the patron's agreement on as many points as possible, while developing and maintaining an affirmative attitude toward the patron and the product.

Second, the person may ask a patron to explain her objections. This must not be done in a critical or haughty fashion, but must indicate a sincere desire to learn from the objections of the customer. The salesperson must treat all patrons' prejudices and fears with sympathy and alleviate them if possible.

Finally, the sales person may strive to turn the objections into a selling point. For instance, if a customer indicates that he hasn't time, the clerk may suggest that a few minutes' time now may save the customer more time by eliminating a second trip.

Meeting Price Objections. The clerk may emphasize the value of the article and show the difference between it and less expensive but similar merchandise. He may demonstrate the superior quality and workmanship necessitating higher cost and selling price. A thrifty customer may be convinced of the long-run economy resulting from the purchase of an article of higher quality.

If the clerk is convinced that the patron actually believes he cannot afford the higher-priced merchandise, the clerk may turn to a lower-priced similar article. But, while discussing that article, he ought to keep the higher-priced and higher-quality product in sight in case the customer changes his mind.

In case of a new, high-priced prescription drug, the obvious suggestion is to point to the savings to the patient now possible with the new drug, i.e., he is spared a protracted period of hospitalization with its accompanying expenses and loss of income.

The patron may claim that he can buy the articles more cheaply elsewhere. A pharmacist and his clerks should be acquainted with competitors' prices and know whether there is a real difference in price or quality. He may need to adjust his pricing policy if he cannot defend it in terms of quality or superior services.

In general, the best rules to follow are: (1) be positive and give encouragement; (2) avoid contradictions, superiority, discouragement, overgeneralization, and too much personal opinion; and (3) if the patron does not buy the product, try to cultivate an atmosphere that will induce the patron to return for the goods later.

LIMITING FACTORS

The success of promotional programs is limited by such factors as: (1) the overall market potential and market saturation, which may have been affected by various promotions; (2) the law of diminishing return, which is a formal expression of the aforementioned factor; (3) the chance that special promotions may "borrow" from future sales at regular prices; (4) the possibility of increased pilferage resulting from the crowded conditions; and (5) the possibility of having unsold merchandise that may have to be sold at less than sale price, or not at all.

Evaluation of Promotion

Most pharmacists no doubt would like to know whether their promotional campaigns are successful. Some are less concerned about measuring the results of the money they spend on advertising and promotion, but they spend the money out of a sense of being competitive. They somehow feel they need to spend 1 to $1^1/_2$ percent of their sales on advertising and promotion because most pharmacy proprietors and managers feel that is what is required to be competitive. This is indicative of the intuitive, nonscientific approach to pharmacy management and practices. For pharmacists who are concerned with the results achieved from the advertising budget, the measuring of results is not an easy task. The institutional type of advertising produces results much more slowly, but its effects last longer than the merchandising type of promotion and vice versa. There are techniques available that will provide some measure of the results achieved through advertising and promotion.

GENERAL METHODS

The general method of measuring the results of promotion involves measuring the increase in sales over a base line previously established. The sales of the same period a year before generally are insufficient to serve as base line data. Some event, such as a special sale, a flu epidemic, or extremely bad weather, could have influenced the sales for that period of the previous year. This possibility should be investigated and adjustments made as necessary. The pharmacist must establish the sales growth trend resulting from general economic growth and from the pharmacy's own sales growth data resulting from its own relative market strength.

Once the overall annual sales growth trend for the pharmacy has been established, seasonal adjustments should be computed for each month and week, especially for those weeks or months with large sales variations, such as December. This is accomplished in the following manner. Let us assume that the last five years have been used to establish the annual sales growth trend. Using the figures for the last five years, we compute a monthly, or weekly, sales index as follows: (1) compute the average sales for each month, or week, for the last five years; (2) compute the average annual sales for the past five years; (3) divide the average annual sales by 12 to compute a hypothetical average monthly sales figure for the past five years; and (4) divide the actual monthly sales of each month by the overall monthly average to determine the average monthly variation from the overall monthly average for each month. Let 100 represent the overall monthly average, and the average sales for each month will be represented by an index number in relation to 100.

An example will illustrate the technique. Let us assume the overall monthly sales averaged $20,000 over the last five years. Further, let us assume that the average sales for December for the last five years were $22,400. Dividing $22,400 by $20,000 gives a quotient of 1.12; thus, December has a monthly seasonal index of 112 after multiplying 1.12 by 100, a 12 percent variation from the overall monthly average. If the average sales for June for the past five years were $18,000, then the index for June would be 90 ($18,000 ÷ $20,000 = .90 and .90 × 100 = 90).

Accurate records of advertising and promotion budgets and expenditures are necessary to determine whether extra expenditures for a particular month, week, or special event had an effect on the sales for a particular period. Allowance should be made in computing seasonal (monthly or weekly) indices or adjustments. If the annual five-year growth trend and the seasonal, monthly, or weekly indices are developed during a period of typical or normal advertising and promotion expenditures, then the base line data should be adequate to measure a significant sales increase resulting from a special promotional campaign supported by increased expenditures.

SPECIAL METHODS

There are some special methods or techniques for measuring the success of a special promotional campaign. By placing in an ad a coupon that is to be detached and presented to receive a discount or a prize, the pharmacist can determine how effective the ad has been. The ratio of the number of "redeemed" coupons to the total market potential would be indicative of the degree of success of the promotion. Different types of promotion or advertisements could be compared as a measure of the effectiveness of promotion or the design of the advertisement.

Perhaps a better technique is to require the name and address to be completed on a coupon in a newspaper advertisement, circular, or direct mailing for a drawing for a prize. By charting the addresses on the redeemed coupons, the pharmacy manager can measure the market penetration as well as the geographic location of the market. He can also determine whether he has made contact with new patrons.

Summary

Extending the advertising and promotional program through the point of sale is essential. No advertising program is complete without it. An ad cannot make the sale, only the salesperson can. Unfortunately, many pharmacists fail in their advertising campaigns precisely at this critical point. Their salespeople frequently do not know what is going on, are limited in their ability to do the job, or are not properly motivated to do the job. Therefore, a final admonishment should be made to pharmacists/managers regarding a successful promotional program. It should include the following: develop the budget, establish the objectives, prepare the theme, select the media, and, most important, do not forget that salespeople make the sale!

The role of advertising and promotion in our economy has become controversial. Many say that advertising is an unjustifiable social cost which does nothing more than switch people from one brand of merchandise to another. Others who support advertising claim that it does provide a service to our society, and it does justify all the expenditures made. Furthermore, they argue that advertising also keeps the economy strong by encouraging expenditures, which in turn increase or keep employment high. The controversy over advertising continues, and there certainly is merit in both arguments. It may be true that advertising cigarettes does nothing more than encourage people to elect between several equally bad alternatives. On the other hand, advertising does increase consumption and demand in our free economy.

Rather than pursue the argument whether advertising and promotion are worthwhile expenditures of funds, the general philosophy of this chapter rests on the following assumptions: (1) the pharmacist/manager's competitors will advertise, (2) if the pharmacist intends to make a go of his enterprise, he, too, must advertise, and (3) advertising is an additional cost of doing business. As for the moral or ethical considerations of advertising, the general tenor of this chapter is to consider advertising and promotion as a means of communicating information that will have a positive effect on the health and well-being of the public. Other references should be consulted for additional information on promotion.[3-8]

REFERENCES

1. Consumerism vs. professionalism: a panel discussion. *J. Amer. Pharm. Assoc., NS 12,* 356–66, 1972.
2. *Communicating the Value of Comprehensive Pharmaceutical Services.* Report of the Dichter Institute for Motivational Research, Inc., Washington: Amer. Pharm. Assoc., 1973.
3. *How to Win Friends and Influence Customers.* New York: Sterling Drug Co. (Co-sponsors—NARD, Chicago), 1962.
4. Farr, G., Huffman, D. C., and Ryan, M. R. (Eds.): *Professional Promotion for Pharmacy Managers.* Memphis: Amer. Coll. Apoth., Aug., 1973.
5. *How To Promote Your Retail Pharmacy.* Chicago: NARD, 1969.
6. Sawyer, W. E.: Sell as Customers Like It. 7th printing, New York: Dell Publishing Co., 1971.
7. McMahon, J. L., Baldwin, J., and Sawyer, W. E. (Eds.): *Sales Management.* Vol. 1, New Brunswick, N.J.: Johnson & Johnson and Co., 1971.
8. Huffman, D. C., Jr., and Smith, H. A.: *Building A Successful Pharmacy Practice: A Case Study.* Memphis: Amer. Coll. Apoth., 1972.

REVIEW

1. What are the five general objectives of pharmacy promotion?

2. Discuss the differences between institutional and merchandising promotions.

3. Which types of pharmacies can best utilize the institutional and the merchandising type of promotions?

4. Describe the several modes of promotion.

5. Discuss the promotional plan.

6. Discuss how a pharmacist can develop a promotional budget and a calendar of events.

7. Discuss the five steps in implementing a promotional plan.

8. Define advertising.

9. What are the three basic types of merchandising advertisement?

10. Discuss the major types of media available for advertising and their use for different types of pharmacies.

11. Discuss the steps in preparing an advertisement.

12. Outline the basic psychologic principles of display and advertisements keyed to the acronym AIDA.

13. Discuss the various types of displays and how they are best used.

14. What are some of the major factors influencing the type of merchandise used in displays?

15. Outline the steps in constructing a display.

16. List several examples of types of miscellaneous promotions, both professional and nonprofessional.

17. Describe professional personal selling.

18. What are the five fundamentals of professional personal selling?

19. Discuss the methods of answering patrons' objectives generally and price specifically.

20. What are the factors limiting the success of a promotional program?

21. Discuss the methods of evaluating promotion.

22. Discuss the ethical aspects of advertising by pharmacists.

23. Who are the critical people at the end point of the chain of events in the promotional program?

14. *Financial Analysis and Management*

Once a pharmacist has established his pharmacy, he is faced with the task of managing the various components in a manner that fosters growth and maximizes profit in the long run. All aspects of management are important to a successful practice. Some phases of management focus on the initial establishment of a practice, whereas other phases are either a continuous process, for example personnel administration, or a continuing periodic process, such as financial and profit analysis. A thorough financial and profit analysis is a necessary precursor to the discovery of problem areas and of the nature and causes of problems.

Analysis Objectives

Profit and financial analysis is directed toward one or more of several objectives. Obviously, one of these is the *profit* objective. Another objective is the *liquidity* objective. Liquidity, as the term is used in financial management, indicates the ability of a firm to meet its current debts without jeopardizing its existence or profit potential. Another important and related objective is *solvency.* Solvency is defined as the capability of meeting current debts and recallable long-term debts from available current assets and avoiding bankruptcy in the meantime. Another objective is a good *financial* and *credit position.* This objective balances all the owner's assets, his equity or net worth, against all the debts, both long- and short-term. It is desirable that the owner's equity equals or exceeds the total liabilities if at all possible. *Efficient operation* is the fifth objective.

The objectives are self-explanatory for the most part. The interrelationships that exist among these objectives are less obvious. Profit is necessary under most conditions to achieve the other objectives, and conversely, achievement of the other objectives enhances the prospects of profit. Greater liquidity usually increases the solvency, which, in turn, enhances the financial position in time.

There are several financial ratios that indicate achievement of the various objectives, or the failure to achieve them. Some ratios are more indicative and significant than others; however, a conclusion relative to a problem should be supported by several ratios pointing to the problem area. Some ratios point toward more than one objective and to more than one problem area. In addition, the analyst must look beyond the ratios themselves to the actual data and the economic and social environment of the pharmacy for a final determination.

Definitions and Standards

Some ratios are derived from the profit and loss statement, while others are derived from the balance sheet, but the most significant ratios are derived from a combination of the two financial statements. The various terms and classifications of the two financial statements are defined in this section.

LIQUIDITY AND SOLVENCY RATIOS

Current Ratio. To determine this ratio one divides the current assets by the current liabilities. It is an old and time-honored ratio which is indicative of solvency. The minimum desirable ratio is 2:1. The *Lilly Digest* average for 1972 was 3.2:1. This ratio means that if the current assets exceed the current liabilities by a margin of 2 to 1, sufficient cash, together with credit if necessary, should be available to meet current debts due within a year.

Acid Test Ratio. One can arrive at this ratio, which is often referred to as the *liquidity ratio,* by dividing the current assets less the inventory value (at cost) by the current liabilities. The minimum desirable ratio is 1:1. The *Lilly Digest* average for 1972 was 1.1:1. This ratio is a more rigorous test of the pharmacy's ability to meet its current obligations. When inventory has to be sold under adverse conditions, it frequently is sold at a sacrifice in value. Thus, inventory is not included in this ratio.

While it may be that accounts receivable may not receive dollar for dollar if sold to a financial institution, it is the usual practice to balance accounts receivable against accounts payable. Therefore, cash plus accounts receivable should equal accounts payable at the very least. This assumes accounts receivable will be collected at about the same rate as current debts become due.

Net Working Capital (NWC). This term is the excess of current assets over current liabilities. The amount of working capital varies with the size of the pharmacy and more particularly with the sales volume. As a rule, older pharmacies have a greater amount of net working capital than do newer ones. Also, net working capital usually is somewhat less than net worth, but the two values are close in a well-established pharmacy. The most definitive statement one can make about net working capital is that it should fall within the range of 50 to 60 percent of total assets, with an average of approximately 55 percent for established pharmacies.

Inventory To Net Working Capital. This ratio, which is often abbreviated as Invt./NWC, is simply the ratio of inventory to the net working capital. It usually is expressed as a percentage. The ratio normally falls within the range of 75 to 125 percent, with a desirable target of about 90 to 100 percent. *The Lilly Digest* average was 95 percent for 1972. The ratio is indicative of two aspects of management—liquidity and inventory imbalance. If an inordinate amount of net working capital is invested in inventory, the pharmacist may experience difficulty in meeting current debts. Under normal conditions, the ratio obviously is indicative of efficient use of capital. On the one hand, too little inventory results in out-of-stock situations and loss of sales, while too much inventory decreases the rate of return on the investment. A high Invt./NWC ratio correlates positively with a large difference between current and acid test ratios, both of which are indicative of a liquidity problem.

FINANCIAL POSITION RATIOS

The Ratio of Current Liabilities To Tangible Net Worth. This ratio indicates the pharmacy's capability to meet its current obligations by utilizing all of its net worth or capital equity if necessary. This ratio normally is expressed as a percentage. Obviously a high percent, above 80 percent, is undesirable and indicative of *undercapitalization.* Undercapitalization is another term for a poor financial or credit position, which frequently is accompanied by liquidity and solvency problems. A ratio less than 50 percent is desirable. The 1972 *Lilly Digest* average was 41 percent. It should be emphasized that tangible net worth was used in computing this ratio, which simply means that goodwill was not included among the assets. This is customary in calculating financial ratios.

The Ratio of Funded Debt To Net Working Capital. This percentage is calculated by dividing the sum of the long-term liabilities (those debts not due within a year) by the net working capital. The ratio is normally expressed as a percentage. This ratio is indicative of two aspects of financial management. A low percentage indicates a good financial position and ability to borrow money if necessary. A high ratio indicates a poor financial position and that the interest charge on the debt will continue to diminish working capital and net profit. This ratio may range from zero to over 100 percent. A value above 50 percent is undesirable. The 1972 *Lilly Digest* average was approximately 22 percent. If a pharmacy's net worth and net working capital are such that the pharmacy is in a sound financial position, a limited amount of funded debt (10 to 20 percent of NWC) with a reasonable interest rate is desirable. It is assumed the pharmacist will be able to use the borrowed capital to generate net profit in excess of the interest charge. This technique is referred to as the use of capital leverage.

Ratio of Total Liabilities to Net Worth. Again, this ratio indicates the overall financial and credit position of the pharmacy. It is indicative of whether a pharmacy can meet its financial obligations in due course of its operation. It also indicates the distribution of the capital between owners and creditors. The ratio is usually expressed as a percentage. If total debts exceed net worth, a ratio above 100 percent, the pharmacy is quite vulnerable to sharp changes in its operation, such as a sudden or prolonged drop in sales or a rise in expenses. Fifty percent or less represents a desirable target value. *The Lilly Digest* average was approximately 60 percent in 1972.

Ratio of Fixed Assets To Net Worth. The ratio is indicative of the degree to which scarce capital has been invested in assets, which precludes alternate use of the capital. This ratio is expressed as a percentage. A percentage of 75 or more indicates that too much money is tied up in fixtures and other fixed assets and not available as working capital. Such a condition is often accompanied by a large long-term note with the concomitant high interest charge, which reduces profit and further encumbers management. A figure as high as 50 percent may represent too much investment in fixed assets. *The Lilly Digest* values ranged from 17 to 36 percent with an average of approximately 20 percent for 1972.

PROFITABILITY RATIOS

Percent of Net Profit to Net Sales. This ratio is the one most frequently used to indicate the profitability of a pharmacy. It is not, however, the best indicator. Profit before income tax, rather than after income tax, is used for a better comparison among pharmacies with varying income tax rates. Net profit does not include the proprietor's salary. Corporations frequently report net profit after corporate income tax has been deducted, and this should be taken into consideration when comparing corporations with other types of legal organizations. *The Lilly Digest* average for independent pharmacies ranged from 3.6 to 5.8 percent over the past decade. The average percent net profit to sales as reported in *The Lilly Digest* in 1972 was 3.6 percent for independent pharmacies and 4.8 percent for chain pharmacies. A target percentage should be 5 percent or greater.

Percent of Net Profit To Net Worth (NP/NW). This percentage is most indicative of the overall profitability and operational efficiency of any single ratio under usual conditions. This ratio relates *net* profit to the *net* investment in the pharmacy and thus measures how well funds, as supplied by the owner(s), are being utilized. *The Lilly Digest* average was approximately 19 percent in 1972. A 20 percent or better figure is considered a realistic target. In a new pharmacy with a relatively small net worth, this ratio may distort the profit picture. In corporations with a considerable amount of outstanding preferred stock, debentures, and long-term notes, the use of net worth or stockholders' equity as the denominator may distort the picture also. For these reasons the next ratio should be used to supplement the NP/NW ratio.

Percent of Net Profit To Total Assets. This ratio has come into greater use in recent years for the reasons cited above. The rationale for using this ratio is that it measures the efficient use of *all* the assets under the control of management. The formula for calculating this ratio is known as the duPont formula.

$$\frac{NP}{Net\ Sales} \times \frac{Net\ Sales}{Total\ Assets} = \frac{NP}{Total\ Assets}$$

The first ratio in the formula has been discussed already and the second will be discussed later and shown to represent the velocity of utilizing assets. When the two ratios are combined, both *profitability* and *efficiency* are being measured. A minimum desirable value is 10 percent. *The Lilly Digest* value for 1972 averaged approximately 12 percent.

Net Profit Per Dollar of Inventory. This ratio is calculated by dividing net profit by the ending inventory. The ratio is expressed in the following manner: $.20/$1.00. While some might suggest using the average inventory as more comparable to the time span the net profit was earned, the more important consideration is the most current valuation of the inventory. The ratio measures both profitability and the efficient use of inventory. Proper management and control of inventory is one of the most challenging aspects of management. This ratio is indicative of how well this is being accomplished. The range of this ratio for independent pharmacies as reported in *The Lilly Digest,* when data were arranged by sales volume, was $0.04 to $0.24 per $1.00. The average was

$0.21/$1.00. The minimum desirable value is $0.20/$1.00. The average for chain pharmacies as reported in the *NACDS–Lilly Digest* was $0.34/$1.00 for 1972.

EFFICIENCY RATIOS

Inventory Turnover Rate (TOR). The TOR is calculated by dividing the cost of goods sold (CGS) by the average inventory (Avg. Invt.) at cost. The average inventory is computed from the beginning and ending inventory for the accounting period. The ratio may be calculated from sales and average inventory at retail value. This widely used ratio is indicative of efficient purchasing and inventory control. A minimum desirable ratio is 3, that is, the average inventory value is purchased and sold three times a year. The practical maximum TOR is 24. Under the current policy of issuing monthly statements during the last few days of the month with payment not due until the tenth of the following month, a pharmacist with good inventory control theoretically could operate on the average monthly cost of goods sold. Only one-half of this amount would be the average inventory investment, providing 24 TOR/year. However, a more realistic target falls within a range of 10 to 12. With computerized inventory control, EOQ and frequent cyclic billing, the maximum efficient TOR may reach 24 turns per year in the future. *The Lilly Digest* average for independent pharmacies was 3.8 in 1972. Chain pharmacies as reported in *NACDS–Lilly Digest* for 1972 registered 5.2 on the average.

Ratio of Net Sales To Inventory. This ratio is only a modification of the inventory turnover rate, in which sales are substituted for cost of goods sold. The ratio obviously will be greater by the amount of gross margin. Again, this ratio is indicative of inventory management with a minimum desirable figure of 5. The target value is in the range of 15 to 18. *The Lilly Digest* average was approximately 6 in 1972.

Net Working Capital Turnover. One can calculate this turnover rate by dividing sales by the net working capital (NS/NWC). It is indicative of the efficient use of working capital. Like other turnover ratios, there is a desirable range, not just a single critical value, which is 4 to 8 turnovers per year. The *Lilly Digest* average was approximately 6. If the value is low, below 4, it is indicative of either low sales and inefficient use of working capital or too much working capital for the sales generated. This may be the result of too much inventory and/or accounts receivable in relation to the sales volume. This condition is known as *undertrading.* If the value is very high, over 8, the opposite condition is the case—too little working capital for the amount of sales, which frequently is caused by excessive trade credit. This is known as *overtrading* due to *under-*

capitalization. New pharmacies can expect to have a rather high net working capital turnover during the first few years. The *Lilly Digest* average in 1972 was 5.6.

Capital Turnover Rate. This ratio is calculated by dividing net sales by net worth (NS/NW). This ratio is similar to the one above except all of the net capital (total assets minus total liabilities) is used. The desirable range is 3 to 8. *The Lilly Digest* average was 5.1 in 1972. This ratio normally is somewhat less than working capital turnover because net worth usually is greater than net working capital. Again, new pharmacies normally have a higher turnover rate during the first few years. A high value, above 8, definitely is an indication of *undercapitalization,* a case in which the firm is being financed by excessive credit, both short- and long-term. It is also indicative of *overtrading.* A low value indicates just the opposite, a sluggish, inefficient operation.

Average Accounts Receivable Collection Period. This value is a useful figure in identifying good or poor credit management. The figure indicates how long, on the average, it takes for the outstanding accounts receivable to be collected during the course of the usual accounting period. The average collection period is computed in the following manner: (1) credit sales for the year are divided by the outstanding accounts receivable at the end of the year to arrive at the average accounts receivable turnover rate, and (2) the 365 days of the year are then divided by the accounts receivable turnover rate to ascertain the average collection period in days. An example will illustrate the procedure: Annual charge sales were $120,000 and the outstanding accounts receivable were $10,000. (1) $120,000 \div $10,000 = 12 turnover rate. (2) 365 days $\div$ 12 = 30.4 or 30 days to the nearest whole day. Since credit is usually granted on a monthly basis, a 30-day average collection period is considered a reasonable period. A period up to 40 days is acceptable, while a 60-day average collection period indicates attention should be given to credit management.

Average Time To Pay Accounts Payable. This value measures how well the pharmacist is meeting his current obligations. It also may indicate whether the pharmacist is receiving his cash discounts. The value is calculated as follows: (1) All purchases of merchandise are divided by the outstanding accounts payable at the end of the accounting period. This determines the accounts payable turnover rate. (2) Then 365 days are divided by the accounts payable turnover rate and this gives the average collection period for accounts payable expressed in days. Again, a value of 30 days is very good and indicates that cash discounts normally are being received. A longer time period, for example 60 days, is not good and indicates the pharmacy is operating on "borrowed" trade capital and may not be solvent.

Methods of Analysis

There are several methods of financial analyses. After analyses, interpretation of the significance of the financial ratios and related values follow. The first step is to compute the financial ratios and arrange them in a *matrix* or *paradigm* in which those ratios that point toward management objectives or problem areas can be identified. Next, an internal analysis of data should be made to confirm the identity of specific problem areas, such as inventory or accounts receivable, and to determine if the profit, efficiency, liquidity, and solvency objectives are being met. The analysis of internal data should include a *trend analysis* for the past three years if the pharmacy is that old. Unfavorable trends of a ratio or a set of related ratios are a good indication that steps should be taken to reverse the trends. As stated previously, the raw data in the profit and loss statement and the balance sheet should be examined carefully to identify weak spots and unfavorable trends in the data.

Another method of analysis is to *compare the ratios with external standards.* Some of the best known standards are described and reported in the *Lilly Digest.* It should be noted that averages do not represent the best a pharmacy can or should do, but they represent a base against which to compare a pharmacy's performance as about "average." The analyst should look beyond the pharmacy to the economic condition of the community and the nation for possible causes. Are the economic indicators on the upswing or downswing? What about trends in population, per capita income, business, industrial and agricultural growth? The trend in number of prescribers in the community is another significant indicator. A pharmacist must judge his sales, profits, and pertinent ratios in light of the economic trends.

RATIOS PARADIGM

Table 14-1 illustrates a useful arrangement of ratios to identify specific problem areas and to determine whether management objectives are being achieved. The matrix in Table 14-1 shows the relationship between the various ratios and management objectives. It also indicates those ratios that are interrelated and point toward one or more problem areas. An "X" with "(?)" indicates a probable, but not definitive, relationship.

A study of the relationships in Table 14-1 shows that most ratios point toward more than one management objective or problem area, and that any problem area will be reflected by two or more ratios. As one would expect, any ratio containing net profit as a factor indicates profitability and often efficiency. Those ratios categorized as turnover rates indicate management efficiency and frequently liquidity, solvency, and/or overall

Table 14-1. *Paradigm for Ratio Analysis*

RATIO	Profitability	Efficiency	Liquidity	Solvency	Financial Position
		Management Objectives			
NP/NS	X				
NP/NW	X	X			
NP/TA	X	X			
NP/Invt.	X	X			
Invt TOR		X			
NS/Invt.		X			
NS/NWC		X	X(?)	X(?)	
NS/NW		X		X(?)	X(?)
Invt/NWC		X	X		
Acid Test			X		
Current				X	
CL/NW			X(?)	X	X
TL/NW				X(?)	X
L-TL/NWC					X
FA/NW		X			X
Avg. A/R CP		X			X(?)
Avg. A/P CP	X(?)	X	X(?)	X	X(?)

financial position. Ratios with inventory as a component reflect the state of inventory management. The average collection periods are indicative of credit problems, but they may also support the identification of other problems. The fixed assets to net worth ratio indicates over-investment in fixed assets.

COMPARISON WITH STANDARDS

The following example of a three-year-old traditional community pharmacy is used to illustrate the application of external standards. It is one of four pharmacies in a small town of 7,000 people with a total trading area of 15,000. There are four physicians practicing general medicine, who are average prescribers. The proprietor is a pharmacist 27 years of age who practiced pharmacy in another pharmacy in this town for three years before starting his own practice. The pharmacy occupies 2,800 square feet of selling area with 340 square feet and $11,000 worth of inventory in the prescription department. The pharmacy dispensed 12,000 prescriptions last year at an average charge of $4.10. Last year's credit sales amounted to $63,000. The first year the pharmacy nearly broke even, and last year the pharmacy realized a net profit of $1,400.

Figures 14-1 and 14-2 are the Income and Expense Statement and the Balance Sheet, respectively, for the third year of operation. Table 14-2 is a comparison of the ratios calculated from this pharmacy with *The Lilly Digest* averages and standards.

Utilizing the ratios and data generated and tabulated in Table 14-2, the analyst should proceed with further analysis and interpretation. Comparison of the computed ratios with standards, averages, and critical values will identify certain financial and managerial problems.

BROWNSVILLE PHARMACY
BROWNSVILLE, KENTUCKY
DECEMBER 31, 1973

Net Sales			$145,000
Cost of Goods & Services:			
Beginning Inventory	$ 30,000		
Purchases	102,000		
Total		$132,000	
Ending Inventory		35,000	
Cost of Goods Sold			97,000
Gross Margin			$ 48,000
Prop. Salary	$ 12,000		
Employee Wages	20,000		
Rent	6,000		
Heat, Light & Power	1,500		
Interest	1,600		
All Other Expenses	2,600		
Total Expenses			43,700
Net Profit			$ 4,300
Add Prop. Salary			12,000
Total Prop. Income[a]			$ 16,300
Income Tax[a]			2,900
Net Discretionary Income[a]			$ 13,400

[a] These figures are not used in computing any of the ratios

Figure 14-1. *Income and Expense Statement*

BROWNSVILLE PHARMACY
BROWNSVILLE, KENTUCKY
DECEMBER 31, 1973

Assets

Current Assets:		
Cash	$ 3,000	
Accounts Receivable	9,500	
Inventory	35,000	
Total Current Assets		$47,500
Fixed Assets:		
Fixtures & Equipment		
(Net after reserve for depreciation)	$16,800	
Total Fixed Assets		16,800
Other Assets:		
Prepaid Expenses	$ 1,500	
Total Other Assets		1,500
Total Assets		$65,800

Liabilities

Current and Accrued Liabilities:		
Accounts Payable	$12,000	
Notes Payable (within one year)	4,000	
Accrued Expenses	7,000	
Total Current and Accrued Liabilities		$23,000
Long-Term Liabilities:		
Notes Payable	$24,000	
Total Long-Term Liabilities		24,000
Total Liabilities		$47,000
Net Worth		18,800
Total Liabilities and Net Worth		$65,800

Figure 14-2. *Balance Sheet*

Table 14-2. *Comparison of Financial Ratios with Lilly Digest Averages and Standards*

	Computed Values	The Lilly Digest Average, 1972	Standard	Position of This Case
Current ratio	2.1:1	3.2:1	2:1	Just above the minimum
Acid test ratio	0.54:1	1.1:1	1:1	Below the minimum
Current debt to NW	122%	41%	50%	Above critical value of 80%
Inventory to NWC	143%	95%	90–100%	Above critical value of 125%
Inventory turnover rate	2.98	3.8	3–12	Below the minimum of 3
Total debt to NW	250%	60%	100%	Above critical value of 100%
Funded debt to NWC	98%	22%	50%	Above critical value of 50%
Fixed assets to NW	89.5%	20%	20–50%	Above critical value of 75%
Net working capital turnover	5.9	5.6	4–8	Within standard range
Capital (NW) turnover	7.7	5.1	3–8	Within standard range
Net profit/$1.00 inventory	$0.12	$0.21	$0.20	Below minimum standard
Net profit to NW	22.9%	19%	20%	Above the minimum standard
Net profit to total assets	6.5%	12%	10%	Below critical value of 10%
Average A/P remittance period	43 days	28 days	30 days	Above critical value of 40 days
Average A/R remittance period	55 days	NA	30 days	Above critical value of 40 days

Profitability. The net profit commands the focus of our attention. In financial jargon, "It's what's on the bottom line that counts." It is obvious that the present pharmacy was not very profitable. This is indicated by the dollar amount of net profit, percent net profit to sales, percent net profit to total (gross) investment in assets, and net profit per dollar invested in inventory. This conclusion is not supported by percent net profit to net worth because net worth is reduced drastically by the large amount of liabilities, both current and long-term. Of course, one must look further to determine the cause, or contributing factors, of the low profits. One may begin with current items and work backward, as it were, but perhaps a better picture can be gained by beginning with the older or long-term items.

Initial Capitalization and Investments. The ratio of fixed assets to net worth at 89.5 percent is much higher than is desirable, even for a pharmacy only three years old. This indicates the strong possibility of over-investment in fixed assets, a common error. It further indicates a small net worth, which is the case in this instance. It also suggests a high amount of liabilities, especially long-term liabilities. By correlating the ratio of funded debt to net worth with the ratio of fixed assets to net worth and considering the dollar values involved, the conclusion becomes apparent—over-investment in fixed assets financed by a large funded debt. This leads to a chain reaction.

Payments on the funded debt reduce the available cash for current operations and thereby causes an accumulation of accounts payable and accrued expenses. In addition, interest charges on these debts further reduce cash, and worse, profits are decreased. This point is supported by the ratios of current liabilities to net worth, total debt to net worth, funded debt to net working capital, and to a lesser degree by the current ratio.

Inventory Management. The problem is compounded by an over-investment in inventory, a $5,000 increase over the previous year. This fact is indicated by the ratio of inventory to net working capital, inventory turnover rate, and a comparison of the current ratio of 2.1:1 with the acid test ratio of only 0.54:1. The acid test ratio does not utilize inventory in the numerator, thus pinpointing the high proportion of capital invested in inventory. Again, the net profit per dollar of inventory is further indication of the problem.

Solvency and Liquidity. The combined economic factors discussed above can be expected to produce an adverse effect on the solvency and liquidity position of the pharmacy. This fact is indicated by the following ratios: current ratio, which is just above the acceptable minimum value; acid test ratio, which is about one-half the minimum value; current debt to net worth; inventory to net working capital; and the average remittance period for accounts payable of 43 days. This latter ratio is indicative of the pharmacist's inability to meet accounts payable on time and earn the cash discount. There is strong indication that the pharmacy is losing up to $2,000 a year in cash discounts, which is nearly one-half the amount of annual net profit.

Four ratios—current ratio, net working capital turnover, capital (NW) turnover, and percent net profit to net worth—seem to indicate a healthy financial condition for the pharmacy. It was noted that the current ratio was just above the minimum. The other three ratios appear normal only because of the fact that low sales and profits are counterbalanced by low net worth and net working capital.

Conclusion. This case illustrates the chain reaction that takes place when a pharmacy is undercapitalized and begins operation at a disadvantage. When this is complicated by poor management, the pharmacy stands to suffer economic loss, even possible bankruptcy. Such is the case with this pharmacy. Large fixed investment financed by a large amount of long-term indebtedness, reduced cash reserves for current operation, and over-investment in inventory (apparently attempting to "buy" himself out of the hole) result in a precarious financial position and reduced profits from interest charges, loss of cash discounts, and salaries and wages which are too high.

The remedy lies in: (1) obtaining some ready cash, if the pharmacist can obtain a bank loan, (2) reducing the inventory as rapidly as possible without jeopardizing sales, and (3) reducing expenses, especially salaries and wages. The extra cash can be used to reduce accounts payable and accrued expenses which will permit the pharmacy to realize cash discounts and increased profits.

TREND ANALYSIS

It is possible, indeed it frequently happens, that a firm may be making a profit and be in a precarious financial position with its creditors. Conversely, a firm may operate at a loss for a relatively short period of time and still maintain a sound financial position with its creditors; however, it should be obvious that a deficit operation cannot continue indefinitely. Trend analysis will identify those problems that develop gradually over time.

Of the several methods of financial analysis, year-to-year trend analysis is perhaps the best single technique. This technique, however, is strengthened significantly by the use of comparative data from *The Lilly Digest.*

ILLUSTRATION OF TREND ANALYSIS: A CASE STUDY

Data for three consecutive years were selected from a traditional community pharmacy and are shown in Figures 14-3 and 14-4 to illustrate year-to-year analysis. The values were rounded for ease of computation. The pharmacy, in its sixth year of operation, is located in a community of 3,500 inhabitants. There is one other pharmacy in the community, and there are approximately 7,500 people in the trading area. The size of the

	3rd Yr.	%	4th Yr.	%	5th Yr.	%
Sales						
Prescription	$ 50,700	39.0	$ 56,000	40.0	$ 61,500	41.0
Other	79,300	61.0	84,000	60.0	88,500	59.0
TOTAL	$130,000	100	$140,000	100	$150,000	100
COST OF GOODS SOLD	84,500	65.0	89,600	64.0	94,500	63.0
GROSS MARGIN	$ 45,500	35.0	$ 50,400	36.0	$ 55,500	37.0
EXPENSES						
Proprietor's salary	$ 11,700	9.0	$ 12,600	9.0	$ 13,500	9.0
Employees' wages	14,300	11.0	16,800	12.0	19,500	13.0
Rent	2,600	2.0	2,600	1.9	2,600	1.7
Heat, Light & Power	1,300	1.0	1,400	1.0	1,500	1.0
Legal & Accounting Fees	390	0.3	420	0.3	450	0.3
Taxes (except on income)	1,950	1.5	1,960	1.4	1,950	1.3
Insurance	780	0.6	840	0.6	900	0.6
Interest Paid	740	0.6	520	0.4	380	0.3
Repairs	390	0.3	560	0.4	750	0.5
Delivery	520	0.4	700	0.5	900	0.6
Advertising	1,690	1.3	1,960	1.4	2,250	1.5
Depreciation	1,800	1.4	1,800	1.3	1,800	1.2
Bad debts charged off	130	0.1	280	0.2	450	0.3
Telephone	390	0.3	420	0.3	450	0.3
Miscellaneous	1,730	1.3	2,340	1.7	2,580	1.7
TOTAL EXPENSE	$ 40,410	31.1	$ 45,200	32.3	$ 50,400	33.6
NET PROFIT (Before Taxes)	5,090	3.9	5,200	3.7	5,100	3.4
TOTAL INCOME	16,790	12.9	17,800	12.7	18,600	12.4
Income Tax	2,260	1.7	2,510	1.8	2,720	1.8
NET PROFIT (After Taxes)	$ 2,830	2.2	$ 2,690	1.9	$ 2,380	1.6
TOTAL INCOME (After Taxes)	$ 14,530	11.2	$ 15,290	10.9	$ 15,880	10.6

Figure 14-3. *Comparative Income Statement Data*

pharmacy is 65 feet by 30 feet with the prescription department occupying 300 square feet.

Sales, both prescriptions and other, show a favorable trend. The percentages of prescription sales and gross margin also show a favorable trend. Gross margin nearly always increases with increased prescription sales. Net profit has *not* increased proportionally, however. Expenses have increased proportionally more than gross margin, providing a slight dollar increase in net profit but a percentage decrease. Employee wages, repairs, delivery, advertising, bad debts and miscellaneous expenses are significant because these expenses are variable or semivariable costs, and can be controlled and brought into a better relationship with sales. Although advertising and delivery are variable or semivariable expenses, these expenditures are needed to sustain sales growth.

This pharmacy is still in the critical *growth profit interval* (G-P-I) of operations—time in which expenses are becoming stabilized while sales are still increasing. The period before a profit is realized is the *growth loss interval* (G-L-I). The problem in this case is to hold employee wages to about $20,000 a year, reducing bad debts to about $300 a year and miscellaneous expenses to approximately $2,000 a year, while increasing sales another 5 to 10 percent. Of course, all the other expenses must be kept at about the present level.

The income statement will not provide all the information necessary to reveal the "soft spot" in a practice. Comparative data from the balance sheet and other data provide additional signs of mismanagement. Let us examine the comparative balance sheet data for this pharmacy.

While net working capital increased steadily ($21,450, $22,610, and $23,330), there were some undesirable trends among the current items. Cash steadily decreased, while accounts receivable, inventory, accounts payable, and accrued expenses increased. Although net working capital increased, it became increasingly less accessible and manageable. Let us

ASSETS	3rd Yr.	4th Yr.	5th Yr.
Current Assets			
Cash	$ 6,500	$ 5,600	$ 4,500
Accounts Receivable	5,200	7,000	9,000
Inventory	23,400	26,600	30,000
Total Current Assets	$35,100	$39,200	$43,500
Fixed Assets			
Fixtures & Equipment	13,000	11,200	9,400
(net after depreciation)			
TOTAL ASSETS	$48,100	$50,400	$52,900
LIABILITIES			
Current Liabilities			
Accounts Payable	$ 7,800	$ 8,190	$10,420
Accrued Expenses	1,300	4,200	6,000
Notes Payable (within one year)	4,550	4,200	3,750
Total Current Liabilities	$13,650	$16,590	$20,170
Long-term Liabilities			
Notes Payable	7,800	4,470	2,620
TOTAL LIABILITIES	$21,450	$21,060	$22,790
NET WORTH	26,650	29,340	31,720
TOTAL LIABILITIES AND NET WORTH	$48,100	$50,400	$52,900
RELATED DATA			
Sales	$130,000	$140,000	$150,000
Credit Sales	54,000	63,700	65,700
Beginning Inventory	22,600	23,400	26,600
Average Prescription Charge	3.60	3.75	3.85
Number of Prescriptions	16,095	17,610	19,219
Turnover Rate	3.7	3.6	3.4

Figure 14.4. *Comparative Balance Sheet Data*

examine the interrelations among these items and certain items of the income statements.

Increased credit sales without proper management produced an increase in accounts receivable and bad debts. Inventory build-up caused a reduction in the turnover rate and an increase in accounts payable. Increased expenses produced a backlog of accrued expenses. All of these reduced the cash available for paying bills and earning cash discounts and reducing the notes payable.

As previously stated, trends are useful to determine the direction a practice is taking and reveal a deteriorating situation. An analysis of the data for one year will not. Financial ratios are especially useful for trend analysis and this is illustrated in the present case.

The current ratio for the third, fourth, and fifth years was 2.57, 2.36, and 2.15 respectively. A current ratio above 2.0 is considered to be above the minimum safe level. Similarly, the following ratios evidenced an unfavorable trend:

Inventory to Net Working Capital:	109%	117%	129%
Net Profit to Net Worth:	19.1%	17.7%	16.1%
Net Profit to Total Assets:	10.6%	10.3%	9.6%
Net Profit Per Dollar of Inventory:	$0.22	$0.21	$0.18
The Average Time to Remit Accounts Payable	30 days	32 days	39 days
Inventory Turnover Rate	3.7	3.6	3.3

Four other ratios were outside the acceptable range for each of the years, and they also manifested an unfavorable trend. The acid test ratio, which should not fall below 1:1, was 0.85, 0.75, and 0.66 for the respective three years. The ratio of current liabilities to net worth should not exceed 50 percent. It increased from 51.2 percent to 63.6 percent over the three years. The average collection period for accounts receivable should be maintained at about 30 days. This ratio increased from 35 days to 40 days to 50 days during the three-year period. Finally, net profit to net sales ratio was unsatisfactory and decreased each year.

When the data from this pharmacy are compared with data from *The Lilly Digest,* this pharmacy on balance compares favorably with the exception of employee wages and bad debts. After analyzing this case, it may be concluded that the proprietor, encouraged by the apparent success of the pharmacy during the first three years, employed more help than was necessary and failed to watch closely his credit extension. These are two items that can readily get out of control. Under present economic conditions, a conventional community pharmacy should keep the payroll, including the proprietor's salary, at 20 percent of sales or less; the payroll for this pharmacy was 22 percent of sales the previous year. The average prescription charge was below *The Lilly Digest* average, and this may be a source of additional income depending on the competitive condition of the market.

Summary of Case Study. This pharmacy illustrates improper management of credit, inventory, employee wages, and bad debts. A selective, controlled reduction of inventory to $16,000 could easily support a sales volume of $160,000 a year. This would free sufficient cash to liquidate notes payable and accrued expenses and reduce accounts payable to $9,000. Better management of credit and expenses generally will not produce as spectacular results, but it will increase profits and place the pharmacy in a much better financial position. If the pharmacist would reduce the expenses to 31 percent of sales and increase the prescription charge by five cents on the average, the resulting net profit would be nearly $10,000. This amount of net profit would produce a net return on sales of 6.7 percent and a net return on the net investment (net worth) of 31.5 percent. This would represent a profitable operation and a stable financial position.

BREAK-EVEN FINANCIAL ANALYSIS

Break-even analysis focuses on cost factors as reported in the profit and loss statement. The objective is to determine the point at which the pharmacy breaks even. The break-even point may be determined in terms of sales volume or time in months. Sales volume is most often used. Break-even analysis assists the pharmacist in making decisions that affect costs and/or sales in his pharmacy.

Break-even analysis is based on the anticipation of a probable future performance and assumes certain mathematical relations and a cost classification based on past experience. The analysis determines the outcome of a decision that changes one or more variables. With this analysis, certain questions can be answered and decisions made more intelligently. Some examples of such questions follow. What will be the profit or loss with a change in sales volume? What additional sales volume will be required to cover certain additional fixed costs of modernizing? How will the addition of another staff pharmacist affect the profit, or what are the necessary sales to cover the additional expense? What will be the effect on profit of reducing the percent gross margin? What will be the effect on profit of a change in a fixed rent to percent-of-sales rent?

Procedure for Break-Even Analysis. The following steps provide the procedure and framework for break-even analysis.

STEP 1—Classify all operating expense items into two groups: (a) *fixed* and (b) *variable.* Some expenses are semivariable, that is, they contain fixed elements, but vary with sales to some extent. For example, as the number of prescriptions dispensed and delivered increases, the expenditures for gasoline, oil, and repairs increase, but the depreciation, taxes, and insurance costs remain the same.

STEP 2—Determine the amount of *variable expense* as a *percent of sales.* For the purpose of this analysis, the following expense items are classified as *variable expenses,* even though they may be fixed to an extent for a given pharmacy: advertising, bad debts, employees' wages, and miscellaneous expenses. Employee wages and miscellaneous expenses are semivariable, but they are classified as variable expenses for the purpose of delineating all expenses into two categories.

STEP 3—Determine the amount of *fixed expenses* in *dollars.* Fixed expenses include proprietor's salary, rent, heat, light and power, accounting and legal fees, taxes, interest paid, repairs, insurance, delivery, depreciation, and telephone. Delivery expenses, and perhaps others, are actually semi-fixed, but they are classified as fixed expenses for convenience.

STEP 4—Determine the *marginal income ratio.* This is done by subtracting the percent of variable expenses from the percent of gross margin. This is the percentage of sales left to cover the fixed expenses and net profit, if any.

STEP 5—Compute the sales volume at the *break-even point.* This is done by dividing the amount of fixed expenses by the marginal income ratio. At this point no profit or loss is realized.

This procedure is illustrated by the following example:

Fixed expenses	$ 27,000
Variable expenses	14.4% of sales
Gross margin	36.2% of sales
Marginal income ratio	21.8% of sales (36.2% − 14.4%)
Break-even point	

$$\frac{\$\ 27,000}{.218} = \$123,853$$

This technique may be applied to any fixed investment or expense. Modifications are necessary when the technique is applied to a variable expense. Break-even analysis is based on historical percentages and data, which may change during the experimental year. These changes are usually minor for a well-established pharmacy because of the inherent stability of the pharmaceutical profession.

It should be noted that cost of goods sold is a *variable* cost, but it figures only indirectly into the computation of the break-even point. This is true because it is the *gross margin* that is available to meet the fixed and variable expenses and to provide a net profit, if any.

Application of Break-Even Analysis. Miller's Pharmacy is located in a town of 10,000 people and a total trading area with a 20,000 population. There are four other progressive, modern pharmacies in this town. This pharmacy is old and has not been remodeled in several years. The sales volume is $180,000. The pharmacist would like to know approximately how much additional sales will be required to pay for remodeling, which will cost $4,000. Table 14-3 gives the pertinent data derived from his last profit and loss statement.

Figure 14-5 shows the break-even point when these parameters are plotted.

Since the marginal income ratio is 0.22 expressed as a decimal, the additional sales needed to pay for the remodeling are $18,182 ($4,000 ÷ 0.22). This amount of sales will pay for the additional cost incurred for remodeling and permit the same net profit as for the year before, assuming all other factors remain constant.

Summary

Financial management requires thorough analyses, and financial analyses should be guided by analysis objectives. Some eighteen financial ratios or values should be computed and compared to standard and/or average values to further the analysis process. By relating these various financial ratios to one or more of the analysis objectives, specific financial and managerial problem areas may be identified.

After these initial calculations, analysis may proceed with one or more methods. The first method logically is to arrange the various ratios in a paradigm. In this manner, those ratios which manifest a specific objective or problem area can be readily identified. When two or more ratios point to the same problem or weakness, they usually confirm the problem. This is an internal analysis. Next, the analyst will compare the ratios to external standards and averages for further confirmation. When data for

Table 14-3. *Data for Break-Even Analysis*

	Dollars	% of Sales
Sales	$180,000	
Gross margin	64,800	36.0
Fixed expenses	28,800	- - - -
Variable expenses	25,200	14.0
(Total expenses)	(54,000)	(30.0)
Marginal income ratio	- - - - -	22.0
(Net profit)	(10,800)	(6.0)

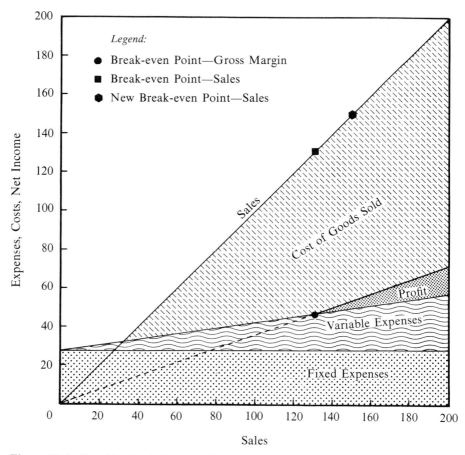

Figure 14-5. *Graphic Break-Even Analysis*

two or more years are available, a trend analysis will not only confirm a problem area, but it will also point to impending problems.

Break-even analysis is used to predict the outcome of certain decisions. More specifically, break-even analysis will indicate the amount of new sales necessary to pay for a fixed investment.

Careful interpretation of the various methods of financial analysis often indicates the necessary steps to solve the problem.

REVIEW

1. What are the five objectives of financial analysis and which ratios relate to or are indicative of each?

2. Define net working capital and three ratios that are indicative of liquidity and solvency. Give the acceptable limits or standards and the desired target value, if applicable, of the three ratios.

3. Define the four ratios that are indicative of the financial position of a firm. Give the acceptable limits and the desired target values, if applicable, for the four ratios.

4. What is undercapitalization?

5. What is meant by capital leverage?

6. Define the four profitability ratios. What are the minimum desired values of each? Which two of the four ratios measure both profitability and efficiency?

7. Define the six efficiency ratios. Give the usual acceptable range or value for each.

8. What are the maximum potential and the realistic target values for inventory turnover?

9. Explain why a high turnover rate is undesirable as well as a low value.

10. Explain the significance of net working capital turnover and how it differs from capital (NW) turnover.

11. Explain undertrading and overtrading and relate these to undercapitalization and overcapitalization.

12. Explain the significance of the average accounts receivable collection period and the average time to pay accounts payable.

13. Give the appropriate data; calculate all of the ratios discussed.

14. Describe each of the methods of financial analysis: Internal using Paradigm; Comparison with External Standards; Trend Analysis; and Break-even Analysis. Using real data from a pharmacy, hypothetical data, or average data from *The Lilly Digest,* apply each of the above analyses.

15. Control Mechanisms

Control mechanisms include a wide variety of techniques that fall into one of two general categories, budgetary and nonbudgetary controls. The former deals primarily with financial controls, the latter with a variety of functions and activities that lend themselves to extra-budgetary controls. This does not suggest that these latter activities are devoid of financial implication. On the contrary, they definitely do have financial implication, but the functions cannot be controlled by budgets alone.

Any control mechanism is composed of two primary elements: (1) procedures or guidelines for controlling activities, and (2) a feedback mechanism to communicate the results in order to assess the effectiveness of the control mechanism. These two elements have been previously depicted in Figure 3-1. Control mechanisms are necessary at several levels of the firm, as is control of the firm itself in relation to society. Management by objectives (MBO) provides the broad framework for overall control without the oppressive influence of most of the older approaches to management and control.

Through MBO, realistic goals and objectives are established that are consistent with the goals of society and the economic environment in which the pharmacy operates. Measurable criteria are established to determine which objectives are being achieved and to what degree. This provides the broad and basic framework for all the control mechanisms. The organizational structure, legal form, and policies can then be formulated within the basic framework provided by MBO. Objectives, policies, and the various coordinating and control mechanisms form an integrated management system.

Budgets are related to, and form a necessary part of, the *financial control* of any organization. However, overall control encompasses a wider scope, reaching beyond the activity reflected by financial data alone. *Overall control* includes every aspect of an organization—objectives, policies, personnel, professional activities, inventory, credit, fixed assets, and security. Some of the mechanisms necessary to control the various aspects of management have been discussed in previous chapters, including objectives, policies, personnel, and inventory. Many of these facets of management are reflected by the financial data and the ratios derived from them.

Nonbudgetary Controls

The personnel area of management has been discussed in Chapter 8. It is only necessary here to reiterate how MBO—when extended to all managerial, professional, and supervisory or key employees—provides an excellent control mechanism. Implicit in MBO are good two-way communications, a philosophy of participatory management, and measurable criteria to determine when objectives are, or are not, being met. Such criteria should consist of performance measurements such as sales increase, expense decrease, and mutually agreed rating scales for less tangible achievements of employees such as improvement and development. It should be noted at this point that nonbudgetary control is complementary to budgetary control. Since inventory control was adequately discussed in Chapter 10, only a reminder that inventory control is a part of the overall control procedure has been included in this chapter.

PROFESSIONAL FUNCTIONS

Control of professional functions is an important area of nonbudgetary control. One specific example is the control of drugs and pharmaceuticals subject to the drug laws. The control of these items exceeds ordinary inventory control methods and includes the necessity of accurate records of receipt and dispensing of all substances subject to these laws.

The monitoring and control of the utilization of all prescription and nonprescription maintenance drugs falls within the scope of the control of professional functions. The proper management of all facets of drug utilization—over- or under-utilization, allergic reactions, drug-drug interactions, and drug-food interactions—requires the use of a medication record system. The professional and public health reasons for maintaining a medication record system have been well documented.[1-5]

A medication record system that provides appropriate control over drug utilization as enumerated above should include certain criteria. First, an individual record should be maintained for each patient. Only then can the pharmacist efficiently monitor the drug utilization of the patient. Individual patient records are also more efficient for insurance purposes. Second, the record should include nonprescription drugs used as maintenance medication. Third, the record should include personal and health data as exemplified in Figure 15-1.

The medication record cards should be filed alphabetically by family with the head of the family first, followed by the remainder of the family filed in the order of spouse and then children from the oldest to the youngest. The card for the head of the family should be of a different and distinct color.

There are economic considerations of medication record systems. Smith reported a cost-to-effectiveness ratio of 1 to 2.54 for a medication record system.[6] In other words, each dollar spent to implement, maintain, and promote the medication record system yielded $2.54 in net profit during the first year following its implementation. The same study found

NAME							BIRTHDATE			
ADDRESS										
CHRONIC DISEASES										
ALLERGIES: Drugs-						Foods-				
IMMUNIZATION DPT										
Polio						Typhoid				

Date	℞ No.	Drug	Str.	Form	Amt.	Prescriber	Price	Renewal Dates		

Figure 15-1. *Medication Record System Card*

that the cost of the system was approximately 3.5 cents per prescription dispensed.

In a study of the use of medication profiles in one of the Appalachian Regional Hospital outpatient pharmacies, it was estimated that it cost 5 cents per prescription to maintain the system.[7] The significance of the study,[8] however, was the effectiveness of the medication record system in controlling utilization of drugs, especially over-utilization. Over-utilization was by far the greatest problem, followed by under-utilization. Over-utilization was more prevalent among patients whose drugs were financed by a third party. Conversely, under-utilization was more prevalent among private patients. Misuse of drugs of all types was more prevalent among those aged 65 years and over. Over-utilization occurred more often among users of psychotherapeutic and antihypertensive drugs when compared to eight other categories. These differences were significant as indicated by the chi-square test.

CREDIT CONTROL

The decision by the independent pharmacist to offer credit to selected patrons is almost automatic. The practice is widespread, and refusing credit, at least to good risk customers, would place a pharmacist at a distinct disadvantage. Credit is widely practiced among most retail establishments and it is expected by the general public. Because of the nature of pharmacy in providing health maintenance and even lifesaving drugs and services, it has a long history of offering credit to those who request it. Although it is true that some of the larger chain drugstores and discount houses with prescription departments do not yet offer charge service, in recent years some of these establishments have provided credit through one of the several charge cards.

In an economic sense, the decision to establish a credit program involves a cost-benefit analysis. In other words, the earnings in net profit derived from the extra sales resulting from the charge service must be compared with the potential earnings from the working capital funds tied up in accounts receivable at the going interest rate. In computing the net profit from the charge sales, the additional expense of bookkeeping, administration, collection, and bad debts resulting from extending credit should be included. Such computation is not an easy task for many pharmacists.

In a 1964 study of 26 pharmacies in a Midwest city with a population of 100,000, the average accounting cost was 2.7 percent of the average credit sales of $80,530.[9] In another study, Doerr and Evanson reported an average accounting cost of 3.9 percent on $32,428 credit sales.[10] These findings compare favorably with the estimated cost of 3 to 5 percent on credit sales reported by Kelly and Lawyer.[11] In the 1964 study, bad debts averaged 0.2 percent of total sales, the figure reported in *The Lilly Digest* annually for many years, and 0.84 percent of charge sales.

It might appear on superficial analysis that credit sales were not profitable, since the average net profit reported in *The Lilly Digest* for 1964 was only 5.1 percent of sales.[12] However, without the charge sales, which averaged almost one-third of total sales in one study, many of the pharmacies would have lost money. This is true because the marginal income produced by credit sales exceeded the marginal cost of these sales. The excess of marginal income over marginal cost was more than could have been derived from the interest on the money invested in accounts receivable.

The *first step* in setting controls for a credit sales program is the decision to extend credit at all. An actual cost-benefit analysis or an intuitive estimate is implicit in this decision. Once the decision has been made, control procedures should be established. Controls should be predicated on the following questions: What type(s) or form(s) of charge accounts will be utilized? What limitation, if any, will be placed on the amount of credit? What collection procedures will be used? Finally, what criteria will be used for charging off bad debts?

Types of Charge Accounts. What types of charge accounts should a pharmacist use? There are four types: (1) the ordinary open account, (2) the installment account, (3) the budget account, and (4) the revolving account. The *open account* is the most common in pharmacy practices. It simply involves charging merchandise and services when purchased, with payment due when the bill is sent to the customer, usually at the end of the month. In the past, pharmacists seldom charged interest or a service on delinquent accounts. In recent years, however, a service and/or interest charge of 1 to $1^1/_2$ percent per month has been assessed on the unpaid balance after the regular 30-day credit period has elapsed.

The *installment credit* plan is seldom used in pharmacy, although it is sometimes used by some pharmacists for expensive items such as a hospital bed. A down payment of 10 to 30 percent is collected, and the remainder is paid in equal payments, usually monthly, over a period of six months to a year. Again, an interest or service charge may or may not be used for installment credit.

The *budget account* is simply a short-term modification of the usual installment plan. Usually, a larger down payment is required, and the balance is paid in equal installments within a period of two to four months. This plan is used for substantial purchases, such as a wheelchair. A service charge may be used at the discretion of the pharmacist.

The *revolving account* has become popular in recent years, especially with department stores. Pharmacists have not used this approach to a great extent, but some chain drugstores are using this method. The revolving account permits the consumer to purchase up to a designated limit, for example $300, and the consumer pays a specified amount each month, for example $50 to $100. A service charge as high as $1^1/_2$ percent per month is paid on the unpaid balance.

Credit cards are popular today, and many pharmacists believe that they should participate in these plans. Any or all of the above credit plans are available from one or more of the various credit card services. In every case, a service and interest charge, usually $1^1/_2$ percent per month on the unpaid balance, is charged the consumer. With many of these plans the pharmacist (or other vendor) is charged a service fee for delinquent accounts. This charge is imposed to cover interest and collection cost, and may range from 3 to 5 percent.

An informal plan is the so-called *lay-away plan.* The consumer pays a nominal amount to have the pharmacist hold an item to be purchased by a designated time. If the customer does not purchase the item by the designated date, he forfeits the initial payment. This is often used at Christmas time to hold an item intended as a gift.

The pharmacist must decide first of all whether to offer credit to his patrons and then which credit plan or combination of credit plans to use. It should be obvious that the greater the number of credit plans used, the more difficult it will be to control credit.

Investigating the Credit Applicant. Investigation of the credit applicant is the *second* and most *critical* step in credit control procedures. Several sources of information may be used to gather pertinent information, including a credit application form, the local credit bureau, banks, and other creditors. The credit application form should request the following types of data:

1. *Personal data*—name, address, how long the applicant has lived in the city or county, age, and names of the members of his or her family.

2. *Employment*—the employer, position, immediate supervisor, previous employer, and names of other employed members of the family.

3. *Bank*—the name of the bank or banks the applicant patronizes.

4. *Other firms* at which the applicant has charge accounts.

After the applicant has completed the credit application form, he should be told when he will be notified of his credit status. After examining the information on the application, the pharmacist should check with the credit bureau to determine whether the applicant has been reported delinquent by any of his other creditors. Every pharmacist who contemplates considerable charge sales should belong to the local credit bureau; otherwise, the information requested from the bureau will be rather expensive. Members of the local credit bureau usually are sent weekly bulletins, which list poor credit risks and other related information. It is a good policy to check with two or more other creditors to determine more precisely the payment record of the applicant. The banks are reluctant to provide much financial information about a client because they consider this to be confidential information. However, they do provide some general information that can be useful in deciding the credit risk of an applicant.

Form letters should be carefully composed for acceptance or rejection of a credit applicant. Both letters should be as pleasant in tone as possible. The acceptance should indicate your appreciation to the person for selecting you as his family pharmacist and enumerate all the special services and merchandise lines you feature. The credit policies and terms should be explained in such a manner that the patron will understand and accept them.

It should be noted at this point that as a professional person, licensed to provide critical health services, the pharmacist should not let his credit policies preclude the dispensing of a prescription on credit *in an emergency.*

Monitoring Charge Accounts. This procedure is an important phase of credit control. There are two basic techniques of monitoring charge accounts: *account age analysis* and the *average collection period of accounts.* The latter technique was described in Chapter 14. Ideally, the average collection period should not exceed 30 days, but a 40-day average period is not too critical. An average collection period of 60 days or more is too high and indicates concerted steps should be taken.

The average collection period is a control check on the credit management as a whole, but it does not indicate which accounts are delinquent. Account age analysis will indicate the status of each account in terms of rate of payment related to rate of credit. Account age analysis provides information on the overall balance at the end of the month, the amount purchased and paid during the past month, and the amount that has been due 60 days, 90 days, and over 90 days. Some account age analyses classify the amount due 120 days and over.

As a general rule, debts more than 90 days old are difficult to collect. As a significant portion of a current balance is revealed by the age analysis to have been due for 90 days or more, steps should be taken to collect the account. Depending on the history and circumstances of the particular client and the general reputation of the people in the trade area, debts of 60 days' duration may be considered as doubtful in terms of collection.

A related question concerns the time when a pharmacist has to write off an account as a bad debt. As a general rule, a time period of one year is reasonable. If an account, or a significant portion of it, has been due for a year, and all attempts to collect have failed, it would be wise to write off the account as a bad debt and take the income tax advantage.

Collection Procedures. Although investigating and selecting charge customers is the most critical phase of the credit control procedure, efficient collection procedures are the *most difficult* phase. A system should be devised to prevent credit extension from getting out of hand and to treat all patrons fairly. Again, the cost-benefit analysis approach should be used in determining how far one is willing to go to collect a debt. For example, it is unprofitable to spend $25 to collect a $10 account.

A good collection procedure should include the following steps. *First,* an invoice or "charge ticket" for each charge purchase should be given the customer at the time of the purchase, and two copies of the invoice retained in the pharmacy. Regular statements should be mailed to all charge customers. The statement should include a duplicate copy of each invoice or "charge ticket" for all purchases listed on the invoice. Statements normally are mailed monthly; however, in rural areas statements may be mailed quarterly, semi-annually, or sometimes annually. Statements are sent less frequently in the rural areas because rural patrons receive most of their income once or twice a year, when they sell their major cash crop, and because charge sales generally constitute a smaller percentage of total sales.

As a *second step,* some pharmacists stamp a notice of "past due" on the second mailing of the statements. Other terms used are "Please remit (or pay) promptly," or "Kindly send us your check for this statement." This type of reminder generally is used only if a significant payment has not been made during the previous month.

The *third step* in the collection procedure is to send a personal letter requesting payment of the past due bills. This type of letter should be firm, but not offensive. According to Steinmetz et al.,[13] this type of letter should have two objectives: "(A) Bring the debtor to a conviction that the bill must be paid, and (B) secure the debtor's action by the shortest possible route and still retain his goodwill." The same authors further state that "the collection letter should start out as a reminder, then become firmer, and as a last resort indicate drastic action."[13] However, several other authorities recommend three different letters emphasizing the same three separate points stated in the order above. The last letter, however, should end on a conciliatory note after indicating whatever drastic action is contemplated. Sometimes the telephone is used in place of the initial letter to provide a more personal touch. A set of prototype letters is provided here:

First Letter

Dear Mrs. Jones:

It has come to my attention that your account (in the amount of $_____) is past due. We are pleased to have had the opportunity to serve you and extend credit as an additional service. As you know it costs our pharmacy a great deal to provide our many services and this is especially true of our credit service.

Will you not pay your bill promptly in order that we may continue to serve you and our other clientele as efficiently and professionally as we have in the past? Your thoughtful consideration of this matter will be appreciated.

Sincerely yours,

Second Letter

Dear Mrs. Jones:

This is the second reminder of your past due bill in the amount of $_____ including the interest charge. I cannot overemphasize the seriousness of this matter. Failure to pay your bill has added to our operating cost and could jeopardize your credit status in our community. I urge you to remit the above amount within the next ten days.

Sincerely yours,

Third Letter

Dear Mrs. Jones:

I regret to say that our previous appeals have failed, and you have not responded in any manner to our request that you pay your bill. If you do not pay your account within ten days, I will turn your account over to a collection agency. Needless to say, I am reluctant to do this, but you have left me no alternative.

We have cherished your patronage in the past and will continue to do so if you will pay your account in full, or arrange to pay a substantial amount now and the remainder within an agreed period of time.

I trust you will act promptly on this proposition and re-establish our long-standing and mutually beneficial relation.

Sincerely yours,

The *final* and *most drastic step* is to utilize a free-lance collector, a regular collection agency, or an attorney to collect the bill. The pharmacist has more control over the proceedings if he uses an attorney, but it usually costs him more. A regular collection agency normally is the most efficient because these organizations are specialists in this particular activity.

As a final note to the collection procedure, it is the consensus of most experienced people that the customers are more likely to continue to give a firm their patronage after they have been coaxed, pressured, or forced to pay their bill. There are two reasons given for this theory. First, people stop patronizing a place after they have accumulated a sizable bill because they are embarrassed to face the proprietor. After the bill has been paid, this barrier is removed and they often return to the pharmacy for their pharmaceutical needs. Second, the pharmacist often gains additional respect for his forthright business-like practices. As a professional person and humanitarian, a pharmacist should give proper consideration to hardship cases. Historically, this has been one of the hallmarks of the pharmaceutical profession.

STORE SECURITY

Burglaries and Robberies. Security has become one of the major problems in pharmacy with the increase in both burglaries and robberies, which have been motivated primarily by the need for dependence-producing drugs. With the passage of the Controlled Substance Act in 1965, and the more stringent law, the Comprehensive Drug Abuse Prevention and Control Act in 1970, "street drugs" have become more difficult to obtain. Consequently, there has been an increase in robberies and burglaries of pharmacies to obtain these drugs, reaching "epidemic" proportions in the last five years.

First, the burglaries and robberies began in the large metropolitan cities, but they soon spread to the rural towns throughout the United States. The problem has become so serious that a bill has been introduced in Congress to make burglaries and robberies of pharmacies a Federal offense. Some pharmacies have been burglarized more than six times.

Pilferage. Pilferage is another serious problem for pharmacists. It costs them more than burglaries and robberies combined; however, it does not have the attendant danger of homicide or serious injury and the social problem of drug abuse and dependence.

Pilferage is committed by both employees and "outsiders." The former source of pilferage can be controlled by good personnel administration practices, especially with good selection techniques and appropriate compensation. Some pharmacists use the polygraph in selecting employees or in suspected cases of pilferage.

Security Measures. As previously mentioned, good employee selection procedures and personnel relations can control, if not completely eliminate, the problem of pilferage by employees. Controlling pilferage by the public is much more difficult. The use of large mirrors in the front of the pharmacy has reduced pilferage only to a nominal degree.

A system of closed-circuit television cameras and monitors has proved to be effective in reducing pilferage. One small drugstore chain of 35 units has installed a closed-circuit television system with excellent results.[14] The system usually is installed on a lease and purchase agreement. The cost averages between three and four dollars per day per pharmacy over a period of 36 months, depending on the number of cameras and monitors required. This cost includes the rental and service for four cameras and one to three monitors. One monitor is placed in or near the prescription department, and one is placed in the center of the pharmacy. This latter monitor is used for its psychologic effect because customers can see people over the entire pharmacy as the scene switches from one camera view to another. At the end of 36 months, the system may be purchased for a nominal fee of about $100.

The cost for an individual pharmacy is considerably more. However, a cooperative group or a group of pharmacies in a city or a cluster of neighboring towns could negotiate a favorable contract based on the economics of servicing the equipment. In either case, the pharmacist will have to pay for service calls after he purchases the system.

Most pharmacists have burglary and robbery insurance, but these policies are usually cancelled after two or three burglaries or robberies. There are several variations in burglary alarm systems. Originally, an alarm (bell) sounded when the circuit around the door and safe was broken. This was refined to a remote alarm at the nearest police station but silent in the pharmacy. This was designed to apprehend the burglars before they finished the burglary. An infrared sensitive device and a noise sensitive device have been incorporated into the newer systems. Like participants in the cold war, the burglars have learned to avoid every alarm innovation.

Probably the simplest and most effective technique available is the dispersal of controlled drugs throughout the prescription department and frequently relocating them together with a remote alarm. Before the burglars can find enough drugs to make the burglary worthwhile, the police can apprehend the culprits. After all, arrest and conviction are much more effective than the sophisticated gadgets, which most burglars learn to foil.

The 1973 September issue of *Pharmacy Times* listed 20 techniques to improve security. The major items have been discussed above, but the various other techniques, such as checking that the pharmacy is free of customers before it is locked each night, are common sense, and worthwhile practices.

Budgetary Control

Any budgetary control procedure requires a working knowledge of basic accounting concepts and procedures. Accurate records are necessary to the successful operation of any organization, either profit or nonprofit. In fact, the evidence indicates a close relationship between inadequate accounting records and business failures.[15] A well-designed accounting system is necessary for a budgetary or financial control system. It also serves other purposes. An accounting system has four objectives. The first objective is to provide the financial information necessary for bank or trade credit. The second objective is to provide the basis for income tax returns. The third objective is to protect the firm's assets from careless errors and frauds and to provide a systematic method of depreciation of fixed assets. The fourth objective is to serve as a basis for financial and business planning. It is the latter two objectives that are the primary focus of the remainder of this chapter.

The control budget is divided into two primary sections, the income or revenue section and the expenditures section. The latter is further divided into fixed and variable costs (defined in Chapter 14).

Usually nonprofit organizations develop an expenditure budget based on goals or planned services and hope the revenue will be sufficient to meet the budget. This is not the case in institutional pharmacies, generally speaking, because the pharmacy, along with the clinical laboratory and the X-ray department, are the departments that most consistently show an operational surplus.

REVENUE COMPONENT OF THE BUDGET

This portion of the budget is both the most critical and most difficult to project. Yet it is a vital and necessary part of budgetary planning for both profit and nonprofit organizations, if either a balanced budget or profit is to be achieved. Projection of revenue usually is based on data from past experience. Too frequently the projection for the next fiscal year is based on the change between the year ending and the previous year. This is sound under stable conditions. The simplicity of this approach ignores two important variables, one internal and one external.

Internal Variable. This variable is the growth curve of the pharmacy. One normally would anticipate a rapid growth rate for a newly established pharmacy. An in-depth location analysis will provide a basis for the early growth rate projections, which should be adjusted annually according to the actual sales data. Of course, if a large error is made in estimating the potential volume and growth rate, not only will the adjustment be large, but relocation should be considered, especially if the error was made on the optimistic side. Normally, the early growth rate of a pharmacy begins to plateau in about four to five years, followed by a normal growth pattern corresponding to the general economic conditions of the market.

External Variable. This is the overall economic growth curve or decline of the market in which the pharmacy is located. The market conditions include a multitude of factors, such as the general economic condition of the country as measured by the gross national product (GNP), local economic variations, and both seasonal and random or nonpredictable fluctuations. Local economic variations may include strikes, new industries, droughts, and the like. Seasonal variations have little or no effect in predictions covering a period of more than one year. Random, nonpredictable variations include such factors as epidemics, unusual weather, an increase or decrease in prescribers, and the introduction of a new drug for the treatment of a disease for which no adequate treatment previously existed. Obviously, these nonpredictable factors cannot be used in the projection of the revenue or sales portion of the budget.

The pharmacist can use the GNP growth trend to make appropriate adjustment in his pharmacy's growth trend, based on a broad consensus among the professional economists concerning the national trend. The pharmacist should take note of the local economic trends and development and make appropriate adjustments in his income projections.

Income projections should be based on at least five years' data when available. One can use as a guide a well-established pharmacy under normal economic growth conditions, or *The Lilly Digest* average sales during a similar period. A straight-line equation is used to establish the trend. Table 15-1 shows the average sales volumes, as reported in *The Lilly Digest*[16] for the years 1967-71.

The data may be used to illustrate income projection. The technique is the simple least-squares method for a five-year trend using the middle year as the origin or pivotal point of the trend line.[17] The equation is:

$$Y' = a + bx$$

where: Y = the actual sales
 Y′ = the estimated sales volume for the respective years
 x = the deviation in terms of the number of years from the mid-year
 a = the average annual sales for the period
 b = the rate of change in the sales volume or the slope of the trend line.

The computations are as follows:

$$a = \frac{\Sigma Y}{N} = \frac{\$1,058,500}{5} = \$211,700$$

$$b = \frac{\Sigma xY}{\Sigma x^2} = \frac{\$118,500}{10} = \$11,850$$

Substituting in the equation, Y′ = a + bx, the estimated sales volume for 1972 is calculated as follows:

$$Y'(1972) = \$211,700 + 3(\$11,850) = \$247,250$$

EXPENDITURE COMPONENT OF THE BUDGET

The expenditure component of the budget is composed of two parts, variable expenses and fixed expenses.

Table 15-1. *Sales Forecast for 1972 Based on 1967–71 Data*

Year	Y*	x	x²	xY	Y′
1967	$188,500	−2	4	$ − 377,000	$188,000
1968	199,000	− 1	1	− 199,000	199,850
1969	214,000	0	0	− − − − − −	211,700
1970	221,500	+1	1	221,500	223,550
1971	236,500	+2	4	473,000	235,400
− − − −	$1,058,500	0	10	$118,500	− − − − − −

* Rounded to nearest $500.

Variable Expenses. Since variable expenses, by definition, vary proportionally with sales, it would appear that they could be projected by multiplying the percentage for each by the projected sales. This procedure is acceptable, however, only after each expense item has been analyzed carefully and compared with some standard, such as a comparable group of pharmacies as reported in *Heart of the Lilly Digest.* The percentages of the several variable expenses change with the level in sales volume, as shown by a study of *The Lilly Digest.* Based on data from this source, a range of percentages for the several variable expenses applicable to most pharmacies has been constructed.

Employees' wages	10.0–12.0%
Advertising	1.0– 1.5%
Bad debts	0.1– 0.3%
Miscellaneous expenses	2.0– 2.5%
Total	13.1–16.3%
General average	15.0% (rounded nearest 1%)

Fixed Expenses. Fixed expenses are constant for a given fiscal period, normally a year, but they may increase with time as the pharmacy grows significantly in sales volume, or by enlarging the facilities or services provided. Unless a significant change has taken place, the pharmacist may plan for the same fixed expenses as budgeted and/or expended the previous year. Sometimes, however, on close examination, he may see the need to alter certain items.

Some fixed expense items are not absolutely fixed, but vary with sales. Delivery costs, for example, vary to a degree with an increase in sales, but the larger portion of the costs—depreciation, insurance, property taxes, and repairs—is fixed for the most part, at least for a given year. Although inventory can be expected to increase with sales, and thus the insurance premium and property tax on inventory, insurance premium and property tax on fixed assets would decrease because of depreciation. This decrease in insurance and property tax through depreciation usually equals or exceeds the increase due to increased inventory.

Most pharmacists pay a fixed rent per month. Some pay rent as a percentage of sales. In this case, rent is certainly a variable expense. This situation occurs more frequently in medical clinic buildings and large shopping centers. Normally, the lessor requires a minimum monthly rent which covers sales up to a designated amount; then the lessee pays a percentage rent, which again may decrease at various intervals up to a specified sales volume. The latter feature, a decreasing percentage rent with increasing sales volume, should be included in all percentage rent leases, and the pharmacist should negotiate for an upper dollar limit on the rent.

Nearly all other expenses are fixed, at least in a given fiscal period. The proprietor's salary should be realistic—the amount one would have to pay a manager to perform comparable work.

Budgeting Depreciation

Depreciation is a significant and unique expense. It is unique in that the expense is not a cash outlay, but rather a deduction allowed by the Internal Revenue Service (IRS) for the depreciation of fixed capital investments. Because of its unique features, and the various formulas of depreciation permitted by IRS, this topic will be discussed in considerable detail.

BASIS FOR DEPRECIATION

There are basically *three reasons* for allowing depreciation of an asset. *First,* the asset may be subject to physical wear with use and time, or depletion in the case of natural resources such as coal, oil, and gas. *Second,* the asset may become obsolete because of changing technology and other changes. *Third,* depreciation of fixed capital investment *encourages investment and economic growth.* This is the basic reason double allowances and other fast write-off procedures for the first year's depreciation are allowed, especially during a period of economic recession or depression.

DEPRECIATION CRITERIA

The nature of the property determines: (1) whether an asset qualifies for depreciation, and (2) the duration of the period of depreciation. There are *three* criteria that the asset must meet to be eligible for depreciation. *First,* the life of the property must be definite and exceed one year. Thus, *real property* (land) cannot be depreciated.

Second, the property must be used in the enterprise for the production of income, but *inventory* held for sale cannot be depreciated. However, this does not mean that deteriorated or unsalable inventory may not be written off at the end of a fiscal period.

Third, intangible property can be depreciated *only* under certain conditions. The cost incurred in obtaining an intangible asset, such as a copyright or a covenant not to compete, may be depreciated at uniform rates over a period of time negotiated with the IRS. The value of goodwill, trade names, or trademarks is not eligible for depreciation.

COMPONENTS OF DEPRECIATION

The fundamental steps in setting up a depreciation schedule are: (1) determining the value basis for depreciation; (2) determining the useful life of the asset; (3) determining the salvage value of the asset; and (4) determining the maximum deduction allowed.

Value Base. The cost of the property ordinarily is the basis for determining the *value base* for computation of the depreciation. If a non-business property is converted to business use, for example, a used personal automobile, the fair market value (blue-book value in this instance) would be used as the value base for calculating depreciation from the date of conversion to business use. If a pharmacist purchases a building in which he operates his practice, a valuation of both land and the building must be made since the land may not be depreciated. In those cases in which a pharmacist leases a building and improves the value of the building through remodeling, he may depreciate the cost of the remodeling over the established life of the improvements.

Useful Life. The Internal Revenue Service maintains a Table of Useful Lives of Depreciable Property. An abbreviated version is available as "IRS Bulletin F" from the Superintendent of Public Documents in Washington. Most fixtures and furnishings have a useful life of ten years. Refrigerators, for example, have a useful life of twenty years. Some equipment lasts only about five years. If a pharmacist's experience indicates a useful life other than the standard life, he can have this established for the particular fixture or equipment in his pharmacy by appropriate documentation of his prior experience with the particular property. The estimated useful life of a given asset may be modified at the end of a tax year, if the pharmacist can produce convincing evidence as a basis for changing the length of the useful life.

Salvage Value. The salvage value of an asset is the estimated value or sale value of the asset at the end of its useful life. This estimation is made at the time the asset is purchased or acquired, and it is indicated in the depreciation schedule on the next income tax return. This value depends on the nature of the property and the length of the useful life, which is affected, in part, by the replacement policy for the asset. If the pharmacist intends to keep the asset for its full inherent useful life and indicates this in the depreciation schedule, the pharmacist may deduct from the salvage value the cost of removing and transporting the property to a junk dealer.

Maximum Depreciation. The maximum depreciation allowance is the value base minus the salvage value. It is also the aggregate of annual deductions. A pharmacist should deduct the allowable depreciation each year; otherwise, he will lose it. A depreciation allowance cannot be carried over to future years. However, it is possible to get variable depreciation by selecting from among several methods of calculating depreciation.

DEPRECIATION METHODS

Four different methods for calculating depreciation are accepted by the IRS. In addition, there are some modifications allowed through negotiations. In fact, the IRS states that any reasonable method of depreciation is permitted if negotiated and applied consistently. One frequently used modification is the additional first-year depreciation allowance, that is, allowing twice the normal deduction above the regular amount. This extra depreciation allowance is not a permanent rule, but it is used to encourage investment and expansion during economic recessions.

Straight-Line Method. The simplest method of calculating depreciation is the straight-line method. The salvage value is subtracted from the cost of the asset (or the value base) and the difference is divided by the number of years of the asset's useful life.

Declining Balance Method. This method is a little more complicated than the straight line method. With it, the salvage value is not deducted from the cost before the depreciation is calculated; however, the pharmacist cannot deduct depreciation below the salvage value. With this method, the amount of depreciation allowed is deducted from the cost, and the balance is used as the basis for computing the next year's depreciation allowance. Thus each year the basis for calculating the deduction is the declining balance, and hence, the name of the method. The rate of deduction is the straight-line rate and remains the same for the life of the asset. Under certain conditions, $1\frac{1}{2}$ to 2 times the straight-line rate of deduction is allowed. To qualify for this method, the asset must have a useful life of three years or more and be acquired, constructed, or renovated after December 31, 1953.

Sum-of-the-Years-Digits Method. The principle of this method is the application of a progressively smaller fraction (ratio) to the cost or other value base after subtracting the salvage value. This method can be applied to an individual asset or to a group of assets with the same useful life. The denominator of the fraction is determined by adding all the digits representing the years of the useful life of the asset(s). For example, a useful life of ten years would give a denominator of 55 $(10 + 9 + 8 + 7 + 6 + 5 + 4 + 3 + 2 + 1 = 55)$. The denominator can also be computed by the formula of $\dfrac{n^2 + n}{2}$, where n = years of useful life $\left(\dfrac{10^2 + 10}{2} = \dfrac{100 + 10}{2} = 55\right)$. The numerator is simply the number of years of useful life remaining at the beginning of the year for which the deduction is being computed.

Remaining Life Plan. The fourth method of calculating depreciation is the remaining life plan, which is a modification of the sum-of-the-years-digits method. The fraction increases each year, while the base for computing the deduction decreases in a manner similar to the declining balance method. This method incorporates concepts from the declining balance and the sum-of-the-years-digits methods, but the results are the same as the latter. The purpose of this method is to permit a fast rate of depreciation of assets with different useful lives. Each asset with a different useful life remaining is computed separately.

The denominator of the fraction is the sum of the digits of the remaining years of useful life, while the numerator is the number of years of remaining useful life. For example, if an asset has five more years of useful life, the denominator is 15 and the numerator is 5, providing the fraction $^5/_{15}$. This fraction is multiplied by the balance or unrecovered cost of the asset. A comparison of these four methods is shown in Table 15-2.

CHOOSING THE BEST METHOD

The choice of the method of depreciation depends primarily on the projected total income (net profit plus proprietor's salary for proprietorship or partnership). During the early years of a pharmacy, various conditions may exist that would cause a pharmacist to select a particular method of depreciation. First, let us assume the pharmacist's location analysis indicated a good potential for the location with rapid growth, yielding some net profit the first year and a significant net profit during the second year. If the pharmacist had a minimum amount of capital, he would need to generate as much cash as possible to meet his obligations. He will want to deduct the maximum depreciation during the early years to minimize the income tax liability. This will provide additional funds to meet either short- or long-term liabilities. The pharmacist should select the declining balance method of depreciation, since this method provides the fastest rate of depreciation. The slight penalty of unrecovered cost is a small price to pay for the advantage.

On the other hand, if the pharmacist has adequate capital and the location analysis indicates a slower but steady rate of growth with a significant amount of net profit in about the third or fourth year, the pharmacist would benefit most by the slower but steady depreciation rate of the straight-line method.

If the status of a pharmacy falls between these two extremes, the pharmacist should select the sum-of-the-years-digits or the remaining life plan. However, these latter two methods provide a much faster rate of depreciation than the straight-line method. Thus, by selecting the most appropriate depreciation method, the pharmacist can control one of his most significant fixed costs to his greatest advantage.

Table 15-2. *Comparison of Four Methods of Depreciation*

	Straight-Line Method				Declining Balance Method			
Year	Base*	Rate	Depreciation	Accumulated Depreciation	Base*	Rate	Depreciation	Accumulated Depreciation
1964	$10,000.00	10%	$1,000.00	$1,000.00	$11,000.00	20%	$2,200.00	$2,200.00
1965	10,000.00	10%	1,000.00	2,000.00	8,800.00	20%	1,760.00	3,960.00
1966	10,000.00	10%	1,000.00	3,000.00	7,040.00	20%	1,408.00	5,368.00
1967	10,000.00	10%	1,000.00	4,000.00	5,632.00	20%	1,126.40	6,494.40
1968	10,000.00	10%	1,000.00	5,000.00	4,505.60	20%	901.12	7,395.52
1969	10,000.00	10%	1,000.00	6,000.00	3,604.48	20%	720.90	8,116.42
1970	10,000.00	10%	1,000.00	7,000.00	2,883.58	20%	576.72	8,693.14
1971	10,000.00	10%	1,000.00	8,000.00	2,306.86	20%	461.37	9,154.51
1972	10,000.00	10%	1,000.00	9,000.00	1,845.49	20%	369.10	9,523.61
1973	10,000.00	10%	1,000.00	10,000.00	1,476.39	20%	295.28	9,818.89†

	Sum-of-the-Years-Digits Method				Remaining Life Plan			
Year	Base*	Rate	Depreciation	Accumulated Depreciation	Base*	Rate	Depreciation	Accumulated Depreciation
1964	$10,000.00	10/55	$1,818.18	$1,818.18	$10,000.00	10/55	$1,818.18	$1,818.18
1965	10,000.00	9/55	1,636.36	3,454.54	8,181.82	9/45 (1/5)	1,636.36	3,454.54
1966	10,000.00	8/55	1,454.55	4,909.09	6,545.46	8/36 (2/9)	1,454.44	4,908.98
1967	10,000.00	7/55	1,272.73	6,181.82	5,908.98	7/28 (1/4)	1,272.78	6,181.76
1968	10,000.00	6/55	1,090.91	7,272.73	3,818.24	6/21 (2/7)	1,090.92	7,272.68
1969	10,000.00	5/55	909.09	8,181.82	2,727.27	5/15 (1/3)	909.09	8,818.77
1970	10,000.00	4/55	727.27	8,909.09	1,818.23	4/10 (2/5)	727.30	8,909.07
1971	10,000.00	3/55	545.45	9,454.54	1,090.93	3/6 (1/2)	545.47	9,454.54
1972	10,000.00	2/55	363.64	9,818.18	545.46	2/3	363.64	9,818.18
1973	10,000.00	1/55	181.82	10,000.00	181.82	1/1	181.82	10,000.00

*The base is the cost less salvage value or the declining balance depending on the method used.
†This method allows a maximum depreciation of $9,818.89, and an unrecovered cost of $181.28 above salvage value.

Summary

Management controls can take many forms, both budgetary (financial) and nonfinancial, indirect budgetary controls. Many of the controls are inherent in the total management system, especially if management by objectives is the basic managerial method used. In addition, many of the controls have their roots in other phases of management—location analysis, capital planning, accounting systems, financial analysis, purchasing and inventory control, organizational form and structure, personnel administration, and the philosophy and policies of management.

Controls are accomplished through three primary mechanisms—management objectives with measurable criteria for each, a well-designed accounting system, and a two-way communication system based on openness, fairness, and integrity. As stated in previous chapters, a firm that utilizes MBO and good personnel policies will have little problem in controlling a pharmacy.

REFERENCES

1. Schwarting, A. E.: Presentation made to American Association of Colleges of Pharmacy, April 1971.
2. Seidl, L. G., Thornton, G. F., and Smith, J. W.: Studies on the epidemiology of adverse drug reactions III: reactions in patients on a general medical service. *Bull. Johns Hopkins Hosp., 119*:229–315, 1966.
3. Schimmel, E. M.: The hazards of hospitalization. *Ann. Int. Med., 60*:100–110, 1960.
4. Gardner, P., and Leighton, L. E.: The epidemiology of adverse drug reactions—a review and perspective. *Johns Hopkins Med. J., 126*:77–87, 1970.
5. Huffman, D. C., Jr.: Managerial Aspects of Patient Medication Record Systems. Paper presented at the American Pharmaceutical Association Academy of General Practice of Pharmacy in Boston, Massachusetts, July 26, 1973.
6. Smith, H. A.: Application of cost-effectiveness analysis to patient record systems. *J. Amer. Pharm. Assoc., NS13:* 13, 14, 1972.
7. Billups, N. F., and Glascock, L. M.: Personal communications.
8. Solomon, D. K., Baumgartner, R. P., Glascock, L. M., Glascock, S. A., Briscoe, M. E., and Billups, N. F.: Use of medication profiles to detect potential therapeutic problems in ambulatory patients. *Am. J. Hosp. Pharm., 31:*348–54, 1974.
9. Smith, H. A., et al.: Few pharmacists use cash registers fully. *American Druggist,* p. 55, May 24, 1965.
10. Doerr, D. W., and Evanson, R. V.: Consumer Credit Practices in Pharmacies. Paper presented to the Section on General Pharmacy Practice, Amer. Pharm. Assoc., New York, 1964.
11. Kelly, P. C., and Lawyer, K.: *How To Organize and Operate A Small Business.* 3rd ed., Englewood Cliffs: Prentice-Hall, Inc., p. 501.
12. Chagaris, C. A.: *The Lilly Digest,* Indianapolis: Eli Lilly and Co., 1964, p. 5.
13. Steinmetz, L. L., Kline, J. B., and Stegall, D. P.: *Managing the Small Business.* Homewood: Richard D. Irwin, Inc., 1968, p. 559.
14. Mudd, F. P.: Director of Pharmacy Operations, Begley Drug Co., personal communication.
15. Steinmetz, et al., *op. cit.,* p. 249.
16. Slavin, G. F.: *The Lilly Digest,* Indianapolis: Eli Lilly and Co., 1972, p. 16.
17. Pearson, F. A., and Bennett, K. K.: *Statistical Methods.* New York: John Wiley & Sons, Inc., 1945, p. 79.

REVIEW

1. Explain the concept and the mechanisms of total control.

2. Discuss the methods of control of professional activities.

3. Discuss credit control procedures and explain each specific mechanism.

4. Describe how the four types of charge accounts, credit cards, and lay-away plans operate.

5. Describe the process of investigation of credit applicants.

6. Discuss the monitoring of charge accounts, including the necessary calculations of the two basic techniques for monitoring accounts.

7. Describe efficient collection procedures fully.

8. Explain why forced collection of debts improves patrons' relations in many instances.

9. Explain the necessity of a good accounting system to budgetary control.

10. What are the objectives of a good accounting system?

11. Explain the influence of internal and external variables on the revenue portion of a budget.

12. Given an appropriate set of data, construct a budget including: (1) income section, projected with the least-squares method; (2) variable expense section, determined by using the average variable expense ratio of a typical pharmacy; and (3) fixed expense section, determined from data given.

13. What are the necessary criteria for an asset to qualify for depreciation?

14. What are the three reasons given for allowing depreciation deductions?

15. Explain the four methods of computing depreciation, list the four steps necessary for setting up a depreciation schedule, and compute a depreciation schedule by each of the methods when given the basic data.

16. Explain the basis for selecting the various methods of depreciation.

16. *Risk Management and Insurance*

The purpose of this chapter is twofold. The *first objective* is to acquaint the student with the basic nature of risk and insurance mechanisms and to discuss logical approaches to the management of risk. The *second objective* is to introduce the basic coverages available that may be needed in a particular situation.

Risk Management

TYPES OF RISK

A pharmacist invests his time (including his education), effort, and capital into his private practice in the hope of producing a reasonable salary and net profit. Obviously, there are risks involved when such a venture is undertaken. Risks arise from the uncertainty of the future and are of two basic types.

The first type is *market risk*, sometimes referred to as *dynamic risk* because of its changing character with changing market or economic conditions. The degree of market risk varies from ordinary risk, which is associated with most business enterprises, to high risk. The former is called *entrepreneur* risk; the latter is called *speculative* risk. The second type is called *exogenous* or *static* risk because the risk arises outside the market or economic environment and is difficult, if not impossible, to control or prevent in many instances. Fires and windstorms are examples of this type of risk.

A pharmacy with a favorable location analysis, adequate capital, and a well-educated and experienced manager certainly would be classified as an ordinary entrepreneur risk. Even so, the pharmacist needs to take precautions to minimize both the market and the exogenous risks. Consistent with this objective, it is vitally important that he maintain adequate insurance coverage to provide protection against an unpredictable financial loss, which could seriously jeopardize the future success of his firm. For example, fire hazard is an ever-present danger that demands attention. Furthermore, liability coverage is also necessary to avoid losses evolving out of third-party claims against the business. Such claims can arise in cases of patrons injured on the premises, negligent employees, or use of the pharmacy's product or service. Attention should also be given to such perils as business interruption, theft, the death of key personnel, and a host of others.

APPROACHES TO RISK MANAGEMENT

It is appropriate at this point to discuss the various methods of handling the risk of financial loss in a pharmacy.

Risk Avoidance. First of all, it is possible that risk may be avoided. However, such a situation is most unusual in the case of market risk, since such risk can only be avoided before the choice to enter business is made. Hence, avoiding risk is simply avoiding the exposure.

Risk Assumption. Certain risk can be assumed or is assumed. For example, a lack of funds to purchase insurance may force the individual to assume the risk. On the other hand, risk may be assumed out of ignorance or the stubborn unreasonableness of the individual. An example is the case of a businessman who, recognizing his need for fire insurance, fails to realize that the standard fire contract, without the extended coverage endorsement, provides inadequate coverage.

It is possible that the decision to assume risk is the best decision, especially in cases of overinsurance. In other words, it is possible for the firm to become insurance-poor by simply having so much coverage that the total amount of premiums puts a strain on the financial position of the business. Another method for assuming risk is to self-insure. Self-insurance involves the establishment of a fund within the business to handle the possibilities of financial loss in relation to a particular peril or hazard. For example, many pension funds that offer both retirement and death benefits may actually be handled through a fund set up by management to meet the various types of liabilities as they arise. Finally, it may be necessary for the businessman to assume risk simply because the insurer will not write coverage for the particular situation. For example, credit insurance is not available at the retail level; hence all risk in regard to poor accounts and bad debts must be assumed by the businessman himself.

Reduction of Hazards. A third method of handling risk involves reducing the hazard of the risk. This approach to risk management involves an awareness on the part of the pharmacist as well as his employees that proper safety precautions are beneficial to all parties concerned. Loss prevention programs and a general recognition of proper safety precautions are important in the proper management of risk, for in many cases, the insurance company recognizes the value of such action and reduces insurance premiums.

All small businessmen should recognize also that losses can be reduced or minimized, should accidents occur, by such measures as fire extinguishers, fire escapes, and an efficiently operating sprinkler system.

Shifting the Risk. The pharmacist may be in a position to shift risk by such arrangements as subcontracting, the use of surety bonds, and simply adopting the corporate form of organization. For example, through subcontracting, the person or persons contracted to perform a particular task will be responsible for adequate performance. In the case of surety bonds, the surety or the bonding company simply guarantees that a particular individual will perform in a prescribed manner. The corporate form of organization represents a risk shift situation in that it offers the limited liability feature.

Risk Reduction Through Insurance. Finally, the pharmacist must recognize that risk can be reduced. The principal means of reducing risk is through an insurance contract. Since insurance is the primary way to reduce risk, it would be enlightening to contrast insurance with gambling, an example of a risk that can be avoided. Insurance and gambling have the opposite effects in economic terms. The economic difference between gambling and insurance is based on the theory of marginal utility. The theory, in simple terms, rests on the concept that each additional unit of any economic good has a decreasing value with the accumulation of that good. Thus, $100 is less valuable to a person if he has $600 than if he has only $500. For example, if two people have $500 each and gamble $100 on a fair and even bet, the person who loses $100 experiences a greater economic loss in contrast to the $100 economic gain. The marginal utility of $100 in relation to the $600 of the winner is less than the marginal utility of $100 in relation to the $400 of the loser. The overall net effect of a gamble is a reduction in marginal utility. Insurance works to reduce risk and increases the overall marginal utility. This theoretical basis of insurance is explained in more detail in Marshall's economic treatise entitled *Principles of Economics.*[1]

Insurance Principles

DEFINITIONS OF INSURANCE

When financial loss involves the negligence of another party, the loss is shifted by society through the common law to the person responsible. When the loss evolves out of an act of God, the burden of loss must be assumed by the injured party. Regardless of the shift in the burden of loss or the assumption of the burden of loss, the loss is likely to cause someone serious financial difficulty. The insurance mechanism represents an effective solution to this problem by providing a private contractual arrangement allocating the burden of individual losses to members of a group who are exposed to similar losses. The insurance mechanism does not merely represent an accumulation of funds to meet uncertain losses, but, by virtue of the insurance contract, also spreads the risk.

The insurance mechanism is able to operate efficiently through the application of the law of large numbers. In other words, the greater the number of exposures, the more nearly will the actual experience approach the probable results expected. As the number of exposure units increases, events appearing to be caused by chance occur with amazing regularity. Thus, the law of large numbers, the law of probability, provides the basis for the social benefit of the insurance mechanism.

Economic Definition. The insurance contract is defined as an economic device for reducing risk by combining a sufficient number of exposure units in such a manner as to make their individual losses predictable collectively but not individually. The predictable loss is then shared by all group members, and this simply means that certain small "losses" in the form of insurance premiums are exchanged for the possibility of a large loss that any given individual in the group may experience. The insurance company is in business to indemnify the injured party, that is, to compensate for the loss of injury sustained. Thus, the function of the insurance company is to determine whether a financial loss has occurred, and if so, to place the injured party in the same position as he was prior to the loss.

Legal Definition. In addition to the aforementioned socioeconomic definition of insurance, there is the legal definition of insurance. In legal parlance, insurance is a contract whereby a company or group undertakes to indemnify a person or firm against loss, damage, or liability arising out of an unexpected or uncontrollable event or contingency.

Accounting Definition. The accounting definition may be stated in the following terms. Insurance is a technique whereby a person or firm substitutes a small, fixed, and regularly occurring cost for a larger and uncertain cost.

REQUISITES OF INSURABLE RISK

For the insurance mechanism to operate effectively, there are certain requisites of an insurable risk.

Common Peril. First of all, there must be a large group of homogeneous units exposed to the same peril. This condition is necessary for the application of the law of large numbers and to provide a situation in which the probable deviation of actual loss from predicted loss is small enough to be offset by reasonable premium additions.

Definite Loss. The loss must be definite. This means the loss must be difficult to counterfeit, and it must be subject to value determination. Insurance companies have run into some difficulty in this respect in writing sickness insurance, disability insurance, and burglary insurance because in these areas the company is somewhat susceptible to fraudulent claims.

Substantial Loss. A large loss must be involved. This requisite is based on the assumption that pharmacists and other people find it feasible to assume small losses.

Accidental Event. The loss must be of an accidental nature. This simply means that such losses as the depreciation of capital assets, shoplifting, expected bad debts, or other forms of market risk are not insurable.

Feasibility. The insurable risk must involve an economically feasible cost. In other words, the chance of loss must be small enough to permit assessment of a reasonable premium level. Efforts by insurance companies to satisfy this requirement of a feasible cost are evident in the widespread use of deductibles. This requisite is also the reason for the slow development of prescription coverage under private insurance policies. Younger and healthier individuals do not need the coverage, and therefore the premiums for the older and less healthy people would have to be high. Drugs and pharmaceutical coverage have been included in major health insurance policies, union negotiated insurance coverages, and certain government programs in recent years because such policies cover a broad spectrum of people. These pharmaceutical coverages came about to meet the special needs of certain groups of people and because of the realization of the positive cost-effectiveness ratio of drugs and pharmaceutical services in relation to other categories of health care services.

Loss Dispersion. The risk must be such that it is unlikely to produce a financial loss to the majority of the exposed units simultaneously. Insurance companies protect against this possibility by distributing their underwriting efforts geographically and by prescribing certain minimum standards of conformity for exposure units. When the risks are great, insurance companies spread the risk with cross or shared insurance by underwriting only a portion of the total risk. In other words, the primary insurer reinsures a portion of the risk with several other companies. Insurance companies also protect themselves against this possibility through the use of certain clauses in the insurance contract. For example, the standard fire policy contains the war exclusion clause, which suspends coverage under conditions of war, insurrection, rebellion, revolution, or action taken by the government to stem the possibility of such activity.

Actuarial Soundness. A seventh requisite of an insurable risk is the requirement that the chance of loss be determinable. This means that statistical information and data must be available in adequate quantities to permit the application of the law of probability, which in turn will yield reliable estimates of expected losses. The mathematical technique of calculating the pure premium rate (exclusive of administrative costs and profits) for a given risk is based on the statistical probabilities derived from historic data related to the frequency of the incidence and costs of the losses. This special technique is known as actuarial science.

FORMULATING THE INSURANCE PROGRAM

The pharmacist typically is ill-equipped to formulate his own insurance program and should resort to the help of a competent insurance agent or insurance broker. The agent or broker approaches the problem by considering the nature of risk in the particular situation as it relates to the type of pharmacy, the location of the firm, the personnel involved, the market situation, and the general characteristics of the physical properties. A sound program of insurance coverage encompasses both *required* and *optional* types of coverage. For example, certain types of coverage, such as workmen's compensation and auto insurance, represent required coverages, whereas business interruption or burglary insurance may be considered optional.

Hall et al. made a survey of the use of insurance by owners of pharmacies in the Southwest.[2] The survey indicated that the majority of pharmacists were well covered in the traditional areas of fire, extended coverage, and liability, but inadequately covered by insurance for employees and business life insurance.

In selecting those types of coverage that are optional, the insurance broker or agent is extremely helpful in eliminating or avoiding unnecessary types of coverage. From an analytical point of view, the decision to provide a particular coverage is based on the relationship between the cost of insurance and the probability of loss. It is safe to assume that in the majority of cases the pharmacist would be unable to make this type of analysis. Furthermore, the insurance agent or broker can be helpful in recognizing situations that require actions that will minimize the cost of insurance or the loss. For example, the use of a deductible would be of benefit in terms of the cost of the insurance when applied to certain types of coverage. On the other hand, certain changes in the physical property, such as the installation of a sprinkler system or improvement in the construction, may have a significant influence on premium rates.

The questions of how much insurance is enough, what types of coverage are required, and how much coverage is adequate all demand the careful attention of an experienced, competent insurance agent or broker. The pharmacist cannot afford to use his good judgment alone. The pharmacist should select an agent he can trust, provide him with all the information necessary to arrive at proper advice, and give all his insurance business to him. Not only will this encourage him to give the best advice, but it is also economical. The pharmacist should give the agent the necessary time and keep him informed of any significant change in the value of the pharmacy's assets, especially inventory. This, of course, requires complete and accurate accounting records. In case of a loss, the agent should be notified promptly. The pharmacist should review his insurance coverage with his agent at least annually. For this reason it is better if there is a single all-encompassing policy, or a common expiration date if there is more than one policy.

Types of Insurance Coverage

The major types of insurance coverage available to the pharmacist are described only briefly. A basic knowledge of the coverages available will enable the pharmacist to communicate more intelligently with his agent or broker.

FIRE INSURANCE

A type of coverage that certainly should be required in every case is the standard fire insurance policy, which covers direct loss to all physical property, including leasehold improvements, resulting from fire or lightning and the removal from the premises of goods endangered by the perils of fire and lightning. The basic fire policy of and by itself, however, is grossly inadequate and requires the endorsement of additional forms of coverage. These forms fall into two basic categories: (1) forms covering additional perils and (2) forms covering additional losses.

Extended Coverage. Coverage under the standard fire policy can be considerably enhanced by the addition of the extended coverage endorsement. This endorsement extends the coverage of the basic policy to include direct loss to physical goods resulting from the perils of windstorm, hail, explosion, riot, civil commotion, damage by aircraft or other vehicle, and smoke and smudge damage. The extended coverage endorsement has two distinct advantages. First, by including these additional perils within one policy, the cost is considerably lower than it would be if each of the additional perils had to be added separately. Second, the extended coverage endorsement tends to avoid or eliminate any disagreement as to the particular cause of loss. For example, assume that as a result of fire an explosion takes place. Without the extended coverage endorsement, the problem would be to determine the amount of loss resulting from the fire and the amount of loss resulting from the explosion. Obviously, with the extended coverage endorsement there would be no question as to the amount of loss resulting from the individual perils, since both fire and explosion are covered.

In addition to the extended coverage endorsement, there are a number of other allied endorsements that fire insurance companies are permitted to write that may or may not be appropriate in a particular case. Among the additional coverages available are building collapse, earthquake, flood and rain (under certain conditions and places), sprinkler leakage, and fire legal liability insurance.

CONSEQUENTIAL COVERAGE

As previously noted, the standard fire policy only covers direct loss, and yet in many cases the pharmacist finds himself exposed to indirect or consequential loss situations. The following forms are available to cover such additional loss situations and may be endorsed to the standard fire policy.

Business Interruption. This coverage is available to cover loss of profits as well as to cover fixed charges, which continue to be assessed despite the fact that the pharmacy is forced to discontinue operations as a result of a fire loss or a direct loss resulting from some other covered peril.

Profits and Commissions Insurance. This endorsement is available to cover a situation in which, although the business operations are not entirely suspended, a loss of profit occurs. For example, if a fire in early December destroys a lot of Christmas merchandise, a loss of profit would be apparent despite the fact that the business may not be entirely suspended. It is important to note at this point that the business interruption form only covers loss of profit and fixed charges in a situation in which operations are entirely suspended; hence the profit and commissions form would be necessary to cover a partial loss situation that does not totally suspend operations.

Extra Expense Coverage. Insurance is available to cover a situation in which additional costs are incurred as a result of doing business under unfavorable conditions. In other words, as a result of a loss, it may be necessary for the business to incur additional costs in avoiding suspension of operations. For example, if a pharmacy suffers a fire loss that forces them to rent or lease a building and additional equipment temporarily to avoid the suspension of business, the extra expense form would cover the added cost.

Rental Endorsements. Additional insurance may be endorsed to the standard fire policy if the pharmacist has rental or leased properties, for example, offices above the pharmacy. With the first endorsement, the rental insurance forms indemnify the insured for rent revenues that are not forthcoming because of a fire loss. With the second endorsement the insurance would protect the pharmacist who is forced to continue lease payments despite the fact that a fire loss has temporarily interrupted business operations. Obviously the rental insurance endorsements are valuable additions to the standard fire policy in a situation in which the business involves the renting of rooms or apartments.

Demolition Insurance. This form of endorsement is available to cover the situation in which an expensive fire loss occurs and a building or buildings must be totally reconstructed. In such a case, demolition insurance is the answer because it can be written to cover not only the cost of tearing down the remains of the destroyed building, but also the increased costs of reconstruction resulting from certain city ordinances or requirements that call for a particular type of construction.

Indirect Damage Insurance. This type of insurance covers consequential loss from damage to physical properties that indirectly results from a fire or other perils covered under the standard fire policy and the extended coverage endorsement. Consequential loss insurance is available in two basic forms. One form covers damage to goods resulting from temperature change or a change in other physical conditions. For example, it may well be that a fire loss results in the deterioration of drugs or a malfunction of a refrigeration unit which in turn results in damage to perishable items that require refrigeration. The other form covers damage to one of a set of items. For example, it may be that a combination of three products which was sold and used as a unit would suffer an indirect financial loss because fire damaged one part of the combination set, and the remainder of the set would certainly not maintain its proportional value if the entire set was not available.

Replacement Cost Insurance. Replacement cost insurance covers the actual cost of replacing damaged property without deduction for depreciation. In other words, the replacement cost endorsement actually violates the principle of indemnity, which states that the function of insurance is to place the insured party in the same relative position that he maintained prior to the loss. Replacement cost insurance provides a valuable and desirable type of coverage, because ordinary indemnification on the original cost less depreciation normally does not provide the insured party with adequate funds for replacement. For example, assume that a pharmacy has fixtures that are 10 years old and based on an original cost less depreciation, they have a present value of $3,000. Assume further that the fixtures are totally destroyed by fire and that under the standard fire policy indemnification only $3,000 will be paid. It is safe to assume that the $3,000 would be grossly inadequate in providing comparable fixtures. In such a situation the replacement cost form would be a valuable addition to the standard fire policy.

In summary, the standard fire policy, of and by itself, only provides coverage for direct loss resulting from fire and lightning, and hence must be supplemented by various forms that tend to broaden the coverage. First, the standard fire policy can be extended to include additional perils, either in a package form through the use of the extended coverage endorsement or on a peril by peril basis. Second, the standard fire policy can be endorsed to cover various types of indirect loss situations.

CASUALTY INSURANCE

It is necessary for the pharmacist to use certain insurance policies written by casualty insurance companies. This category includes third-party liability, employer's liability, and other types of liability insurance. Third-party liability insurance protects the insured party against monetary penalties arising out of his negligence. Coverage is available to pay claims from court action, the cost of defense and investigation, and also first-aid and medical expenses. It is important to note that liability insurance does not in any way protect the insured against injury to himself, his partner or partners, his employees or any person or persons engaged in maintenance or alteration work on the premises. These are covered by other types of insurance. The usual forms available in the professional and/or business liability area are briefly described below.

Owners, Landlords, and Tenants Liability Insurance. The owners, landlords, and tenants liability form covers bodily injury or property damage sustained in or about the building or business premises. The policy covers negligence or alleged negligence of the insured party. It also covers medical payments. The owners, landlords, and tenants policy does not cover elevator, professional or product liability, or liability arising out of alterations, new repairs, or demolition activity at the place of business.

Elevator Liability. Elevator liability insurance is optional and can be endorsed to either the owners, landlords, and tenants policy or a contractors liability policy, or it may be acquired separately. This policy includes any liability of the insured party resulting from the operation of elevators, escalators, or hoists, and it covers bodily injury, property damage, collision coverage, and medical payments. The pharmacist may have little use for this type of coverage unless he owns the building, but he should be sure his landlord has the coverage in order to preclude any possibility that he may be held responsible. This is especially important to a pharmacy or apothecary located above or below the ground floor, in which case elevators may be used to enter the pharmacy.

Contractual Liability. Often the leasing or rental of business properties creates a situation in which contractual liability exists. For example, the tenants of an office building are liable for accidents that may occur in the hallways or on the stairways of the building. Also, a pharmacist may be held liable for accidents that occur on the sidewalk in front of a pharmacy. Therefore, the pharmacist should determine whether his landlord's insurance covers injuries occurring on the sidewalk or in the vicinity of the building, and if not, it would be advisable to have this extra protection. The reality of this type of liability is illustrated by the following case. A pharmacist, the lessee of the building, was held liable for the injuries sustained by a person who was walking in front of the pharmacy when the front plate glass window suddenly exploded. Many city ordinances require the owners of buildings to keep the sidewalks in front of their buildings safe, and this liability devolves to the person leasing the building.

Contractors Protective Liability Insurance. According to the law, a general contractor is liable for the actions of subcontractors, and similarly any individual hiring another person as an independent contractor to work on the premises is liable for the actions of the independent contractor. The obligation of the owner to protect the public cannot be shifted. Hence, there are situations in which the owner of a building can become liable to the public for the actions of independent or subcontractors. The owners and contractors protective liability insurance policy is intended to meet this need by providing the same basic coverages as the owners, landlords, and tenants policy. This type of situation could involve the subleasing and subcontracting of the operation of a department in a pharmacy, such as a fountain or some special skills department.

Product Liability Insurance. An important area of liability insurance that demands the pharmacist's attention is product liability. Product liability insurance is intended to cover liability for injuries sustained by any person or damage to any property caused by accident and arising out of the handling or use of goods or products manufactured, sold, handled, or distributed by the insured. The product liability form only covers the use and consumption of products off the premises; therefore, it excludes fountains in a pharmacy. Where there is consumption of products on the premises, such as fountains, a special endorsement to the policy is available.

The pharmacist should understand the basis of product liability, its importance, and its relationship to professional liability. Product liability arises out of a contractual relationship between a pharmacist and his client. When a pharmacist sells a product to his patron, he gives a guarantee or warranty, either expressed or implied, that the product is suitable for its intended purpose, if it is for human consumption. If the pharmacist either expressly states, or implies by his actions, that a product (and this is especially true in the case of a drug) has particular beneficial characteristics or values, he may be held legally liable if an injury is sustained by the person who used the product while relying on the pharmacist's judgment. If the injury results from a faulty or inadequate product, the complaint normally is based on the breach of warranty associated with the sales contract.

Professional Liability Insurance. Professional liability insurance is of great concern to the pharmacist because it offers protection to the professional man in connection with services rendered or services that should have been rendered but were not. The insurance covers the cost of defense as well as damages. All pharmacists, both proprietors and employees, should carry the necessary professional liability insurance to complement the pharmacy's product liability clause, which is commonly referred to as the "druggists liability policy." The two types of coverage are analogous to the situation of damage resulting from either a fire or an explosion or both—the pharmacist is covered in either instance.

Professional liability insurance is especially useful for a pharmacist who consults with a hospital or nursing home, works in several pharmacies as a "relief" pharmacist, works as a hospital pharmacist, or is an employed pharmacist in a pharmacy that may have inadequate coverage for the employed pharmacist under the pharmacy's regular product liability or "druggists liability insurance." A pharmacist can purchase professional liability insurance through the American Pharmaceutical Association group policy, which covers $200,000 per claim and up to $600,000 per year. The American Druggists' Insurance Co. now offers and actively promotes professional liability insurance.

Pharmacists and students should not view the problem of professional liability in a negative or passive manner. The modern pharmacist has a positive duty to perform professional services as a result of the expanding roles of the pharmacist and the increasing expectations the public has of pharmacists. With physicians becoming more pressed to use their time wisely because of an increasing patient load, the pharmacist is expected to fill some of the resulting void in patient consultation. For example, it is rapidly becoming the standard of pharmacy practice, if indeed it is not already, that the pharmacist should warn the patient against driving or manipulating heavy machinery while taking an antihistamine or a sedative purchased either on a prescription or over-the-counter. The same is true of nasal rebound from over-utilization of a nasal decongestant, the proper use of laxatives, and drug interactions. All of these situations place a positive duty on the pharmacist to provide the necessary professional consultation when dispensing these drugs.

Injuries resulting from a failure to perform a professional service that is considered to be a standard of practice are subject to liability suits just as readily as those resulting from the dispensing of an incorrect drug.

"All-Risk" Liability Insurance. For small pharmacies, there is a comprehensive general liability policy available that can be used in lieu of either the owners, landlords, and tenants policy or the contractors policy. The comprehensive general liability form provides an all-risk type of coverage for small businesses in that it covers bodily injury and property damage at specific locations as well as at operations not specifically mentioned. In addition, product liability, professional liability, and contractual liability can be endorsed to the comprehensive general liability form.

SPECIAL TYPES OF COVERAGE

There are several special types of insurance that every pharmacist-proprietor should consider and, in most instances, purchase.

Automobile Insurance. The pharmacist undoubtedly needs automobile insurance coverage. Automobile or vehicular insurance involves elements of casualty or liability insurance as well as insurance against damage to the vehicle itself. There are sufficiently unique features in this type of insurance to warrant its separate treatment.

For the pharmacist who uses his private passenger car for business purposes, the insurance companies provide liability coverage in addition to collision insurance for both private and business use. The basic policy usually covers accidental bodily injury and property damage arising from the ownership or use of the vehicle, and it also protects the insured's vehicle either for specified perils or on an all-risk basis. The legal liability section protects the insured in any vehicle driven by him or his agent for business purposes, covering such items as first-aid and medical expenses, cost of bail bond, cost of defense, cost of judgments, and court costs. The policy may also cover those situations in which another vehicle is temporarily used because of a breakdown, service, theft, or total destruction of the original vehicle. If the vehicle is stolen, a daily compensation is provided for necessary transportation.

Glass Insurance. If the pharmacist has a great deal of glass in the pharmacy building, he will find that the standard fire policy provides inadequate coverage, and comprehensive glass coverage is recommended. Glass insurance can be written to cover not only the loss of the glass itself, but also the frames, and the cost of removal and repair. Also, injury resulting from broken glass may be covered. This type of coverage is relatively expensive, and it should be cautiously considered as an endorsement.

Crime Insurance. Protection against burglary, robbery, and theft of merchandise, fixtures, or other equipment owned or held by the insured is available through the mercantile open-stock burglary policy. This policy is available to pharmacists to cover direct losses or damage when the pharmacy is not open. The mercantile interior robbery policy provides the same coverage for the same premises while the pharmacy is open. For insurance purposes, the distinction between robbery and burglary is a simple one. Burglary involves forced entry, and thus could only take place when the pharmacy is closed. Robbery, on the other hand, does not involve forced entry, and thus it occurs when the pharmacy is open. In addition to the burglary and robbery coverage, the pharmacist may have need for the mercantile safe burglary policy, which covers the forced entry into a safe. Other forms that may be required in particular situations are exterior messenger robbery policy which covers the insured or the insured's representative if robbery takes place while he is away from the pharmacy, and provides protection for money, securities, or other properties outside the premises. The money and securities broad form policy gives a much more complete coverage, on or off the premises, for securities or money for deposit, records, and accounts, which are either limited in coverage or omitted completely from the standard mercantile burglary and robbery forms.

The owner of a small pharmacy may satisfy his needs with the store-keepers burglary and robbery policy, which is an "all-risk" type of coverage. This form covers inside robbery, outside robbery, safe burglary, the loss of money and securities in limited amounts, mercantile open stock, and finally, damage that results from actual or attempted robbery or burglary. This type of coverage, sold in units of $250, would be feasible only in the case of small pharmacies.

INSURANCE FOR EMPLOYEES

Workmen's Compensation. The laws of the several states and territories of the United States require that an employee is entitled, without consideration of personal fault, to indemnification for all economic loss due to accident or disease resulting from his employment. Thus, the pharmacist as an employer is required to have workmen's compensation insurance. The basic benefits under workmen's compensation include disability pay, medical and surgical benefits, rehabilitation and re-education benefits, and death benefits. It is customary, if not required, that the employer insure his liability under the workmen's compensation law with a private insurance company.

Bonding. A bond is a written contract under which one party binds himself financially for the performance or honesty of another. The three parties to a bonding arrangement are the principal who will perform, the surety who guarantees that the first party will fulfill his obligation, and the obligee, to whom the promise is made. If the principal does not perform, the surety must pay the obligee. The surety is a type of insurance company.

There are two basic types of bond—the *fidelity bond*, which guarantees the honesty of the principal, and the *surety bond*, which guarantees the performance of the principal of an agreed task or obligation.

Fidelity bonds, which guarantee the honesty of the employees, are available on an individual or a blanket bond for all employees. They can be made to cover a particular person by name, a group of people by name, a particular position in the firm, or group of positions in the firm. For example, a pharmacist could bond the position of accountant, without specifying the particular individual performing the duties of the accountant, or he may bond the particular individual regardless of what functions this individual performed in the business.

Pharmacists have little need for surety bonds; however, a general knowledge may prove to be useful, especially if he should have a building constructed for his use. The latter type of bond does not apply to employees in the usual sense. Surety bonds, which guarantee the performance of the principal, can also be purchased on an individual or blanket basis by position or name. The types of surety bond which the pharmacist may find useful include the supply bond, the construction bond, and the completion bond, which are all forms of the basic contract bond that guarantees fulfillment of an obligation.

Employee Group Insurance. If a pharmacist hires several employees, he may want to develop an employee group insurance plan. Group plans are available for life insurance, accident, accidental death, dismemberment, hospitalization, medical care coverage, and annuities. The benefits of employee group plans should be apparent. First of all, such plans enable employees to secure insurance that would otherwise be available only at a high cost. Also, such plans offer employees insurance coverage that otherwise might not be insurable on an individual basis. This is true because the insurance company is only concerned with the average results of the group and not individual results. Each group of employees has its own eligibility rules, usually based on period of service, occupation, and wages. These group insurance plans can be set up on a contributory or noncontributory basis, and membership can be optional. Pharmacists who are members of state or national organizations may become part of a large group insurance plan, often at greatly reduced rates. This is one of many advantages of joining pharmaceutical organizations. There is a potential feature of group insurance policies through associations that has not been fully exploited for the mutual benefit of all concerned. This feature is the extension of insurance coverage to all employees who have been employed in a member pharmacy for a designated number of years, with the privilege of reciprocity among member employers thereafter.

CO-INSURANCE

Broadly speaking, any type of deductible is a form of co-insurance. Deductibles may take one of several forms: (1) the insured pays a designated amount referred to as "first dollars" or a corridor deductible before the insurance covers the loss; (2) the insured pays a designated percentage of the loss, for example 20 percent; (3) the insured pays a fixed amount of a recurrence of each incidence of a loss, for example, $1.00 each time a prescription is dispensed; and (4) sometimes the deductible takes the form of a combination of (1) and (2) or (1) and (3).

In a more restricted sense, co-insurance clauses are attached to fire and extended coverage insurance policies commonly encountered in the practice of pharmacy. The policyholder, in consideration of a reduced rate, agrees to carry insurance equal to a certain percentage of the *actual value* of the property insured—usually 80 percent or more. If the insured fails to carry the designated amount of insurance, he becomes a co-insurer, and he can collect only that proportion of his loss which the amount he carries bears to the amount required. For example, if the value of the property is $50,000 and the insured agrees to carry at least 80 percent insurance, the amount of insurance required to comply with the co-insurance clause is $40,000. If, however, the policyholder carries only $30,000 worth of insurance and has a partial loss, he is a co-insurer and can collect only three-fourths of the loss because he is carrying only three-fourths of the amount required to comply with the clause. If the loss is $20,000, the insured will collect $15,000 and will have to bear the $5,000 loss himself. If the policyholder carries the required amount of insurance, he collects the full amount of his loss up to the amount of the policy. If there is a complete loss in the above example, the insured collects $40,000, the full value of the insurance policy.

Since most fires and related or extended damages seldom cause a complete loss of the property insured, the pharmacist should seriously consider the co-insurance clause.

The formula below is used to calculate the insurance company's liability under a co-insurance clause.

$$Li = \frac{C}{R} \times L$$

where: C = the amount of insurance carried;
R = the amount required under the co-insurance clause;
L = the loss sustained; and
Li = the insurance company's liability.

Business Life Insurance

BASIC INFORMATION

Nature of Business Life Insurance. Business life insurance is life insurance used to protect a business, or the family of a businessman, from the financial loss that results from the death of someone associated with the business, usually the proprietor. Many billions of dollars worth of this protection is now in force, giving assurance of business continuity to the firms and full value of the business equity to the family of the deceased. There is no basic difference between business life insurance and regular life insurance used for personal and family needs. Both provide insurance on the lives of individuals. But the protection set up by business firms does involve many more complex details to meet legal, financial, tax, and technical problems.

Implementation. A pharmacist contemplating the establishment of a business life insurance plan faces technical problems that require advice. He should consult *four experts* who can make certain that every aspect of the firm's interests is being safeguarded. These experts include the firm's *attorney, accountant, trust officer* of its bank, and *life insurance agent.* The insurance agent provides the technical advice concerning the arrangement of policies, while the others provide additional essential information on which the plan is based. They will double check the plan when completed and assume the responsibility for carrying out the legal and banking details. Many life insurance agents who specialize in business life insurance are familiar with the whole range of problems, but they prefer to have their client's lawyer, banker, and accountant included in the consultation. The owner of a pharmacy, devoting his energies to make his practice a success, is not usually in a position to analyze his insurance needs or prescribe the correct policies or policy arrangements to meet those needs. Such a prescription calls for the highly specialized knowledge and technical advice of experts.

Tax Factors. Taxes, both income and estate, are involved in many business life insurance arrangements. These should be taken into consideration in order that the plan will not involve unnecessary additional taxes. On the other hand, too much weight should not be given to the tax angles, as they are constantly changing, and a plan set up today on the basis of a certain tax advantage may prove to be disadvantageous next year.

Reserves for Emergencies. Most business life insurance plans utilize life insurance that has cash value that grows over the years. This cash value provides the firm with a valuable reserve for emergencies in the event of any sharp dislocation in business conditions. When necessary, the cash value of the policy can be used as the basis for loans. When, for one reason or another, this type of policy is not possible, term life insurance may be used.

TYPES OF BUSINESS LIFE INSURANCE

Key-Man Insurance. Almost every pharmacy has one or more men upon whom it depends heavily for its major success. Frequently it is the proprietor or manager. It may be the employed pharmacist, upon whose shoulders rests a major responsibility of the pharmacy and whose technical efforts are vital to the firm's success. It may be any employee whose death would be a considerable loss to the business. Key-man insurance is indicated for anyone whose death would cripple the business, or at least cause a setback until a replacement is secured. Such insurance provides insurance benefits at the death of this vital employee in order that the firm will have resources with which to employ and train a successor in the competitive market and to cushion the loss of profits in the meantime.

Proprietorship Insurance. Life insurance protection for the sole proprietor provides his dependents or heirs with cash representing the sound valuation of the business at his death and ensures continuity of the pharmacy. This is *as yet an undeveloped and widely neglected area of protection,* probably because the need is considered to be in the province of personal life insurance. Even in sole proprietorships, there are special considerations that should be recognized when writing the business life insurance policy. Adequate and specific provisions must be made to meet the conditions of a will or trust agreement concerning sales or liquidation of the business when such is desired. These include the selection of the beneficiary to fit the particular situation, and the question of who is to pay the premiums for a particular plan.

There is no set pattern; each case has to be determined on its own merits. One plan may call for sale of the pharmacy to specified employees, with the purchase money provided by the insurance. Another plan may provide that the pharmacy be run by the executor or the heirs, and in still another case, a trust company may be named as beneficiary and management control may be established. Many a small pharmacy has foundered after the death of the sole owner merely because he did not take the proper steps while alive to ensure its continuance. Numerically, pharmacies of the individual proprietor type predominate, comprising approximately 50 percent of all units engaged in the practice of pharmacy. The sole proprietor who is interested in selling his pharmacy to one or more of his employees should consult with an attorney and a life insurance underwriter about the advantages of combining a pension or profit-sharing plan with a purchase agreement, funded by life insurance on the life of the pharmacy owner.

Partnership Insurance. In the absence of legal safeguards to avoid dissolution, a partnership automatically dissolves at the death of any of its partners. This results in cessation of normal partnership activities, and the surviving partners become what is known as "liquidating trustees." They cannot do any new business, but must confine themselves to winding up the affairs of the partnership. If they continue the business, they may become personally liable for any losses incurred should the assets not cover such losses. There are several ways to avoid these difficulties, one of which is an adequately financed *buy-and-sell agreement* providing for the purchase at a pre-arranged valuation of the deceased partner's interest. An attorney will draw up the necessary papers carrying out the wishes of the partners. After a buy-and-sell agreement has been executed, the next step is to fund the arrangement, which can be done effectively through business insurance. It enables the surviving partners to reorganize at once and continue in business; it liquidates the interest of the deceased partner without loss; it enables the beneficiaries of the deceased partner to secure full, fair value for his interest in the firm at once and with a minimum of trouble; and it lends support to the credit standing of the firm.

Corporation Insurance. A corporation is not as directly and immediately affected by the death of a shareholder as is the partnership by the death of a partner, but unfortunate consequences are a distinct hazard. Unlike the partnership, the corporation is not terminated at the death of an owner. However, with the transfer of the deceased stockholder's shares, new stockholders, new to management and possibly an unknown element, may enter the picture. The death of a principal stockholder may deal a severe blow to the firm's credit. There are several ways to handle the problem, one of which is an *adequately financed stock sale and purchase agreement,* drawn up by the firm's attorney. This too may be funded by insurance. An adequate corporation insurance program on the lives of its principal shareholders provides retirement of their interest at death. It gives the deceased shareholder's heirs full value for his interest at once and reduces the shock of changes in ownership. This is of special concern to the small corporation with a few shareholders whose interests keep them close to the management of the business. Frequently, ownership and management are one and the same. The great bulk of the country's corporations are in this category. Large numbers of them are small, closely held businesses which adopted the corporate form primarily for its legal, tax, and continuity advantages. By so doing, however, these owners have not escaped the death hazards that affect any business organization. Life insurance can provide the corporation with funds to purchase the interest of a stockholder at his death.

Periodic Analysis and Evaluation of Program

Once established, the business life insurance plan should receive a careful periodic evaluation by experts. Financial conditions change, tax laws vary in their effects, valuations of the interests of the owners are never constant—just to mention but a few of the changing conditions that can affect the plan. It is important that the details of the plan be kept up to date at all times. Revaluations should be made whenever necessary in connection with buy-and-sell agreements and partnership and corporation policies. Every new revenue act suggests a need for a special checkup to make certain the tax angles are still adequately covered. At least once each year, the plan should go through a careful screening by the life insurance agent.

Since each state regulates insurance through its insurance statutes and regulations, the insurance agent, properly licensed, should be utilized at least annually for an analysis and evaluation of the insurance program.

Summary

Providing for appropriate and adequate insurance coverage must be of primary concern to the pharmacist. Failure to recognize the various needs for insurance protection leaves the pharmacist susceptible to conditions in which one unpredictable, accidental event can cause financial disaster and wipe out the benefits of many years of hard work.

The pharmacist is advised to deal with an independent insurance agent or broker because he has available a wider range of insurance policies and endorsements by dealing with a number of different companies. There are two types of insurance companies, mutual companies and stock companies. In the mutual company, the policyholders are the owners and the "profits," if any, are returned to the policyholders as dividends, rebates, or reductions in the cost of the premiums. A stock company is owned by the stockholders and is operated for the benefit of the stockholders just like any other stock company. Most of the life insurance in America is written by mutual companies, whereas about 80 percent of the business insurance is written by stock companies. One of the most active stock companies in the pharmaceutical profession is The American Druggists' Insurance Co. The majority of the shares of this company are held by pharmacists. The pharmacist's insurance package should be custom-tailored in consultation with his agent.

CITED REFERENCES

1. Marshall, A.: *Principles of Economics.* 8th ed., New York: The Macmillan Co., footnote p. 135.
2. Hall, E. J. W., Owen, H. T., and Daniel, B.: The uses of insurance by owners of pharmacies—a survey. *Texas J. Pharm., 1:*90–98, 1960.

GENERAL REFERENCES

1. Memorandum to Small Business No. 1—*Group Life Insurance for Employees.**
2. Memorandum to Small Business No. 2—*The Insured Pension Plan for Employees.**
3. Memorandum to Small Business No. 3—*Group Accidental and Sickness Insurance.**
4. BSB No. 33—*Sole Proprietorship Life Insurance.*†
5. BSB No. 35—*Corporation Life Insurance.*†
6. BSB No. 36—*Partnership Life Insurance.*†
7. BSB No. 125—*Building an Insurance Plan for Your Business.*†
8. Duncan, D. J., and Phillips, C. F.: *Retailing Principles and Methods,* 6th ed., Homewood, Ill.: Richard D. Irwin, Inc., 1963, Chapter 26, pp. 715–739.
9. Steinmetz, L. L., Kline, J. B., and Stegall, D. P.: *Managing the Small Business.* Homewood, Ill.: Richard D. Irwin, Inc., 1968, Chapter 16, pp. 319–336.
10. Greene, M. R.: *Insurance and Risk Management for Small Business.* Washington: Small Business Administration (S.B.A. Management Series No. 30), 1963.
11. Brochure for Pharmacy Graduates published by The American Druggists' Insurance Co., Amer. Bldg., Cincinnati, Ohio 45202.
12. Williams, A. C., and Hedges, B.: *Risk Management and Insurance.* Part II, New York: McGraw-Hill Book Co., Inc., 1964.

REVIEW

1. What are the two basic types of risk and which is insurable?

2. Differentiate between entrepreneur and speculative risks.

3. Discuss the five approaches to risk management.

4. Define insurance as a social device in socioeconomic terms, as a legal instrument in legal terms, and as an accountancy instrument in accounting terms.

5. Discuss the law of large numbers and how it forms the basis of insurance.

6. Identify and describe the seven criteria or requisites of insurable risk.

7. Describe the methods insurance companies have to mitigate the effects of a very large number of losses in a given period of time.

8. Describe the two basic forms or types of *extended coverage endorsements.*

9. Describe seven types of consequential endorsements to the standard fire policy.

10. Describe casualty insurance and the seven types of coverages included under this type of insurance.

11. Discuss what should be included in a comprehensive automobile or vehicular insurance policy.

12. Describe glass and crime insurance.

*All three of the above pamphlets are published by the Institute of Life Insurance, 277 Park Ave., New York, N.Y. 10017.

†All four of the publications may be ordered from the Department of Commerce, Washington, D.C., or from any of its field offices.

13. Discuss employee insurance including bonding, workmen's compensation, and employee group insurance.

14. What is the difference between fidelity and surety bonds?

15. Define co-insurance in the restricted sense and calculate the company's liability when given the appropriate data.

16. Discuss the general purpose of business life insurance and list six specific purposes.

17. Discuss the procedure in setting up a business life insurance program and identify the four experts the pharmacist should consult.

18. Discuss key-man, partnership, corporation, and individual proprietorship business life insurance in terms of purposes and coverage.

17. Current and Future Developments in Pharmacy and Health Care

Social and institutional changes come slowly, but they inevitably come. The manner in which health care in general has been provided since the Flexner Report in 1911 has changed slowly but significantly. Pharmaceutical services have changed probably more during this period, but in a different manner. The Flexner Report caused a revolution in medical education, lifting it from the status of trade schools and placing it in very respectable, university-based educational institutions.[1] Over the period of a relatively few years, physicians were, for the most part, well educated and well trained. After their training they left the group environment where they were educated to practice individually in the place of their choosing. They were highly esteemed and became nearly indispensable people within their respective communities.

Physicians also became a highly organized group through a system of affiliation of local and state societies and one national organization, the American Medical Association (AMA). The strength of this union emanated from the policy that hospital staff privileges were based on membership in the local medical society. Physicians needed hospital staff privileges to properly treat their patients. As individuals, physicians were independent and conservative, and as a group, acting through the AMA, they could control any effort to change their manner of practice. The solo practice of medicine has been termed a "cottage industry" with the connotation of a highly individualized, independent mode of operation.

Pharmacy, on the other hand, improved its educational program much more slowly, and consequently developed professionally very slowly. Although pharmacists were independent, there was much diversity within pharmacy. Together, these factors acted as deterrents to pharmacy's professional development and its political unity.

Changing Modes of Health Care Delivery

EVOLUTIONARY CHANGES

Ironically, it is this high degree of independence and complete freedom to pursue economic goals of physicians that led to one of the basic weaknesses of the profession, *overspecialization*. The economic incentive to specialize is higher income for less work, and especially less confining working hours. Both the availability and accessibility of medical care depend on sufficient numbers and proper distribution of primary care practitioners. (Primary practitioners are the general practitioners, pediatricians, and internists.) In 1940, there were 83 general practitioners and six pediatricians and internists combined—a total of 89 primary care practitioners—per 100,000 population. By 1967, the respective numbers were 32, 17 and 49 per 100,000 people—a 45 percent decrease.[2] The 61 percent reduction in general practitioners enhanced the problem of the shortage of primary care practitioners because these are the physicians most accessible to poor, inner-city, and rural people. The large increase in the number of residencies in hospital since 1940 has been a contributing factor to specialization. In 1941, there were 5,000 residencies in this country; in 1970, there were 46,000 residencies, 15 percent of which went unfilled.[3] Residencies are offered by hospitals not only for the purpose of special training, but also to provide sufficient house staff to cover the various services. Thus the residencies include all medical specialities.

Because of the shortage of primary care physicians due to specialization, and because of the escalating cost of medical care, a crisis in the American health care "system" has developed. Fundamentally, it is the absence of a true system of medical services that is the underlying cause. Terris describes America's health care as three subsystems.[4] One is the pediatrician-internist private system, used by the upper and the more sophisticated upper middle classes. The second is the private general practitioner subsystem, used by the less sophisticated middle class, the skilled laborers, and most rural people. The third is the charity subsystem, presently represented by people in the Medicaid programs.

Over the years attempts have been made to alter the manner of delivering medical care. These efforts have met with little success until the past decade, and even then the degree of change has been modest.

The first effort to alter health care delivery was an attempt to enact a governmental health insurance in New York in 1919.[4] It failed in the House in 1919 and failed completely in 1920 because of the expulsion of five socialist members of the General Assembly. The AMA passed a resolution in support of national health insurance in the mid 1920s, but it was rescinded the following year. The Committee on the Costs of Medical Care recommended a voluntary health insurance program and a hospital-based group practice in 1932.[5] The AMA "filed a minority report which stated, correctly, that 'Voluntary health insurance schemes have everywhere failed' and have been replaced in Europe by compulsory systems."[6] Ironically, the position which the AMA condemned in 1932 has been its official position for the past several years.

Government health insurance originally was part of the Social Security Bill of 1935 until it was deleted as a result of the opposition of the AMA. The Wagner Bill of 1939, based on the principle of Federal support to the states for government health insurance, was similar to a portion of the 1974 Nixon Administration Comprehensive Health Insurance Program (CHIP). Wagner's Bill received little support. The same fate came to the Wagner-Murray-Dingel bills introduced during World War II. President Truman, with the support of labor, attempted to enact a compulsory health insurance program, but it also failed to gain sufficient support.

At one time, most states had laws preventing the corporate practice of medicine. Several states have since rescinded this law, and there are now several corporate medical clinics. Some of these clinics are very efficient and provide quality medical care; however, their services are not inexpensive.

Several states had laws that prevented prepayment group practices unless they were controlled by medical societies. As late as 1966, 17 states had such laws.[7] Now there are a number of prepayment group practices serving millions of people. Prepayment group plans have built-in efficiency and long-term, high productivity-to-costs ratios. Quality of care is usually also high, but not necessarily assured in every aspect of health care.

There have been great advances in the technical aspects of medical care, requiring the use of large hospitals and expensive equipment. These advances were stimulated by Federal grants supporting medical research and technologic developments. The Hill-Burton Act supported the construction of many new hospitals, which resulted in the duplication of facilities. Increased specialization provided the personnel and the incentive, in part, to provide expensive surgical procedures. The increased affluence of society along with the influence of third-party pay organizations increased the demand for medical and surgical services. These events combined to increase the use of hospitals to provide medical care, which resulted in duplication of equipment, inefficiencies, and increased costs.

Up to this point most of the changes in the mode of health care have occurred voluntarily, with public influence operating to increase the demand for services rather than to change the mode of care, or the organization for delivering health care.

A medical care system should exhibit the following criteria: (1) health maintenance, not episodic medical care, should be the basic objective; (2) there should be continuity of care, both in reference to time (longitudinally) and to referrals to various specialties (cross-sectionally); (3) health care should be comprehensive, providing all the preventive, maintenance, acute, and rehabilitive health services; and (4) medical care should be accessible, in terms of both availability of facilities and personnel in all areas and economics—that is, available to people of all income levels.

THIRD PARTY INFLUENCES

Third party influences in health care delivery became significant during World War II, when wages and prices were frozen and the unions negotiated for increased fringe benefits, including medical services. After World War II, private insurance, along with the Blue Cross and Blue Shield organizations, began to sell more health insurance, especially group policies. These activities increased demand for medical and surgical services, but they provided little incentive to control costs. Few policies included drugs and pharmaceutical services.

Not until 1961, when the Kerr-Mills Act was enacted, did government become a significant third party. The Act provided Federal support to states for limited medical care for the indigent. A distinguishing feature of this law was the fact that eligibility required a means test. This placed these programs in the charity classification, with all of the consequential connotations.

Medicare and Medicaid. By 1965 public pressure for better medical care for the indigent and the aged resulted in the passage of two laws, Title XIX (Medicaid) for the indigent and Title XVIII (Medicare) for the aged. Medicaid, patterned after the Kerr-Mills Act, was supposed to produce uniformity in eligibility requirements among the beneficiary classes within a state and provide similar benefits to all recipients of benefits. Drugs were an optional benefit unless the state had provided them under the Kerr-Mills Act.

Title XIX was financed by a combination of state appropriations and a sliding scale of Federal matching funds. The state's share was based on the standard of living within each state and increased with time. Cost control was implemented by some states, but quality control was, for the most part, nonexistent. Many states, even on a cost-sharing basis, were unable to finance adequate, high-quality medical care. The absence of appropriate organizational controls caused Medicaid to be less than satisfactory for both the beneficiaries and the providers of service. Abuses by beneficiaries and frauds by providers occurred all too frequently.

Medicare, on the other hand, was financed by a payroll tax assessed on both employee and employer. A wide range of medical services, excluding outpatient drugs, was provided to beneficiaries at "reasonable" costs or charges. There has been increasing public pressure to include outpatient drugs for Medicare beneficiaries because aged beneficiaries utilize large amounts of maintenance drugs. There was little control over costs and inadequate control over quality, except for the quality control exercised by institutional committees such as the Tissue Committee and the Pharmacy and Therapeutic Committee. Medicare required deductibles and co-insurance as cost control devices, yet government expenditures for Medicare increased progressively. Private insurance and Blue Cross-Blue Shield programs have experienced similar increases in costs for the same reasons.

Other Third Party Programs. Since the passage of Titles XVIII and XIX, several other health insurance programs have been developed by private insurance companies and the Blue Cross and Blue Shield programs. Some of these provide supplementary benefits for Medicare beneficiaries; some policies include outpatient drugs.

The inclusion of drugs in re-negotiated union contracts during the early 1970s has had the greatest impact on pharmacy. The third parties in these instances have been insurance companies, the Blue Cross programs, PAID Prescriptions and Pharmaceutical Card Systems (PCS). The latter two organizations act as fiscal intermediaries and program administrators, but not as insurers. PAID Prescriptions originally was an underwriter, but it later restricted activities to claim processing as fiscal intermediator and program administration. Both PAID Prescriptions and PCS have become proficient in their field. They have contracted with union funds, insurance companies, and Medicaid programs in some states to administer the drug programs. Both organizations have been efficient and innovative and have been able to differentiate the levels of pharmaceutical services and to pay additional fees for patient drug profile systems, emergency prescription services, and other nondispensing services.

Drugs have been the only services that were consistently subjected to cost control. Pharmacists could not negotiate fees because drugs are subject to the antitrust laws. (Drugs move in interstate commerce.) As a consequence, pharmacists have not fared as well as other providers of services under the various third party programs.

Recently, PAID Prescriptions implemented a pilot program in Spokane, Washington, to pay pharmacists for not dispensing a prescription under certain conditions. The pharmacists must participate in continuing education programs. A system of patient medication profiles for the 8,000 people (2,200 families) and a peer review mechanism are also a part of the program. The pharmacists monitor the drugs prescribed for drug interactions, adverse drug reactions, and duplicative medication. When they detect any of these conditions, the prescriber is contacted to reconcile the problem. Then, the pharmacists complete an Adverse Drug Alert Form (in triplicate). One copy is sent to the prescriber, one copy to PAID Prescriptions, and the third copy is filed with the patient's profile. For this professional service, PAID Prescription pays the pharmacist $3.00. After the pilot project, it is anticipated that the underwriter will continue paying for these services. It is anticipated that the money saved by not dispensing the drug, and thus preventing expensive hospitalizations, will pay the service fee many times over.

HEALTH MAINTENANCE ORGANIZATIONS

Health maintenance organizations (HMOs) are modern versions of the prepayment group practice programs. The older established prepayment group plans brought efficiencies to the delivery of medical care primarily through economies of scale. They provided comprehensive service of good quality at reasonable costs; however, quality assurance was not the primary goal. The HMOs are designed to provide comprehensive health services with quality assurance and long-term economy.

The accepted definition of a HMO is: (1) an *organized system* of health care which accepts the responsibility to provide or otherwise assure the delivery of . . . (2) an agreed upon set of *comprehensive health maintenance* and *treatment services* for . . . (3) a *voluntarily enrolled* group of persons in a geographic area and . . . (4) reimbursed through a *prenegotiated* and *fixed periodic payment* made by or on behalf of each person or family unit enrolled in the plan.

An analysis of this definition indicates that HMOs meet most of the criteria of an organized system of health care. It is organized to provide comprehensive health care, including both treatment and maintenance service. The HMO is supposed to provide accessibility and continuity of health services. The prenegotiated, prepayment of a fixed periodic health service charge (premium) provides the incentive for preventive and maintenance health care to achieve long-term economy. Another requirement of HMOs, not in the above definition, is *quality assurance*. This distinguishes HMOs from the older prototype comprehensive group practices. An analysis of the HMO Act by the staff of the American Public Health Association lists five substantial weaknesses and five points that should improve health care delivery.[8] Only time will prove whether HMOs will perform as expected.

As of early 1974, there were 125 HMO-like organizations in operation, serving between five and six million people.[9] Several have been approved as meeting the official standards of HMOs. Of 105 medical centers responding to a survey, 16 were already sponsoring or affiliated with HMOs, 18 were planning to start one, and another 24 were giving serious consideration to the possibility of establishing an HMO.[9]

Basic health services must be provided to the HMO enrollees, and a list of other services, including prescription drugs, must be provided on an optional basis for a prepaid supplemental, community-based premium. All of these are contingent upon the required health manpower being available. Efforts to require the services of "clinical" pharmacists in HMOs failed, but some HMOs have included the services of pharmacists along with nurses, social workers, home health aides, and physicians as a *primary health care team*. The basic question for pharmacists is whether the HMO has an in-house pharmacy or contracts with local, community pharmacists.

NATIONAL HEALTH INSURANCE

Efforts to pass a national health insurance law dates back to the 1920s,[5] and limited results were achieved with the passage of Title XVIII, the Medicare law. Serious attempts, with the distinct possibility of the eventual passage of a national health insurance (NHI) law, were reflected by the Kennedy-Mills Bill[10] and the Nixon Administration's Comprehensive Health Insurance Program (CHIP),[11] introduced in both Houses of Congress in 1974. Both Bills represented a distinct compromise from their earlier counterparts, the Kennedy Bill and Nixon Administration Bill introduced three years earlier. A great deal of similarity can be found in the two compromise bills, except in the method of financing. However, expectation of the early passage of a NHI law, because of the compromises and similarities of the two bills, was not achieved. Support for NHI waned, especially from labor and consumer groups who favored the earlier and more liberal Kennedy Bill. Most people, except adamant opponents, predict a National Health Insurance by 1976.

The anticipated impacts of NHI on the practice of pharmacy are:

1. Assuming prescription drugs are included, it will certainly increase the demand for prescriptions.

2. It could have a stabilizing effect on prescription prices, depending on the use of co-payment and co-insurance in the payment mechanism.

3. If the program includes a quality assurance provision, it will improve the level of pharmaceutical services via a patient drug profile system, adverse drug reaction reporting system, monitoring of drug utilization and peer review programs.

4. NHI will require that claims processing be computerized. Computerization will require an accurate, efficient, and relatively inexpensive

computer terminal in most pharmacies. With ready access to a computer, it will be feasible to use the terminal for processing both business and professional data.

5. Depending on the form and provisions of NHI, it probably will consolidate all of the various third party pay programs and simplify the claims handling procedures.

The provisions and features that pharmacists desire in NHI are: (1) most, if not all, prescription drugs with few or no exclusions; (2) individual consideration for the reimbursement of the drug component and the dispensing fee component (the pharmaceutical industry does not support this concept); (3) omission of a co-payment provision, i.e., the patient pays a designated amount (e.g., $1.00) for each prescription with the insurance paying the remainder of the charge; (4) if there is a co-payment, a mandatory co-payment to prevent the discounting of the co-payment for competitive reasons. The National Association of Chain Drug Stores (NACDS) has not strongly supported this position, but there are indications that chain drugstores are not adamant in their position. If the co-payment is designed to spread the cost and is of a significant amount, it is regressive or unfair to the near indigent and middle income whose benefits are not financed by general revenue. Pharmacists are divided on the proposition of a fixed dispensing fee or the "usual and customary charge." The most realistic and most likely answer to this issue is a variable fee relative to the range of services provided and the economic condition of the market. A fixed fee among those pharmacies in a particular market may be the solution.

Somers outlined ten criteria for an acceptable program of national health insurance.[12] An analysis by this author of the discussion of these ten criteria indicates that the ten criteria appeared to be unresolved issues in most instances. The issues (or criteria) are: (1) universal coverage without distinction as to income or contribution, (2) comprehensive benefits, (3) pluralistic and competitive underwriting, (4) consumer free choice as far as practical, (5) adequate and stable income for providers, (6) incentives for efficiency and economy, (7) equitable financing, (8) administrative feasibility, (9) general acceptability to consumers and providers, and (10) flexibility in the face of changing supply and demand factors. Noticeably missing from the list of "criteria" was quality assurance through a mechanism such as a Professional Service Review Organization (PSRO).

PHARMACY FOUNDATIONS

The concept of a pharmacy foundation has been advanced as an overall mechanism by which pharmacists can effectively deal with issues arising from third party programs including HMOs, Medicaid, and PSRO.

One of the hopeful objectives of the foundation was the negotiation of more equitable dispensing fees with various third party payment programs. Pharmacists soon became aware that this was not possible because such action would violate the antitrust laws. As a result of this limitation, interest decreased in foundations, but has since been revived because of other worthwhile functions.

Types of Foundations. Pharmacy foundations may be one of two types. The first type that was organized was the insurer or underwriting type. If the foundation met the insurance regulation of the state, it was free to negotiate fees and other terms of the contract. PAID Prescription began as this type of organization, but it later became primarily a fiscal intermediator, claims processor, and administrator. This type of organization represents the second type of foundation.

There are still many areas of negotiation for the non-underwriting type of foundation. For example, the foundation can negotiate with various third party programs to use one simplified claims form. This would resolve many minor problems for pharmacists and increase their efficiency in dispensing prescriptions in third party pay programs.

Objectives of a Foundation. The *overall objective* of a foundation is to provide a contractual mechanism for pharmacists to provide *comprehensive* pharmaceutical services to patient-clients in a variety of health care settings, for example, HMOs, extended care facilities (ECF), and home health care agencies. The term "comprehensive pharmaceutical services" encompasses many components, both traditional and innovative. The following are components or functions that should be incorporated into the overall objectives of the foundation:

1. Provide for the traditional dispensing function. This can be accomplished through established pharmacies or through an in-house pharmacy under the direction and auspices of the foundation.

2. Develop standards of practice. These standards should include patient consultation concerning the appropriate manner of administering the medication, side effects as appropriate, monitoring the complete drug regimen, storage, and other information deemed desirable in individual cases. A patient medication record system should be included. The prescription charge should be made flexible to cover the various professional services.

3. In cooperation with PSRO, establish the guidelines and the mechanism for peer review to ensure quality pharmaceutical services and appropriate utilization of drugs.

4. Provide, through contractual arrangement, for in-house and/or periodic visits of a pharmaceutical consultant. Such consultation would provide information to physicians, nurses, and paramedical personnel concerning the proper use and storage of drugs. The particular arrangement would be negotiated to best serve each particular organization or group.

5. Perform, or contract for the performance of, research to establish the economic basis for a fee for service—dispensing, consultation, and other services—and/or per capita cost to provide a specified package of services. This is a necessary adjunct to the above functions.

There are *secondary* or *ancillary* objectives or functions which the foundation could perform. These include providing continuing education directly or by acting as a clearinghouse for such programs. The foundation could also provide a range of predetermined consultative services to its members on a fee-for-service basis. In some cases, it may be desirable for the foundation to act for members by developing specifications, gathering bioavailability data, and related activities for the purchase of drugs. Additionally, the foundation could conceivably establish HMOs or other types of organizations by working with a medical foundation. This type of mutual relationship should include reciprocal participation in peer review and other similar activities.

Establishing a Pharmaceutical Foundation. The first step in establishing a pharmaceutical foundation is to consult an attorney for preliminary legal advice and an estimated cost of the legal proceedings. A legal brief or prospectus for the foundation based on the desired objectives and functions of the foundation should be developed.

The second step is to obtain an estimate of the membership fee based upon the estimated cost and number of members necessary to establish the foundation and to carry out the preliminary investigation and research. This could be accomplished with a survey of potential members.

Third, the cadre should draw up a tentative proposal and circulate it to all potential pharmacist members with an invitation to indicate an interest in becoming a member of the foundation. Based on this response, the initial membership fee and a sustaining (annual) membership fee could be established.

Finally, a permanent proposal with membership dues would be circulated to all potential members. Based on the results, the foundation could be established formally, including Articles of Incorporation, Bylaws, and the election of officers.

Activities of the Foundation. Initially, the foundation should employ an administrator, retain an attorney for routine consultation (with a provision for a negotiated contract for more extensive legal services), employ the necessary administrative staff, and arrange for the necessary consultative and research services.

The first task of the research-consultant would be to compile all of the available information on third-party pay organizations, and government programs involving drugs and pharmaceutical services within the market area. Other data would include statistics on diseases and drug utilization by age groups and various other relevant classifications. Research should be undertaken to determine the per capita cost for providing various packages of pharmaceutical services for various groups with different age and employment profiles, and consultants could be used when necessary. Other activities should include peer review as an ongoing process. It would be desirable to establish a clearinghouse for the exchange of information with other foundations.

The establishment of a pharmaceutical foundation is not only feasible and desirable—it might well be the only means of preserving pharmacy practice as we know it today. Any pharmaceutical foundation that is established *must* be designed for long-range goals and not be a crisis-directed effort. Any short-term effort would be an exercise in futility, which has been a characteristic of pharmacy in too many instances in the past.

Computer Technology

Computer technology has almost revolutionized our way of life, affecting nearly every facet of our society. Computers are being used by large and medium-sized chain drugstores, drug wholesalers, and manufacturers, but only a small minority of community pharmacies make comprehensive use of computers. During the last few years, community pharmacies have increased their use of computers, primarily for accounting functions, and a few have used them for maintaining patient medication profiles and inventory control. However, it is predicted there will be increased use of computers within the next few years.

Spokesmen for the Social Security Administration have stated that when prescriptions are included in either the Medicare program or NHI, it will be essential to place a computer terminal in nearly every pharmacy. The basis of this statement is the fact that the number of claims will be so great that the processing unit simply cannot handle the backup paper work resulting from a fraction of one percent error rate. This will not only require a computer terminal in nearly every pharmacy, but the operation of such a terminal must be extremely accurate and relatively inexpensive.

FEASIBLE COMPUTER TERMINALS

A feasible computer terminal like the one we have described is not generally available in 1974, but the components of such a terminal are. Large retailing firms are already using a variation of this terminal. What are these components? First is a new method of coding information which will replace the old numerical and alpha numerical coding. The code is alternately called a line code, bar code or line/bar code. It is simply a number of lines and in-between spaces within a standardized rectangle.

There are three variables in the code—the number of lines or bars, the width of each line, and the width of the space between each pair of lines. One can vary the magnitude of only one unit of the three variables while allowing all the others to remain constant, and thus produce a system of great variability within a small area of space. Numerical or alpha numerical codes will have to be translated to line/bar codes and appear in juxtaposition for verbal communication. The line/bar code must be imprinted with great precision to provide the necessary accuracy.

The line/bar code can be "read" by a photoelectric cell which, in turn, translates it to a magnetic tape within the terminal. The process is almost 100 percent accurate, provided the photoelectric cell traverses from one end of the bar to the other. If this does not happen, nothing is translated or transcribed on the magnetic tape and a light appears signaling a repetition of the stroke. The data on the code can be transcribed in machine language, in contrast to Fortran or Cobal languages, thus reducing the number of steps and increasing the efficiency and accuracy of processing the data.

The identification of the pharmacy would be encoded within the terminal, and the date would be set and encoded at the beginning of each day. The terminal can be programmed to receive the data from the line/bar code in any order and transcribe it in a set format for transmitting to the computer. Transmission is accomplished inexpensively during the night hours when the computer and the telephone lines have a relatively light load.

BENEFITS OF COMPUTERS

The benefits that can be derived by the processing of data with a computer range from many professional functions to basic business functions. The application is most effective when rapid, repetitive computations and rapid retrieval of accumulated data as information are required.

Professional Applications. A special typewriter can be designed and attached to the computer terminal to perform additional functions, including typing the prescription label and the information on a patient medication profile card. The terminal would have to be programmed to perform these tasks. I believe the increased efficiency can be expected to reduce the cost of these two functions sufficiently to justify the initial investment and continuing costs of this innovation.

Accounting Applications. The pharmacist can computerize his entire accounting procedure or only major components, such as accounts receivable and accounts payable. To computerize the accounting procedures would require an adaptation of the cash register. The cash register, in turn, would be connected electronically to the computer terminal. The line/bar code would be used for product identification, the supply source, and customer identification. For the latter purpose, the social security number would be converted to a line/bar code. In addition, a complete financial analysis could be performed by the computer.

Inventory Control. Using the computer, the pharmacist could achieve the ultimate in inventory control. He could have a perpetual control for each product with an automatic reorder point determined by programming the EOQ model into the system. The EOQ could be updated as demand fluctuated over time or with seasons. Out-of-stock situations would be reduced to a minimum.

Future Health Care Systems

The form and characteristics of any future health care system or systems depend primarily on the provisions of a future national health insurance. Based on the provisions of NHI bills now in Congress, HMOs will have a favored status in future NHI schemes. However, ours is a pluralistic society with a tendency to protect major socioeconomic institutions representing a wide spectrum of interests. Our legislative process is a grand form of collective bargaining in which the essential interests of major political and social groups are preserved through compromises. Special interest groups protect their interests through strong organization and the art of lobbying—a lesson pharmacists have failed to learn. Given the nature of our legislative process and the wide range of special interest groups that will be affected by NHI, most of the ten criteria proposed by Somers,[12] and enumerated above, will be met to some degree at least. Quality assurance is likely to be incorporated into any future NHI program. At present, we have national legislation to develop and test the feasibility of HMOs, which will have considerable impact on the characteristics of any future health care system.

REQUISITES OF FUTURE HEALTH CARE SYSTEM

The requisites of a future health care system(s) differ from those noted by Somers for NHI,[12] since they are for a *system* of health care, not just a NHI program. These requisites are:

1. Any future health care system will have to accommodate existing social and health care institutions, and these institutions will have to make the changes necessary to transform these fragmented institutions into a *system.* This applies to individual consumers and providers of services.

2. It must use the ultimate in technology, especially computer technology, to handle the great amount of data involved.

3. It must provide for maintenance of a comprehensive health data bank capable of providing a complete health profile for each person.

4. Complete confidentiality of health information must be assured.

5. Freedom of choice of providers of service by consumers must be preserved.

6. There must be necessarily some central control to provide uniformity in general administration and application of rules as well as assurance of quality of care.

7. The system will have to be regionalized to deal with complexities of health care delivery and the associated problems.

These requisites will permit the system to deal more realistically with variations in geographic, economic, social and health problems. Another important reason for regionalizing the health care delivery system is to reduce it to manageable units, and thus avoid diseconomies of scales that surely would result with a huge monolithic system encompassing the entire country.

REGIONAL ORGANIZATION

The system must be organized on a regional basis for efficient management and also, to accommodate to special needs of the various geographic areas. Each area should be organized as a comprehensive Regional Health Data Center (RHDC). Each RHDC should be governed by a council, democratically elected and broadly representing all types of providers and consumers. Appropriately trained administrators should be used to permit full use of primary care professionals in the most productive manner possible. The RHDC must be organized to serve as both a communication and referral network as depicted in Figure 17-1. The RHDC should provide the following features:

1. Each individual's health data and information profile should be programmed as a hierarchy in order to permit access to a level of information that is pertinent to the level of service of a particular provider. This is necessary to preserve *confidentiality* of the individual's health record.

2. *Free choice* of provider would be assured by requiring the identification codes of both the consumer and the provider to obtain access to an individual's health record. (This would also support the confidentiality requirement.)

3. The network should include *all* "legitimate" *providers* of services in a *meaningful* way subject to the safeguards of 1. and 2. above.

4. *Referrals* of patients from one level or type of care to another should be a matter of free choice of an *informed* person. This suggests both patient education and appropriate advice by professionals to maximize efficiency and the proper use of manpower.

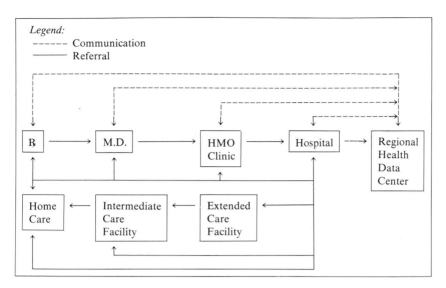

Figure 17-1. *Communication and Referral Network of RHDC*

5. *Entry* into the system should be facilitated by the appropriate use of public health nurses, pharmacists, and other health professionals with various contacts and primary health care roles.

6. The RHDC should be organized to provide *six levels of health care* for the most efficient use of scarce resources. These are: (a) preventive care—health education, immunization, early diagnosis, and promotion of a healthy environment; (b) ambulant care—health maintenance through regular treatment of the chronically ill and necessary periodic examinations; (c) acute care—hospitalization, ranging from intensive care to a lesser level of care requiring hospital facilities; (d) health care in a skilled nursing facility (SNF); (e) less skilled nursing care in an intermediate care facility (ICF); and (f) home health care (HHC) with periodic home visits providing primary care by appropriate teams of paramedical professionals.

All of these levels of care should be organized and coordinated to afford the best possible care at the least possible cost. It is impossible to include all the future developments in health care because such would require clairvoyance. Therefore, only those current and future developments in health care that seemed to me to be most apparent have been included. Pharmacists must become informed now and continue to keep themselves informed on these matters. Moreover, they must unite and organize themselves politically if they hope to play a *meaningful role* in the future delivery of health care.

Conclusion

In conclusion, the words of Congressman Roy summarize the status of health care delivery in this country:[13]

I realize that this (HMO) legislation which I have introduced is not a panacea for all the problems which beset our health system today, for that system is intricate, and its problems are complex. The resolution of the health crisis will require major improvement in many areas: First, manpower; second, facilities; third, biomedical knowledge; fourth, financing; and fifth, organization.

Let me say, however, that this proposal is important, for without a reorganization of our health care delivery system, manpower will continue to be maldistributed and inappropriately employed, facilities will remain poorly located and inefficiently managed, knowledge will fail to affect those who need it most, and additional financing will be inflationary.

REFERENCES

1. Flexner, A.: *Medical Education in the United States and Canada.* New York: Arno Press, Inc., 1910. (Reprinted by Science & Health Publications, Washington, D.C.)
2. Overpeds, M. D.: Physicians in Family Practice 1931–67. *Public Health Reports,* 85:485–494, 1970.
3. Council on Medical Education, American Medical Association; Graduate Medical Education. *J.A.M.A., 218:*1229–1257, 1971.
4. Terris, M.: Crisis and Change in America's Health System. *Amer. J. Public Health,* 63:313–317, 1974.
5. The Committee on the Costs of Medical Care, Medical Care for the American People: *The Final Report of the Committee on the Cost of Medical Care.* Chicago: University of Chicago Press, 1932.
6. Terris, *op. cit.,* p. 313.
7. MacColl, W. A.: *Group Practice and Prepayment of Medical Care.* Washington: Public Affairs Press, 1966.
8. Analysis Examines HMO Act, Asks Increased Consumer Input. *The Nation's Health* (April, 1974).
9. HMO Legislation May Reshape American Medicine. *Change,* p. 51, March, 1974.
10. Senate Bill, S. 3286 and House Bill, H. R. 13870.
11. Senate Bill, S. 2970 and House Bill, H. R. 12684.
12. Somers, A. R.: *Health Care in Transition: Directions for the Future.* Chicago: Hospital Research and Educational Trust, 1971, pp. 136–141.
13. Roy, W. R.: *The Proposed Health Maintenance Organization Act of 1972.* Washington: The Science & Health Communications Group, 1972, p. 19.

REVIEW

1. Discuss the evolutionary changes in health care between the years 1910 and 1960.

2. Discuss the various legislative proposals and acts that have influenced: (a) increased demand for health care, and (b) the restructuring of health care delivery.

3. Discuss how third party pay organizations came into being and the various functions they perform.

4. Contrast the differences in Medicare and Medicaid.

5. Discuss HMOs, and their definition and requirements.

6. What is the major difference between the modern HMO and older HMO-like organizations?

7. Discuss the desired features and the probable impact of National Health Insurance on pharmacy.

8. Describe pharmaceutical foundations, their types, purposes, and activities.

9. Discuss the future applications of computers to pharmacy.

10. Discuss future health care as a system including the requisites, levels of health care, and regional organizations.

Index

Page numbers in *italics* refer to illustrations; those followed by t refer to tables.